Controlling Costs and Changing Patient Care?

The Role of Utilization Management

Committee on Utilization Management
by Third Parties

Division of Health Care Services

INSTITUTE OF MEDICINE

Bradford H. Gray and Marilyn J. Field, editors

NATIONAL ACADEMY PRESS
Washington, D.C.   1989

National Academy Press • 2101 Constitution Avenue, N.W. • Washington, D.C. 20418

NOTICE: The project that is the subject of this report was approved by the Governing Board of the National Research Council, whose members are drawn from the councils of the National Academy of Sciences, the National Academy of Engineering, and the Institute of Medicine. The members of the committee responsible for the report were chosen for their special competences and with regard for appropriate balance.

This report has been reviewed by a group other than the authors according to procedures approved by a Report Review Committee consisting of members of the National Academy of Sciences, the National Academy of Engineering, and the Institute of Medicine.

The Institute of Medicine was chartered in 1970 by the National Academy of Sciences to enlist distinguished members of the appropriate professions in the examination of policy matters pertaining to the health of the public. In this, the Institute acts under both the Academy's 1863 congressional charter responsibility to be an adviser to the federal government and its own initiative in identifying issues of medical care, research, and education.

This project was supported by the John A. Hartford Foundation of New York City, Grant No. 87343-H, and the Pension and Welfare Benefits Adminstration, U.S. Department of Labor, Contract No. J-9-P-8-0067. The Honeywell Corporation provided funds for a roundtable meeting with corporate benefits managers. The views presented are those of the Institute of Medicine Committee on Utilization Management by Third Parties and are not necessarily those of the funding organizations. The Andrew W. Mellon Foundation contribution to independent Institute of Medicine funds was also used to support the project.

Library of Congress Cataloging-in-Publication Data

Institute of Medicine (U.S.). Committee on Utilization Management by
    Third Parties.
      Controlling costs and changing patient care? : the role of
    utilization management / Institute of Medicine, Division of Health
    Care Services, Committee on Utilization Management by Third Parties
    ; Marilyn J. Field and Bradford H. Gray, editors.
        p.   cm.
    Includes bibliographical references.
    ISBN 0-309-04048-5.—ISBN 0-309-04045-0 (pbk.)
      1. Medical care—United States—Cost control. I. Field, Marilyn
    Jane. II. Gray, Bradford H., 1942- . III. Title.
    RA410.53.I58   1989
    338.4'33621/0973—dc20   89-39638
                                                              CIP

Printed in the United States of America

First Printing, October 1989
Second Printing, June 1990

COMMITTEE ON UTILIZATION MANAGEMENT
BY THIRD PARTIES

JEROME H. GROSSMAN,* *Chairman*, President, New England Medical Center Hospitals, Boston, Massachusetts

HOWARD L. BAILIT,* Vice President for Health Research and Policy, Aetna Life and Casualty, Hartford, Connecticut

ROBERT A. BERENSON, Washington, D.C.

JOHN M. BURNS, Vice President, Health Management, Honeywell, Inc., Minneapolis, Minnesota

RICHARD H. EGDAHL,* Director, Boston University Medical Center, Boston, Massachusetts

JOHN M. EISENBERG,* Chief, General Internal Medicine, University of Pennsylvania, Philadelphia, Pennsylvania

DEBORAH ANNE FREUND, Professor and Chair of the Health Care Faculty, and Director, The Center for Health Services Research, School of Public and Environmental Affairs, Indiana University, Indianapolis, Indiana

PAUL M. GERTMAN, President, ClinMan, Inc., Waltham, Massachusetts

ALICE G. GOSFIELD, Attorney, Alice G. Gosfield & Associates, P.C., Philadelphia, Pennsylvania

MICHAEL E. HERBERT, President, Physicians Health Services, Trumbull, Connecticut

NATHAN HERSHEY,* Professor of Health Law, Graduate School of Public Health, University of Pittsburgh, Pittsburgh, Pennsylvania

NEIL HOLLANDER, Vice President, Corporate Health Strategies, Blue Cross of Western Pennsylvania, Pittsburgh, Pennsylvania

KAREN IGNANI, Associate Director, Department of Occupational Safety, Health, and Social Security, AFL-CIO, Washington, D.C.

CAROL ANN LOCKHART, Executive Director, Greater Phoenix Affordable Health Care, Phoenix, Arizona

ARNOLD MILSTEIN, President, National Medical Audit, San Francisco, California

ALAN R. NELSON,* Associate, Memorial Medical Center, Salt Lake City, Utah

ROBERT PATRICELLI, President & Chief Executive Officer, Value Health, Inc., Avon, Connecticut

CYNTHIA L. POLICH, President, InterStudy, Excelsior, Minnesota

---

*Institute of Medicine member

iii

DONALD M. STEINWACHS, Director, Health Services Research and Development Center, School of Hygiene and Public Health, The Johns Hopkins Medical Institutions, Baltimore, Maryland
BRUCE S. WOLFF, Partner, Proskauer Rose Goetz & Mendensohn, New York, New York

STUDY STAFF

KARL D. YORDY, *Director, Division of Health Care Services*
BRADFORD H. GRAY, *Study Director (through December 1988)*
MARILYN J. FIELD, *Study Director (through January 1989)*
SUSAN E. SHERMAN, *Research Associate*
MARGARET WALKOVER, *Research Associate*
DON TILLER, *Administrative Assistant*
WALLACE K. WATERFALL, *Editor, Institute of Medicine*
EILEEN CONNOR, *Consultant*
SHARON ROSEN, *Consultant*

Contents

Preface

The past decade has seen great growth in efforts by purchasers of health care to understand and influence the treatment of patients. In large measure, these efforts reflect purchasers' concerns that their increasing expenditures are not matched by increasing value and even that a significant amount of care is inappropriate and wasteful. Clinicians and researchers, too, are acutely concerned about unexplained variations in practice patterns and lack of evidence of treatment effectiveness. To respond to these concerns, we must focus on how the health care system works as well as how individual patients are served.

Utilization management brings patient-level and system-level concerns together and represents a new nexus of relations among payers, practitioners, hospitals, and patients. Because it is new, at least as broadly applied, and because it is changing rapidly, utilization management needs to be watched.

This report is a preliminary effort in that direction, and the committee hopes that it will inform private and public policymakers alike. Whether the current organizational forms of utilization management remain or subside, the function of managing utilization will remain a central challenge. Therefore, this committee's conclusions and recommendations bear both on generic issues of knowledge and values and on issues specific to current organizations and procedures for influencing patient care decisions.

The first step in this study of utilization management by third parties was a workshop held in the summer of 1987 to identify policy issues and research questions, consider roles for the Institute of Medicine, and discuss the organization and methods of utilization management. This workshop provided initial direction and encouragement for the committee and staff, who held seven meetings between December 1987 and February 1989. In addition to soliciting presentations from knowledgeable persons at committee meetings, the project sought views, data, and ideas through

- 12 site visits to organizations that provide utilization management services (including freestanding firms, insurer subsidiaries, health maintenance organizations, and peer review organizations);
- a June 1988 hearing in which written and oral testimony was presented by over 30 consumer, provider, industry, employer, and other organizations;
- four papers commissioned by the committee from experts in different aspects of utilization management (two of these papers appear in Appendixes A and B of this report); and
- review of published and, in some cases, unpublished literature on the goals, processes, effects, and operating contexts of utilization management.

Additional information was obtained from ongoing discussions with people involved in utilization management as purchasers of utilization management services, suppliers of these services, and subjects of utilization management review, that is, physicians, hospitals, and patients. Reflecting the competitive nature of the utilization management industry, all of the site visits and some other discussions required commitments that the committee would keep confidential any information that would identify the source.

The committee on utilization management plans further work to evaluate the continued course of utilization management and related means of improving the appropriateness and cost-effectiveness of medical services. Other committees and councils of the Institute of Medicine are studying strategies for quality review and assurance, methods for monitoring and improving access for the uninsured, priorities and processes for technology assessment, and problems facing employer-sponsored health benefit plans. This and related work grows out of a continuing commitment by the Institute of Medicine to an agenda of evaluation that encompasses the cost, quality, and availability of health services.

JEROME H. GROSSMAN
Chairman, Committee on
Utilization Management
by Third Parties

Executive Summary

With great speed and relatively little public awareness, a significant change has occurred in the way some decisions are made about a patient's medical care. Decisions that were once the exclusive province of the doctor and patient now may be examined in advance by an external reviewer—someone accountable to an employer, insurer, health maintenance organization (HMO), or other entity responsible for all or most of the cost of the care. Depending upon the circumstances, this outside party may be involved in discussions about where care will occur, how treatment will be provided, and even whether some treatments are appropriate at all.

Such "utilization management" is part of a complex balancing act created by society's struggles with two important questions. First, how do we ensure that people get needed medical care without spending so much that we compromise other important social objectives? Second, how do we discourage unnecessary and inappropriate medical services without jeopardizing necessary high-quality care?

Experience indicates that these questions have no fixed answers. Rather, we find a series of working hypotheses and partial solutions that are continually revised, discarded, and even reinvented as changes occur in medical technology, social values, economic conditions, and other circumstances. In this preliminary report, the Committee on Utilization Management by Third Parties of the Institute of Medicine examines one current working hypothesis—that external review of the appropriateness of proposed medical services for individual patients can improve the way care is provided and, as one consequence, help constrain health benefit costs.

1

The validity of this hypothesis is of interest to everyone involved with health care—patients and potential patients, practitioners and others who provide medical services, employers, unions, insurers, and makers of public policy.

Utilization management has become a growth industry, spurred by purchasers' search for control over rapidly escalating expenditures for health care. One recent survey reported average cost increases from 1987 to 1988 of 14 percent for employers with insured health benefit plans and 25 percent for employers with self-insured plans. In the private insurance sector, many commercial insurers, Blue Cross and Blue Shield plans, and HMOs have seen substantial losses, and some commercial insurers are withdrawing from the group health insurance market.

To the dismay over rising health care costs has been added a growing perception that a significant amount of medical care is unnecessary and sometimes harmful. The studies that have contributed to this perception have also produced some optimism that external review of physician practice decisions could detect unnecessary care, influence physician behavior, and reduce costs without jeopardizing access to needed services. Such review has also appeared to offer an alternative to retrospective denials of claims for benefits and across-the-board cutbacks in health plan coverage.

In this preliminary report, the Committee on Utilization Management by Third Parties examines several questions.

• How effective is utilization management in limiting utilization and containing costs?

• Are there unintended positive and negative consequences of bringing an outside party into the process of making decisions on patient care?

• Are utilization management organizations and purchasers sufficiently accountable for their actions or are new forms of oversight, perhaps government regulation, needed?

• What are the responsibilities of health care providers and patients for the appropriate use of health services?

The focus is on the private sector, in which two-thirds of the nonelderly population are covered directly or as dependents under employer-sponsored health plans. An estimated one-half to three-quarters of the individuals in these plans are subject to utilization management.

CURRENT STATUS OF UTILIZATION MANAGEMENT

Early in its discussions the committee realized that the term *utilization management* has no single, well-accepted definition. As with the labels *cost containment* and *managed care*, different people may mean different things by the term. In this report, the committee considers utilization management as a set of techniques used by or on behalf of purchasers of health benefits to manage health care costs by influencing patient care decision-making through case-by-case assessments of the appropriateness of care prior to its provision.

The dominant utilization management strategy is prior review of proposed medical or surgical services, which includes several related techniques such as preadmission review, continued-stay review, and second surgical opinions. Prior review provides advance evaluation of whether medical services planned for a specific patient conform to provisions of health plans that limit coverage to medically necessary care. Typically, all elective hospital admissions are subject to such review before the patient enters the hospital, all emergency admissions must be reviewed within a short period following admission, and the need for continued hospital care is assessed periodically.

High-cost case management is a more focused strategy that concentrates on the relatively few people in any group who have generated or are likely to generate very high expenditures. The management process involves an assessment of an individual's health care needs and personal circumstances to determine whether extra assistance in planning, arranging, and coordinating a specialized treatment plan will permit appropriate but less costly care. If the individual's health plan does not cover some elements of the treatment plan, individual exceptions to these coverage limitations may be approved.

Empirical evidence on the effects of utilization management is fairly limited and suffers from a number of methodological weaknesses. Despite these limitations, the committee believes that available evidence, taken together, indicates that utilization management has had some impact on health care use and costs. Specifically:

- Utilization management has helped to reduce inpatient hospital use and to limit inpatient costs for some purchasers beyond what could be expected from other factors such as growth in outpatient resources, changes in benefit plan design, and shifts in methods for paying hospitals. Employee groups with higher initial levels of hospital use tend to show more change than groups with lower initial hospital utilization.

- The impact of utilization management on net benefit costs is less clear. Savings on inpatient care have been partially offset by increased spending for outpatient care and program administration. Some of this offset is an expected and acceptable result of utilization management (and other factors), and some is an unwanted consequence of moving care to outpatient settings, where fewer controls on use and price now operate.

- Although it probably has reduced the level of expenditures for some purchasers, utilization management—like most other cost containment strategies—does not appear to have altered the long-term rate of increase in health care costs. Employers who saw a short-term moderation in benefit expenditures are seeing a return to previous trends.

Systematic evidence about the impact of utilization management methods on the quality of care and on patient and provider costs is virtually nonexistent. Purchasers have not demanded such evidence, and researchers have found the measurement of these effects even more costly, time-consuming, and uncertain than the measurement of effects on purchasers' costs. During the course of this study, the committee did not locate documented anecdotes or other information to suggest that prior review programs in the private sector are jeopardizing patient safety. However, the processes of prior review and associated changes in courses of treatment may cause anxiety and inconvenience to some patients. And utilization management does add to the administrative burdens on practitioners and institutional providers and contributes to resentment about reduced professional autonomy and satisfaction. More positively, the committee has some confidence that high-cost case management is easing some financial and emotional burdens on catastrophically ill patients and those who care for them.

Several features of utilization management are important to keep in mind. First, utilization management as it currently operates in the private sector is highly variable, which makes generalizations difficult. Second, until recently utilization management has focused on the site, duration, and timing of medical care. The unnecessary use of the hospital, rather than the actual need for a particular service, has been the main target. The primary strategy has been discussion and negotiation about appropriate care. Refusals to certify benefits appear uncommon, perhaps 1 to 2 percent of cases.

Third, utilization management in the private sector operates under few explicit legal restrictions. There is, however, considerable awareness among review organizations and major purchasers of the legal risks inherent in efforts to influence patient care decisions and operationalize the terms of health benefit plans. And there appears to be growing recognition of the conventional—but not infallible—protections offered against liability by good management, good judgment, good faith, and good documentation.

The lack of good research on the effectiveness and impact of utilization management is a frequent theme in this report, which likewise notes that research on the effectiveness of many medical procedures is also limited. As utilization management expands its review of the actual need for specific procedures, the clinical foundation for such assessments becomes more important. Good research is a critical base for good utilization management. Moreover, the research on feedback and education strategies to influence physician decisions suggests that utilization management criteria will be more likely to win acceptance and change behavior if they are based on clear clinical evidence from respected academic and professional sources.

HOW UTILIZATION MANAGEMENT IS EVOLVING

The continuing evolution of utilization management is most evident in its scope and its operational efficiency. The reasons for these developments are several. First, the initial savings from shifting the site and timing of care have largely been realized, and the survival of review organizations may depend on their continuing ability to affect benefit costs. Second, review organizations are being influenced by researchers' beliefs that much care is still inappropriate and unnecessary. Third, the administrative and other costs of review programs, including physician dissatisfaction and employee confusion, make simplification and efficiency important objectives.

Thus, based on survival instincts and evidence of continuing utilization problems, the emphasis of utilization management is beginning to expand from the site and duration of care to include the actual need for specific types of inpatient and outpatient services. Again, the availability of sound clinical criteria for assessing medical necessity is one constraint on this movement. Legal concerns are another factor.

At this time, the committee does not see utilization management moving toward intentional rationing of clinically necessary medical services. A decision not to approve payment for an unnecessary service is not rationing per se. However, the committee recognizes that there may be instances when review nurses or physicians may apply implicit cost-effectiveness judgments. In high-cost case management, such judgments may be explicit, but the intention is to determine whether services normally excluded from a benefit plan should be covered to permit less costly but still appropriate care for a particular patient.

With respect to administrative costs, frequently mentioned priorities include greater computerization, expanded use of treatment protocols in high-cost case management, and greater targeting of reviews to high-payoff categories of problems and services. In some cases, gains in operational efficiency should reduce administrative burdens on patients, physicians, and institutional providers of care.

ISSUES FOR THE FUTURE

The committee has identified some shortcomings in utilization management or gaps in the knowledge of it that raise concerns about patient protection, particularly given the growing focus on the appropriateness of specific proposed procedures. If the positive potential of utilization management for improving the cost-effective use of health resources is to be encouraged, then the committee believes that several issues need attention.

• Objective methods and resources for evaluating the impact of utilization management on health care costs, use, and quality are limited and must be improved. There needs to be more confidence about what works and what does not and under what circumstances.

• The review criteria used by those engaged in utilization management (including hospitals and HMOs) should be available for outside scrutiny. Physicians, purchasers, and patients should know the basis for judgments about the site, timing, and need for care.

• Systematic investigation of the effects of utilization management not only on purchaser costs but also on patient and provider costs and attitudes should be a higher priority. A more complete picture of costs and benefits is needed.

• The opportunities for patients and physicians to appeal review decisions should be clearly described and free from unreasonable complexity, delay, or other barriers. This is an essential protection for patients.

• The explicit links between utilization management and quality assessment and assurance mechanisms need to be clarified and strengthened. Review organizations should have standard operating procedures for responding to the quality problems they uncover.

RECOMMENDATIONS FOR THE NEAR TERM

The committee believes that utilization management has sufficient promise that a number of short-term and long-term efforts should be made to promote its positive potential and guard against its shortcomings. A prudent course in the near term is for the parties involved in utilization management—purchasers, review organizations, physicians, and patients— to accept greater responsibility for the reasonable and fair conduct of utilization management and the appropriate use of medical care.

Responsibilities of Employers and Purchasers

As financers of both utilization management and health services, employers are in the best position to exert influence on the conduct of utilization management. Although such an effort may be beyond the resources of small employers, larger purchasers should investigate the operating procedures and capabilities of the organization or organizations from which they purchase review services. This review should include organizations such as HMOs that provide prior review and high-cost case management as part of a broader package of services. Purchasers can visit review organizations, request detailed information and references, and seek advice from business coalitions, consultants, and other similar resources. Human resources staff should be trained to respond to employee questions, assist with problems, and handle grievances.

Employers should also examine other aspects of their health benefit plans for impediments to the appropriate use of medical services or the rational payment for these services. Moreover, workers must be clearly informed of their responsibilities and rights. Also, although employers have the right and responsibility to take vigorous actions to manage the costs of employee health benefits, they should respect both the confidentiality of medical information about employees and the primary obligation that physicians have to serve their patients.

Responsibilities of Utilization Management Organizations

Any supplier of services has responsibilities to purchasers that are intrinsic to the concept of a buyer-seller relationship. It is in the business interest of review organizations to anticipate and respond to purchaser demands for information about the organization, its services, and its results. Further, it is in the legal interest of these organizations to manage their activities rationally, to act in good faith, and to maintain careful records.

Although good business and legal judgment should dictate prudent behavior, those who provide utilization management services also have a moral obligation not to harm the patients whose medical care they review and influence. Harm includes discouraging appropriate care and mishandling confidential information. When organizations perform prior review and high-cost case management for individually purchased insurance plans (with no employer sponsorship), they have a particular responsibility to provide good educational materials and appeals processes for beneficiaries who have no employer or other sponsor to act as their agent and aid. They should also develop guidelines for what to do when they discover quality of care problems. With respect to practitioners and individual providers of care, good business sense should dictate that review organizations encourage provider acceptance and cooperation by

- using sound clinical criteria that are open to examination,
- involving the medical community in criteria development,
- minimizing the administrative burdens placed on hospitals and physicians, and
- clarifying and simplifying processes for appealing negative judgments.

The committee is aware that further steps, in particular, making clinical criteria available, raise difficulties given the competitive environment of benefit plan administration. Organizations that have invested their own resources in developing criteria will be reluctant, on the one hand, to make them available to competitors with less initiative and, on the other hand, to reveal some details to practitioners and institutions for fear of their "gaming the criteria" by providing misleading information. Though these are reasonable concerns, on balance, they are outweighed by the need to move toward open criteria and standards.

Responsibilities of Practitioners and Institutions

The committee found the responsibilities of physicians and other health care providers in utilization management the most troublesome to analyze and define, a situation typical of many current ethical and policy issues in health care today. On five basic issues, the committee agreed that health care practitioners and institutions are responsible for

• cooperating with the reasonable efforts of payers, including utilization management, to ensure that payments are for appropriate care within the terms of a patient's benefit plan;
• constructively challenging unreasonable utilization management programs and specific decisions that threaten patient safety or damage patient privacy;
• informing patients about treatment options, risks, and benefits and then considering their preferences;
• seeking to ensure that patients get needed services, which may mean locating an alternative source of care if the patient cannot pay and the provider cannot give free treatment; and
• staying current with scientific literature on the necessity and effectiveness of medical services in their areas of practice.

Although some difficult situations with insurers and review organizations may be more conveniently and quickly dealt with in the short term by misrepresenting patient symptoms, diagnoses, or treatments, the committee believes that it is in the patient's, physician's, and society's interest over the long term for physicians to deal honestly with reviewers and claims administrators and to challenge questionable criteria, procedures, and decisions directly. Manipulation and evasion can have serious risks. Specifically, incorrect information may enter the patient's medical records or insurance history with later negative consequences. Moreover, perceptions by purchasers that physicians are gaming the system undermine professional credibility and stimulate the sorts of auditing, second-guessing, and external oversight to which practitioners object.

Responsibilities of Patients

In many respects, patients and potential patients are the weakest strand in the web of responsibilities for the appropriate use of medical services. When ill, individuals may not be able to act in an informed and prudent way. And whether well or ill, individuals may find both their benefit plans and their medical care difficult to understand and evaluate. Nonetheless, health plan members should try to understand their responsibilities under the plan. The challenge for those involved in health care delivery and financing is to help all kinds of patients make informed decisions about getting or not getting care.

LONGER-TERM RECOMMENDATIONS AND QUESTIONS

As noted earlier, the committee views utilization management as, essentially, a working hypothesis—one of several partial and overlapping strategies for balancing health care expenditures, access, and quality. When knowledge advances, economic conditions change, and social values shift, these partial strategies are revised, integrated, and sometimes discarded. However, even if some of the techniques now employed by utilization management organizations are abandoned or the organizations themselves change, improvements in the criteria for judging appropriate care and for monitoring the provision of care will continue to be relevant. The longer-term recommendations of the committee focus on the foundations for improving effective and safe decision-making about patient care: knowledge development, knowledge utilization, and value clarification. The recommendations cover three areas:

- research on the effectiveness of medical services *and* the effectiveness of utilization management and related techniques,
- formulation and dissemination of guidelines for medical practice and criteria for utilization review, and
- possible oversight of utilization management.

Research on Effectiveness

Utilization management can be no better than the clinical evidence and expertise on which it is based. Although review organizations today may not be effectively using all available research, they are still constrained by the large areas of undocumented impact and clinical uncertainty involving many major medical procedures.

Policymakers are increasingly recognizing that the free market system is unlikely to invest sufficiently in outcomes research and data collection because those making the investment cannot capture all the benefit but must share it with those who have not invested. Since the public gains from investments in such research, public financing and priority setting are appropriate, although they should add to rather than replace initiatives being undertaken by private researchers, health care organizations, and others.

The creation of an agenda to strengthen knowledge of what is effective in medical care is well under way, and the Institute of Medicine is actively involved with many other private and public organizations in developing and implementing this agenda. It is, however, important to have realistic expectations.

In the first place, there are practical and ethical limits on clinical effectiveness research—too few researchers, long time horizons, and numerous procedures where clinicians would balk at research protocols that require withholding treatments generally thought to be useful or providing treatments generally thought to be inappropriate. Second, much care does not really focus on the effectiveness of care in an average setting or population, nor does it evaluate the impact of care on quality of life and many other outcomes that society now considers important. Third, effectiveness research that relies on existing claims and other records, although less expensive and time-consuming than most clinical trials, is not quick or suitable for many questions. Fourth, research cannot resolve some questions, for example, whether use of a specific procedure for a specific problem is prudent given other uses to which limited financial resources could (and would) be put. Fifth, sound clinical research does not automatically affect behavior.

The research on what works in medical care should be complemented by research on how to ensure that such knowledge is used effectively and efficiently. Such programmatic research is, for the most part, a low priority today. It is expensive, methodologically troublesome, and slow to pay off. As part of the overall strategy for containing total health care costs and improving the appropriateness of health care for all citizens, the committee urges federal and private consideration of carefully targeted research projects to test prior review and case management strategies and build methodologies for documenting the effects of ongoing programs.

Practice Guidelines and Review Criteria

Translating effectiveness research into valid, reliable, and usable guidelines for medical practice and utilization management is a complicated undertaking. The committee has identified a number of questions about the process of developing, disseminating, and updating practice guidelines that need attention. They include the following:

• Should there be some kind of oversight of guidelines developed by different sources—a sort of quality review mechanism that assesses both the method and the substance of specific guidelines? What should happen when different sources develop conflicting guidelines?

• To what extent should patient preferences or cost-effectiveness analyses be considered in the development of practice guidelines? How should these issues of value be dealt with in the application of guidelines or in other strategies?

• Should adherence to guidelines provide physicians with protection against malpractice charges? Over the long term, should a role for community or local standards continue?

• What considerations should apply in the translation of guidelines into criteria used in prospective or retrospective review programs?

These questions are relevant to much of the Institute of Medicine's work. Further exploration of these issues is under way and will draw on the expertise of the Committee on Utilization Management by Third Parties, the Committee to Design a Strategy for Quality Review and Assurance in Medicare, the Council on Health Care Technology, and other parties inside and outside the Institute.

Oversight of Utilization Management

The protections offered by caveat emptor, self-regulation, and tort liability, although important, do not respond to all concerns about the impact of utilization management on patients, providers, and overall health care costs. The committee believes that incompetent review organizations need to be weeded out and that some form of oversight seems advisable. However, premature or misguided regulation to accomplish this could stifle worthwhile innovations, lock in ineffective methods, or so paralyze utilization management that purchasers abandon it for more onerous methods of controlling their costs. The experience of the federal government in overseeing peer review organizations (PROs) shows how difficult the oversight function is.

At this time, the committee feels that neither it nor other parties are in a good position to make sound specific recommendations about oversight for utilization management. The committee has posed several questions that it intends to explore further.

• How do we decide whether oversight is necessary and feasible?

• If an oversight mechanism is necessary and feasible, should it be public or private?

• What should be its focus?

• Should utilization management conducted by different kinds of organizations, for example, HMOs, be subject to different kinds of oversight?

• Can anything be learned from government oversight of PROs or the accreditation process managed by the Joint Commission on the Accreditation of Health Care Organizations?

These are not simple questions. Answering them demands more information and more thoughtful debate over how to judge the strengths and weaknesses of utilization management versus those of other strategies to control costs and influence patient care decisions. This, in turn, will depend on better evidence about the impacts of different cost containment strategies. Finally, recommendations about oversight will require more deliberation about the legitimate but sometimes conflicting needs, interests, and values of the parties involved in utilization management.

In a broader sense, the limits of utilization management and any other single strategy, even any combination of strategies, need to be recognized. The issue is not whether utilization management does everything that needs to be done but whether it produces desirable results in reasonable ways at an acceptable cost. Is it, on balance, better to use it than to discard it? How can it be improved, and what other strategies are needed to supplement it? This report provides a progress report and some preliminary views on these issues.

The Institute of Medicine will continue its efforts to better define what role utilization management might play in helping society find an acceptable balance of efficiency, access, and appropriateness in health care. This clearly must be a shared venture. Fortunately, the quest to know what is useful and how to apply it universally are now central issues in medical research and public policy.

1
Utilization Management: Introduction and Definitions

Prior to having the cholecystectomy recommended by her physician, Greta Harrison calls an 800 telephone number to notify the organization that does utilization management for her employer. That organization gets in touch with the surgeon's office to discuss various aspects of the care that is proposed for her. Is hospitalization necessary or can the surgery be done as an ambulatory procedure? How long will the patient need to be in the hospital? In this case, the reviewer agrees that inpatient care is clearly appropriate but questions the plan to admit the patient two days prior to surgery. Since the patient lives in the same town as the hospital and can easily have preoperative tests performed on an outpatient basis, the surgeon agrees to admit her on the day of the surgery.

After Michael Travers is admitted to the hospital following a myocardial infarction, the hospital—aware of his benefit plan's requirements—notifies the appropriate utilization management organization. The length of stay is discussed, but no explicit target date for discharge is set. However, the hospital is then called every third day by the organization, which evaluates information about the patient's need for further hospitalization. The calls continue until Mr. Travers, who has a difficult recovery, is improved enough to be discharged to his home. The physician has not had to adjust the treatment plan but feels irritated at the "red tape" involved. And Mr. Travers has worried on some occasions that payment for part of his hospital stay might be denied.

With their daughter depending on a ventilator to breathe and receiving other hospital care for muscular dystrophy, the parents of Patty Simon are contacted by a case manager for the insurance company that covers the family. The question is whether they and their physician would like to explore arrangements for home care, which is possible in this case but considerably more complex than usual. With the parents' and physician's cooperation, the case manager works out a plan for transfer that includes assessment of the home's wiring (which is adequate for the equipment), provision for two shifts of home nursing care every day, and purchase of appropriate medical equipment and supplies. This requires some expenditures not normally covered by the benefit plan, but the employer agrees with the insurer to make an exception in this case because the arrangements will not only be less costly than hospital care but will also improve the quality of life for the family.

13

With great rapidity and relatively little public awareness, a significant change has taken place in the way some decisions are made about a patient's medical care. Many decisions like those just described, once the exclusive province of the doctor and patient, now have to be examined in advance by an external reviewer, someone who is accountable to an employer, insurer, health maintenance organization (HMO), preferred provider organization (PPO), or other entity responsible for paying all or most of the cost of the care. Depending upon the circumstances, this outside party may be involved in discussions about whether a service is needed, how treatment will be provided, and where care will occur.

This preliminary Institute of Medicine (IOM) report describes the nature of this change in medical decision-making and assesses its impact on patients, providers, and purchasers of medical services. It focuses on the utilization management efforts of the private sector, which provides health benefits for most Americans under age 65.[1]

Prior review of proposed medical care is not entirely new in the 1980s. Review organizations for Medicare were performing some preadmission review in the 1970s, and some private payers made limited use of the technique even earlier. However, widespread application of this approach to managing health care utilization is a phenomenon of the 1980s.

A survey conducted in 1983 reported that only 14 percent of corporate benefit plans required prior approval of nonemergency admissions to hospitals (Equitable Life Assurance Society of the United States, 1983). By 1988, another survey found 95 of 100 large firms had such programs (Corporate Health Strategies, 1988). Perhaps half to three-quarters of employees nationwide are now covered by such programs, up from only 5 percent in 1984 (Foster Higgins, 1987; Gabel et al., 1988).

What accounts for this rapid spread of utilization management through external assessments of the need for proposed medical services? The most obvious factor is rapidly rising health care costs. Purchasers' search for effective ways to limit their financial liability for health benefits stems directly from their belief that costs are out of control.

The trends responsible for this view are painfully familiar to everyone concerned with health care financing. In 1987, the latest year for which statistics are available, total spending on health care reached an estimated $500 billion, up from $234 billion just 5 years earlier (Levit and Freeland, 1988). This spending has been increasing at a rate considerably above the rate of general inflation (Table 1-1), and the share of the gross national product attributed to health services went from 5.9 percent in 1965 to 11.1

---

[1] Public programs have been the subject of several reports in recent years (for example, General Accounting Office, 1983, 1988a, 1988b; Health Care Financing Administration, 1979; Physician Payment Review Commission, 1988, 1989; and Project HOPE, 1987).

TABLE 1-1 Consumer Price Index in the United States (Annual Average, 1967 = 100.0)

Item	1960	1967	1975	1980	1985	1986
All	88.7	100.0	161.2	246.8	322.2	328.4
Medical care	79.1	100.0	168.6	265.9	403.1	433.5

NOTES: Some data are revised. Data for 1960 are based on urban wage and clerical workers. Data for other years are for all urban consumers.

SOURCE: Health Insurance Association of America, *Sourcebook of Health Insurance Data* (1987, 1988). Based on Bureau of Labor Statistics, U.S. Department of Labor, *CPI Detailed Report*, various issues.

percent in 1987. Spending for health care by business as a percentage of the gross private domestic product grew from 1.1 percent in 1965 to 3.4 percent in 1987 (Levit et al., 1989).

High health care costs for employers have been cited as one factor impairing American competitiveness in world markets and a reason why many small firms do not provide health benefits for workers. In 1987, spending for health care by business equaled about 6 percent of total labor compensation compared with about 2 percent in 1965 (Figure 1-1) (Levit et al., 1989). A recent survey of nearly 800 employers of all sizes reported average premium increases from 1987 to 1988 of 11 percent for conventional insurance plans and between 8 and 10 percent for HMOs (Gabel et al., 1989). Another survey cited average increases from 1987 to 1988 of 14 percent for employers with insured programs and 25 percent for employers with self-insured programs (Foster Higgins, 1989). Companies that self-insure assume all or most of the financial risk of paying for covered medical services used by employees and their dependents instead of paying an outside insurance to accept that risk. In the private insurance sector, many commercial insurers, Blue Cross and Blue Shield plans, and HMOs have seen significant underwriting losses—$3.6 billion for commercial carriers and $1.1 billion for Blue Cross and Blue Shield plans in 1988 (Donahue, 1989). Some commercial insurers, for example, Kemper, Provident Mutual, Allstate (for large groups only), and Transamerica Occidental, are withdrawing from the group health insurance market (Meyer and Page, 1988).

To the dismay over rising health care costs has been added a growing perception that much medical care is unnecessary and sometimes harmful. The studies that have contributed to this perception have also produced some optimism that external review of physician practice decisions could detect unnecessary care, influence physician behavior, and reduce costs without jeopardizing access to needed services (Eisenberg, 1986; Schwartz,

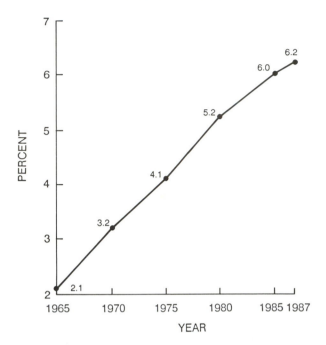

FIGURE 1-1   Expenditures by private industry for health services and supplies as a percent of total labor compensation, 1965-1987. SOURCE: Levit et al. (1989, p. 9).

1984; Wennberg, 1984; Wennberg et al., 1977). In addition, experience has suggested that review of some care prospectively—prior to its provision—would be more palatable and effective than retrospective review has been. This set of perceptions and expectations is, in essence, the hypothesis of utilization management, a hypothesis of interest to patients, practitioners, purchasers, and policymakers.

The IOM Committee on Utilization Management by Third Parties has examined the utilization management hypothesis by asking several questions.

• How effective is utilization management in limiting utilization and containing costs?

• Are there unintended positive and negative consequences of bringing an outside party into the process of making decisions about patient care?

• Are utilization management organizations and purchasers sufficiently accountable for their actions, or are new forms of oversight, perhaps government regulation, needed?

- What are the responsibilities of health care providers and patients for the appropriate use of health services?

The committee's investigatory approach has been described in the preface. Chapters 2 through 5 discuss the committee's findings about why utilization management has become so widespread, how utilization management actually operates and appears to be evolving, and what is known about its effects. In Chapter 6, the committee assesses the current status of utilization management, including its strengths and shortcomings, and recommends near-term and longer-range actions that could help utilization management realize its objectives of controlling costs and reducing inappropriate services without undermining patient access to needed care.

WHAT IS UTILIZATION MANAGEMENT?

In its study of utilization management, the committee found that the term has no single, well-accepted definition. As with the labels *cost containment* and *managed care*, different people may mean different things by the same term. In this report, the committee considers *utilization management* as *a set of techniques used by or on behalf of purchasers of health care benefits to manage health care costs by influencing patient care decision-making through case-by-case assessments of the appropriateness of care prior to its provision.*

Three points about the committee's focus are worth underscoring. First, the committee examines methods that rely on *case-by-case* assessments of care. Second, the focus is on review *prior* to the provision of services. Third, this report stresses actions taken to reduce costs for *third-party purchasers* of care. The first characteristic distinguishes utilization management from methods that analyze aggregate utilization patterns to identify potential problems or that rely on across-the-board limits on health care benefits that take no account of individual patient characteristics. The second characteristic differentiates utilization management from the retrospective review of claims or medical records submitted after care has been provided. The third characteristic directs attention to purchaser-sponsored—rather than provider-sponsored—utilization management efforts, except when providers explicitly share the financial risk with purchasers of care, as they do in HMOs.

The dominant utilization management strategy is prior review of proposed medical services, which includes several related techniques. A second, more focused, strategy is high-cost case management (see Table 1-2).

Prior Review

Prior review provides advance evaluation of whether medical services proposed for a specific person conform to provisions of health plans that

TABLE 1-2 Utilization Management Methods

Prior Review Techniques
  Preadmission Review
  Admission Review
  Continued-Stay Review
  Discharge Planning
  Second Opinion
High-Cost Case Management

---

limit coverage to medically necessary care.[2] Most prior review programs include an integrated set of review steps, not all of which will apply to any single patient. The focus may be on the site of care, the timing or duration of care, or the need for a specific procedure or other service.

The first point of assessment, often called *preadmission review*, may occur before an elective hospital admission. This is what Greta Harrison and her physician experienced in one of the vignettes that opened this chapter. In this case, the review did not challenge the need for the procedure itself or the need for hospital care, but it did challenge the proposed admission 2 days before surgery. The terms *preservice review* and *preprocedure review* are sometimes used to indicate that the focus of review is the need for a procedure, regardless of whether it is to be performed on an inpatient or an outpatient basis.

For emergency or urgent admissions to the hospital when prior review is not reasonable or feasible, *admission review* may be required within 24 to 72 hours after hospitalization to check the appropriateness of the admission as early as possible. The vignette describing Mr. Travers involved this technique as well as *continued-stay review* or *concurrent review*, which assesses the length of stay for both urgent and nonurgent admissions. Reviewers may press for timely *discharge planning* by hospital staff and, in some instances, assist in identifying and arranging appropriate alternatives to inpatient care.

In addition, a patient may be required to get a *second opinion* on the need for certain proposed treatments from a practitioner other than the patient's physician. Increasingly, preadmission review or preservice review is used to screen patients so that referrals for second opinions are focused on patients for whom the clinical indications for a service are dubious.

To encourage patients covered by a health plan to cooperate in the

---

[2] *Medical necessity* is another term that is used differently by different people in different contexts. Some use it generally to cover assessments of the site and duration of care as well as the clinical need for a particular procedure, whereas others use it only in the latter sense. Those who use the term more restrictively tend to apply the term *appropriateness* to the former assessments. For a discussion of legal interpretations of medical necessity, see the paper by William A. Helvestine in Appendix A of this report.

prior review process, a financial penalty, such as higher cost-sharing, may apply when individuals fail to obtain necessary certifications. Chapter 3 provides more details about the mechanisms of prior review.

Although terms like *prior review, predetermination, precertification*, and *prior authorization* of benefits are often used interchangeably, the approval of benefits in advance of service provision may be contingent rather than final. For example, if a retrospective claims review suggests that the information on which the predetermination was based was seriously flawed, payment of a claim may be denied upon further investigation. Or if a utilization management firm does not have access to the details of the benefit plan for a group, it might authorize services not covered by the contract. A review of claims prior to payment might then result in denial of benefits. Since this latter practice usually makes patients unhappy, many utilization management firms try to consider restrictions in a client's health plan in their determinations. Retrospective denials of claims following prior certification appear to be rare, as are refusals to preauthorize services.

High-Cost Case Management

High-cost case management—also called *large case management, medical case management, catastrophic case management*, or *individual benefits management*—focuses on the relatively few beneficiaries in any group who have generated or are likely to generate very high expenditures. This small percentage of individuals—perhaps 1 to 7 percent of a group—may account for 30 to 60 percent of the group's total costs. For the United States as a whole in 1980, 1 percent of the population accounted for 29 percent of total health care spending (Berk et al., 1988).

Case management for individuals with high-cost illnesses is similar to other forms of social and health case management, in that it involves assessing a person's needs and personal circumstances and then planning, arranging, and coordinating the recommended services. It differs in its targets, those very expensive cases for which specialized attention may encourage appropriate but less costly alternative forms of treatment.

In contrast to prior review programs, high-cost case management programs are usually voluntary, with no penalties for patient failure to become involved in the process or comply with its recommendations. (In the third vignette, Patty Simon's parents could have refused the alternative course of care suggested for her.) In addition, more effort is generally devoted to reviewing the patient's particular condition and circumstances and exploring, even arranging, alternative modes of treatment. Finally, exceptions to limitations in benefit contracts may be authorized in advance if this will permit appropriate but less expensive care. For instance, additional home nursing benefits may be arranged so that an individual can avoid further hospitalization. In unusual cases, benefits may be provided for other than health care services, such as construction of a wheelchair ramp or rewiring a patient's home, if these expenditures will allow home care or self-care to be substituted for institutional services at a lower total cost. (The assessment of the wiring in Patty Simon's home would have been covered in this fashion.)

Retrospective Utilization Review

Utilization management techniques, particularly prior review methods, attempt to overcome the disadvantages and unhappiness associated with retrospective review and denial of claims after services have already been provided. Retrospective claims and medical record reviews can, however, support and reinforce utilization management by

• monitoring the accuracy of information provided during prior review and identifying problem areas,

• examining claims that are unsuitable for predetermination (generally those with high volume and low unit costs), and

• analyzing patterns of practitioner or institutional care for use in provider education programs and selective contracting arrangements.

Retrospective utilization review methods have a longer history of general application than do prospective methods (Blum et al., 1977; Congressional Budget Office, 1979, 1981; Institute of Medicine, 1976; Law, 1974). Its strengths and weaknesses have been scrutinized in a number of studies before this one and are not explicitly considered in this report. However, constraints on retrospective review have been a key stimulus for the development of prior review methods. Many of the concerns raised by the committee about the clinical soundness of review criteria, the fairness of procedures, and other matters described apply to both prospective and retrospective reviews.

Other Cost-Containment Methods

The techniques of prior review and high-cost case management are but a subset of the cost-containment methods that can influence decisions about patient care. Other methods, some of which are discussed in Chapter 2 and Appendix B, include the following:

• benefit design (including patient cost-sharing and coverage exclusions), consumer education, and other approaches that shape patient demand for care;

• financial incentives (for example, capitation or bonuses) that are designed to reward physicians or institutions for providing less costly care;

- contracts with health care practitioners and institutions that establish limits on payment for care provided to health plan enrollees;
- use of gatekeeping, triaging, and other devices to manage patient flow to specialists and expensive services; and
- physician education and feedback on standards of care and patterns of practice.

Utilization management shares with the last four strategies a recognition of the physician's central role as the player-manager of the health care team who is responsible for organizing and directing the production process and providing some of the productive input (Eisenberg, 1986). The different strategies for influencing decisions about patient care, however, vary in their emphasis or reliance on different models of control (such as professional self-regulation, informed consumerism, or prudent purchasing), their techniques of influence (such as education, financial incentives, peer pressure, or external oversight), and the parties involved (that is, patients, primary care practitioners, or specialists).

As will be described in Chapter 2, different strategies for cost containment have been tried, abandoned, and revived as third-party financing of health care has expanded. This history reflects both the difficulties of the task and an appreciation that there is no single solution to problems of health care costs, quality, or access. Many strategies have a place, each of which has different strengths and weaknesses and each of which needs monitoring and adjustment as circumstances change and people adapt to various attempts to shape their behavior.

TWO NOTES OF CAUTION

Obstacles to Evaluation

This report laments the limited evidence on utilization management and calls repeatedly for more and better assessments. Nonetheless, the committee is well aware that sound evaluation of utilization management programs faces several obstacles. Some are intrinsic to the research problem, some reflect common organizational behaviors, and some involve particular pressures faced by market-driven organizations. Rigorous evaluation also tends to be quite expensive. In Appendix B of this report, the commissioned paper by Joan B. Trauner notes that evidence about the impact of physician financial incentives on patient care decisions and quality of care is also quite limited.

Intrinsic Conceptual and Methodological Problems

A number of problems in evaluating utilization management and other cost-containment programs are predictable difficulties faced, to one degree or another, in much social and evaluation research (Eddy and Billings, 1988; Wennberg, 1987). One such problem is that there are no uniformly accepted and applied rules for measuring health care utilization or adjusting data for differences in the characteristics of groups being compared. Other methodological difficulties involve (1) data quality and availability; (2) definitions and measurements of program characteristics, group characteristics, outcomes, and other variables; (3) projections of what would have happened without the interventions; and (4) generalizations to other programs and settings.

Common Behavioral Biases Against Evaluation

Under this heading come obstacles to systematic evaluation that are typical of organizations whether they be public or private, for-profit or not-for-profit, big or small (Eddy and Billings, 1988; Hatry et al., 1973; March and Simon, 1958; Suchman, 1967). They include preferences for

• action over evaluation, for example, developing, selling, and running a program rather than seeing if it works;
• quick payoff rather than long-term products or results;
• easy rather than difficult actions (for example, using data on inputs and procedures that are simpler to collect rather than data on outputs or outcomes);
• compelling anecdotes, consensus, or tradition over careful and complex analyses; and
• positive rather than negative results.

In addition, faced with limited resources, managers are frequently reluctant to allocate funds for evaluation instead of wages and benefits, shareholder dividends, or other activities. The committee has no information about what utilization management firms spend on evaluation (for internal use or for clients) or how much different employers invest in systematically assessing the impact of prior review or other cost-containment strategies.[3]

Competition and Evaluation

The normal individual and organizational biases against systematic evaluation may be both mitigated and intensified in competitive environ-

---

[3] The private sector is not alone in providing meager resources for program evaluation. The utilization and quality review components of Medicare's peer review organization (PRO) program have not been very rigorously examined (General Accounting Office, 1988a; Physician Payment Review Commission, 1988). The Health Care Financing Administration does have performance standards for PROs, but they tend to emphasize process rather than outcome and tend to involve measures of impact that are more appropriate for ongoing monitoring rather than systematic evaluation of the review techniques.

ments. Certainly, competition can be a powerful stimulus for internal evaluation of how well a product is working and what makes it work better. Also, clients of utilization management organizations have a strong interest in obtaining reports on results and in shifting their business to other firms if they cannot get such reports.

Balanced against these forces are several threats posed by evaluation. Most obviously, an evaluation may be negative and thereby reduce a firm's chances for retaining clients or winning new clients.[4] Moreover, when an evaluation is publicly available, a firm's competitors gain information that could help them build a case to inform potential clients that the competitor could provide better results or, at least, better reports. Further, evaluations of utilization management programs may provide competitors with statistical norms or even provider-specific information that would not be readily available to them otherwise. Likewise, if firms that invest in relatively sophisticated research and development reveal their work, they may give a free ride for competitors to copy or build on the resulting review criteria, analytic methodologies, or other products. In a new and rapidly evolving industry, this can seem a significant issue for more experienced organizations.

Forces Behind Rising Health Care Costs

The Committee on Utilization Management by Third Parties also recognizes that the forces behind rising health care costs are exceptionally strong and difficult to constrain through moderate means. Many believe that, for the foreseeable future, health care costs will continue to increase faster than costs in the rest of the economy.

- Clinical judgments about the value of treatment for various categories of patients are changing as new treatments or new evidence of treatment impact emerges. For example, women who underwent mastectomy for breast cancer and had no evidence that the cancer had spread were until recently not expected to benefit from chemotherapy, but some new analyses suggest such treatment does increase survival rates. It also increases initial treatment costs (Early Breast Cancer Trialists' Collaborative Group, 1988). Recent guidelines for the use of mammography screening could greatly expand the amount of such screening but some professional sources question whether the guidelines are clinically warranted (McIlrath, 1989).

---

[4] Even when the reported results were positive, the committee encountered considerable reluctance by review organizations to have their analyses published.

• New tests may reduce diagnostic uncertainty but not add any information that aids in treatment decision-making (Kassirer, 1989). Advances in screening techniques may catch individuals much earlier in the course of disease and reduce the numbers who will receive later expensive treatments. The question is, will the costs of screening and early treatment offset the savings? Will real survival rates increase? Researchers involved with cancer point to methods under development to screen for very early traces of dozens of different kinds of cancer, not all of which are more successfully treated if they are detected earlier.

• The work force and the general population are aging, and the use of both acute-care and long-term-care services is higher for people in the older age groups.

• Between 1980 and 2000, the number of physicians has been projected to increase from 171 to 260 per 100,000 population (Graduate Medical Education National Advisory Committee, 1981; U.S. Department of Health and Human Services, 1985). Whether this will bring a surplus of physicians is a matter for debate (Ginsburg, 1989; Schwartz et al., 1989). Nonetheless, one estimate, now many years out of date, is that every additional physician results in $400,000 in additional yearly expenditures for medical services.

• The concern about the millions of Americans who have no routine health insurance coverage is generating various proposals to protect these individuals through, for example, state-sponsored insurance pools, mandated employer-based insurance, expansions of Medicaid, and universal federal health insurance (Congressional Research Service, 1988). What are the short-term costs (and for whom) of increasing access? What long-term costs and benefits can be expected?

Reducing increases in health care costs such that they are much closer to the level of general inflation would appear to demand radical changes in American health policy, either major restructuring of the financing and delivery systems or major cutbacks through large shifts in costs to patients, severe limitations on patients' choices of hospitals and physicians, and explicit rationing of some technologies for all or some individuals. Society may not be willing to make such changes, particularly in the short run (Curran, 1987). It may continue the search, described in the next chapter, for more moderate strategies to control health care expenditures. Utilization management is one such strategy.

It is an unfortunate reality, however, that most cost-containment strategies eventually disappoint their supporters and evaluators to some degree. Even when these strategies seem to reduce costs initially, trend projections do not appear to show an appreciably lower increase in total costs over the longer term (Prospective Payment Assessment Commission, 1989). Given the effort and optimism it generally takes to commit a corporation or a government to a new program, it is not surprising that excessively high expectations often give way eventually to disillusionment. Unwarranted or excessive negativism can, in turn, be counterproductive and lead to premature abandonment of modest but still helpful strategies.

Cognizant of these hazards, the Committee on Utilization Management by Third Parties has tried to approach its initial evaluation of utilization management with reasonable expectations. To this end, the committee has reviewed the development of third-party financing of health care in the United States and the ways in which various strategies to manage costs have evolved. The next chapter summarizes this review.

REFERENCES

Berk, Marc L., Monheit, Alan C., and Hagan, Michael M., "How the U.S. Spent Its Health Care Dollar, 1929-1980," *Health Affairs*, Fall 1988, pp. 46-60.

Blum, John D., Gertman, Paul M., and Rabinow, Jean, *PSROs and the Law*, Germantown, MD: Aspen Systems Corporation, 1977.

Congressional Budget Office, *The Effects of PSROs on Health Care Costs: Current Findings and Future Evaluations*, Washington, DC, 1981.

Congressional Budget Office, *The Impact of PSROs on Health Care Costs: Update of CBO's 1979 Evaluation*, Washington, DC, 1981.

Congressional Research Service, *Health Insurance and the Uninsured: Background Data and Analysis*, Washington, DC, June 9, 1988.

Corporate Health Strategies, *The Health Poll*, Fall 1988, p. 1.

Curran, William J., *The Health Care Cost-Containment Movement: A Reconsideration*, Report of a conference sponsored by Medicine in the Public Interest, Baltimore, MD, March 16 and 17, 1987.

Donahue, Richard, "Health Premiums Soared Past the $100 Billion Mark in 1988," *National Underwriter*, June 5, 1989, p. 1.

Early Breast Cancer Trialists' Collaborative Group, "Effects of Adjuvant Tamoxifen and of Cytotoxic Therapy on Mortality in Early Breast Cancer," *New England Journal of Medicine*, December 29, 1988, pp. 1681-1692.

Eddy, David M., and Billings, John, "The Quality of Medical Evidence and Medical Practice," Paper prepared for the National Leadership Conference on Health Care, Washington, DC, 1988.

Eisenberg, John M., *Doctors' Decisions and the Cost of Medical Care*, Ann Arbor, MI: Health Administration Press, 1986.

Equitable Life Assurance Society of the United States, *The Equitable Healthcare Survey: Options for Controlling Costs*, conducted by Lou Harris and Associates, Inc., New York, August 1983.

Foster Higgins, *Health Care Benefits Survey*, New York, 1987.

Foster Higgins, *Health Care Benefits Survey*, New York, 1989.

Gabel, Jon, DiCarlo, Steven, Fink, Steven, and de Lissovoy, Gregory, "Employer-Sponsored Health Insurance in America," Research Bulletin of the Health Insurance Association of America, Washington, DC, January 1989.

Gabel, Jon, Jajich-Toth, Cindy, de Lissovoy, Gregory, and Cohen, Howard, "The Changing World of Group Health Insurance," *Health Affairs*, Summer 1988, pp. 48-65.

General Accounting Office, *Improving Medicare and Medicaid Systems to Control Payments for Unnecessary Physicians' Services*, GAO/HRD-83-16, Washington, DC, February 8, 1983.

General Accounting Office, *Medicare: Improving Quality of Care Assessment and Assurance*, GAO/PEMD-88-10, Washington, DC, May 1988a.

General Accounting Office, *Medicare PROs: Extreme Variation in Organizational Structure and Activities*, GAO/PEMD-89-7FS, Washington, DC, November 1988b.

Ginzberg, Eli, "Physician Supply in the Year 2000," *Health Affairs*, Summer 1989, pp. 84-90.

Graduate Medical Education National Advisory Committee, *Report to the Secretary*, Vol. 1, DHEW Publication No. HRA 81-6510, Washington, DC, 1981.

Hatry, Harry P., Winnier, Richard E., and Risk, Donald M., *Practical Program Evaluation for State and Local Governments*, Washington, DC, The Urban Institute, 1973.

Health Care Financing Administration, *Professional Standards Review Organizations: 1978 Program Evaluation*, Washington, DC, U.S. Department of Health, Education, and Welfare, 1979, pp. 34-37.

Health Insurance Association of America, *1986-1987 Source Book of Health Insurance Data*, Washington, DC, 1987.

Health Insurance Association of America, *1988 Update: Source Book of Health Insurance Data*, Washington, DC, 1988.

Institute of Medicine, *Assessing Quality in Health Care*, Washington, DC, National Academy of Sciences, 1976.

Kassirer, Jerome P., "Our Stubborn Quest for Diagnostic Certainty," *New England Journal of Medicine*, June 1, 1989, pp. 1489-1491.

Law, Sylvia, *Blue Cross: What Went Wrong?*, New Haven, CT, Yale University Press, 1974.

Letsch, Suzanne W., Levit, Katherine R., and Waldo, Daniel R., "National Health Expenditures, 1987," *Health Care Financing Review*, Winter 1988, pp. 109-122.

Levit, Katharine R., and Freeland, Mark S., "National Medical Care Spending," *Health Affairs*, Winter 1988, pp. 124-136.

Levit, Katherine R., Freeland, Mark S., and Waldo, Daniel, "Health Spending and Ability to Pay," *Health Care Financing Review*, Spring 1989, pp. 1-12.

March, James G., and Simon, Herbert A., *Organizations*, New York, John Wiley & Sons, Inc., 1958.

McIlrath, Sharon, "11 Groups Endorse Mammogram Guidelines," *American Medical News*, July 14, 1989, pp. 3, 35.

Meyer, Harris, and Page, Leigh, "New Era in Utilization Review," *American Medical News*, December 9, 1988, pp. 1, 45.

Physician Payment Review Commission, *Annual Report to Congress*, Washington, DC, March 1988.

Physician Payment Review Commission, *Annual Report to Congress*, Washington, DC, April 1989.

Project HOPE, *A Study of the Preadmission Review Process*, Report prepared for the Prospective Payment Assessment Commission, Chevy Chase, MD, November 1987.

Prospective Payment Assessment Commission, *Medicare Prospective Payment and the American Health Care System: Report to Congress*, Washington, DC, June 1989.

Schwartz, J. Sanford, "The Role of Professional Medical Societies in Reducing Variations," *Health Affairs*, Summer 1984, pp. 90-101.

Schwartz, William B., Sloan, Frank A., and Mendelson, Daniel N., "Debating the Supply of Physicians: The Authors Respond," *Health Affairs*, Summer 1989, pp. 91-95.

Suchman, Edward A., *Evaluative Research*, New York, Russell Sage Foundation, 1967.

U.S. Department of Health and Human Services, *Projections of Physician Supply in the U.S.*, ODAM Report No. 3-85, Washington, DC, Bureau of Health Professions, 1985.

Waldo, Daniel R., Levit, Katherine R., and Lazenby, Helen, "National Health Expenditures," *Health Care Financing Review*, Fall 1986, pp. 1-21.

Wennberg, John E., Blowers, Lewis, Parker, Robert and Gittelshon, Alan M., "Changes in Tonsillectomy Rates Associated with Feedback and Review," *Pediatrics*, June 1977, pp. 821-826.

Wennberg, John E., "Dealing with Medical Practice Variations: A Proposal for Action," *Health Affairs*, Summer 1984, pp. 6-32.

Wennberg, John E., "Use of Claims Data Systems to Evaluate Health Care Outcomes," *Journal of the American Medical Association*, February 20, 1987, pp. 933-936.

2
Origins of Utilization Management

In introducing this report, the committee has emphasized the seriousness of the health care cost problem and the challenges involved in constraining expenditures. The next step is to put the problems and strategies in a historical context. Without understanding how or why utilization management and other cost-containment strategies have developed, policymakers may oversimplify both the difficulties and opportunities they face in managing health care benefits. This chapter

• reviews the development of third-party financing of health services in the United States;
• summarizes early efforts to control costs for health benefits;
• describes the growth of government and private employer involvement in cost containment; and
• identifies some factors behind the change in societal attitudes about medical care and the acceptance of external assessments of the appropriateness of health care use.

THE GROWTH OF THIRD-PARTY FINANCING OF HEALTH CARE

Extensive third-party financing of individual health services is relatively new, emerging in this country largely in the past 60 years. Its development reflects more than a century of scientific progress in the diagnosis and treatment of illness. This progress has stimulated substantial growth and change in health care institutions and professions, raised public expectations about the benefits of medical care, and increased the costs of that care. These developments, in turn, have led to broad-based demands that individuals and families be protected against medical expenses by means other than charity. Although third-party payment was and is among the causes of escalating health care costs, it is also a crucially important social invention to deal with that problem. Some key dates in the move to third-party payment are summarized in Table 2-1. Table 2.2 shows the shift in funding sources for selected medical care expenses over the last 60 years.

Before the 1930s, few Americans had anything resembling modern health benefit plans (Anderson, 1968, 1972; Somers and Somers, 1961). Concerns about medical costs were defined largely in personal rather than governmental or corporate terms. For example, the Committee on the Costs of Medical Care (CCMC) reported in the early 1930s that less than 15 percent of American families bore the burden of more than half of all annual family expenditures for illness (Anderson, 1968). For individuals, medical care expenses were highly unpredictable, ranging at that time "from five dollars to one thousand dollars or more" for a single illness (Rorem, 1982, p. 62). When patients and families (first parties) could not pay these costs, health care providers (second parties) absorbed them with varying amounts of assistance from other organizations (third parties) such as local governments, religious groups, and private charities.[1]

Among actuaries and others involved with the commercial life and casualty insurance industry that had developed in the nineteenth century, there was considerable doubt that medical care was an insurable risk (Donabedian, 1976). A classic text on insurance (McIntyre, 1962) describes traditional conditions for insuring a hazard or risk. The insured event (1) must be susceptible to unambiguous description, (2) must not be something the insured person wants or can control, and (3) must be a relatively uncommon occurrence for individuals but have a predictable incidence for a group. Medical care presents problems in all three areas.

Nevertheless, in the early 1930s, a number of individuals, influenced by the analyses of the CCMC, began a virtual social movement to organize and promote new kinds of "third-party" financing for health care—although they did not use the term explicitly (Anderson, 1968, 1975; Rorem, 1982; Somers and Somers, 1961). They believed that medical expenses—at least, hospitalization expenses—for a group of people could be projected with some accuracy so that a group could do what the individual could not:

---

[1] In 1961, Somers and Somers wrote: "The term 'third party,' usage of which varies from a technical concept of contract law to a popular epithet, means . . . an organization or institution involved in the financing or provision of medical care, other than the two primary parties: the vendor—doctor or hospital—and the patient. For most practical purposes the third party is a private insurance carrier, prepayment plan, or government agency." Today, employers should be added to that list.

TABLE 2-1   Key Dates in the Move from First-Party to Third-Party Payment

1798	U.S. Maritime Hospital Service established; deductions from seamen's pay cover part of cost
1847	First company to issue health insurance organized in Boston
1847	American Medical Association organized
1863	Travelers Insurance Company offers accident insurance
1870s	Employee benefit associations formed; offer small death and disability payments
1883	Germany passes broad social insurance laws
1898	American Hospital Association organized
1910s	Physician service and industrial health plans established in Northwest and remote areas
1912	First model law developed for regulating health insurance
1915	Referenda to establish compulsory state health insurance defeated
1917	American College of Surgeons sets standards for hospitals
1927	Committee on the Costs of Medical Care established
1929	Stock market crash followed by Depression
1929	Ross-Loos group founded (first prepaid group practice)
1929	Baylor hospitalization plan founded (first Blue Cross plan)
1934	Roosevelt puts low priority on public health insurance during planning of Social Security legislation
1937	Blue Cross Commission established
1939	Federal Security Agency (predecessor of U.S. Department of Health and Human Services) established
1940	Predecessor of Group Health Association of America founded
1940s	Federal wage freeze increases union interest in fringe benefits
1945	Kaiser Foundation Health Plan opens to non-Kaiser groups
1946	Hill-Burton hospital construction program established
1946	Blue Shield Commission and Health Insurance Council organized
1949	Supreme Court decisions allow employee benefits to be part of collective bargaining
1951	Joint Commission on the Accreditation of Hospitals founded
1954	San Joaquin County Foundation for Medical Care established
1965	Medicare and Medicaid legislation
1971-1974	Economic Stabilization Program (wage and price controls)
1972	Professional standards review organization legislation
1972	John Deere & Co. begins to self-fund health benefits
1973	Wennberg article on small area variations published in *Science*
1973	HMO legislation passed
1974	Employee Retirement Income Security Act passed
1974	Washington Business Group on Health organized (predecessor)
1978	Labor-Management Group paper on health care costs
1978	General Motors cost-containment reports initiated
1983	Medicare Prospective Hospital Payment legislation passed

SOURCES: Health Insurance Assocation of America (1987); Somers and Somers (1961); Starr (1982); U.S. Department of Health, Education, and Welfare (1976); and Wilson and Neuhauser (1974).

TABLE 2-2 Expenditures for Personal Health Care, Hospital Care, and Physician Services, by Major Sources of Funds, in Percentages, 1929-1987

Year	Type of Care	Direct Patient	Private Insurance	Government
1929	All personal health care (PHC)	88.4	NA	9.0
1950	All PHC	65.5	9.1	22.4
	Hospital care	29.9	17.7	48.9
	Physician services	83.2	11.4	5.2
1960	All PHC	54.9	21.1	21.8
	Hospital care	19.8	36.3	41.3
	Physician services	65.4	28.0	6.4
1970	All PHC	40.0	24.1	34.4
	Hospital care	10.1	36.0	52.5
	Physician services	44.1	34.2	21.6
1980	All PHC	28.7	30.7	39.4
	Hospital care	7.8	38.1	53.1
	Physician services	30.4	42.6	26.9
1987	All PHC	27.8	31.4	39.6
	Hospital care	9.5	36.9	52.5
	Physician services	25.6	43.4	30.9

SOURCE: Adapted from Gibson (1980) and Letsch (1988). Government expenditures include both direct services and public insurance. Figures do not add to 100%.

budget the costs of medical care and share the risk of expense among the well and the unwell.

Real growth in health insurance began during the crisis of the Depression. The federal government rejected health insurance as a priority in developing Social Security legislation, but in the private sector communitywide hospital benefit plans began to be organized for employed groups. These plans collected monthly per-employee payments (premiums) that were independent of individual episodes of ill health. Early premiums ran about 50 to 75 cents per month per member.

Once private health insurance had a chance to prove itself, it quickly became regarded as a necessity and enrollments grew rapidly (Figure 2-1). By the end of World War II, more than 30 million people had private hospital insurance, and employment-based insurance was becoming the norm in major companies.[2] Also, as early as 1940, the movement for prepaid group practices (PGPs) had helped organize enough PGPs, such as Group Health Association of Washington, D.C., to warrant establishment of

---

[2] Although some predecessors of Blue Shield plans, the physician service bureaus in the Northwest, predate the Depression, insurance for physicians services grew more slowly than did coverage for hospital services. In part, this reflected the lesser expense of such services compared with that of institutional services. It also reflected resistance from physicians, many of whom agreed with one leader's 1939 quote from George Washington: "He who would surrender liberty for security is likely to lose both" (Fishbein cited in Rorem, 1982, p. 94).

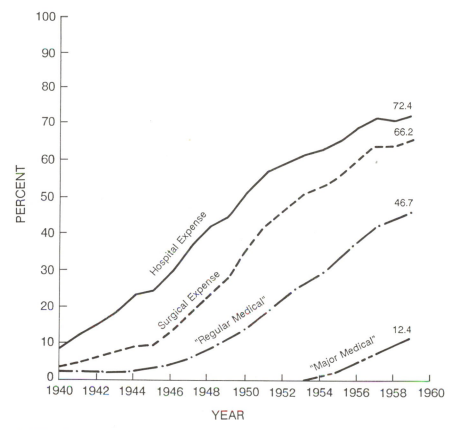

FIGURE 2-1 Private health insurance enrollment. Percentage of civilian population with hospital expense, surgical expense, "regular medical," and "major medical" coverage, 1940-1959. Data are based on end-of-year population and enrollment figures. SOURCES: Somers and Somers (1961). Based on data from the Health Insurance Council and the Social Security Administration of the U.S. Department of Health, Education, and Welfare.

the trade association that eventually became the Group Health Association of America (Somers and Somers, 1961). Insurance coverage continued to expand during the next quarter century, reaching a peak of over 188 million people in 1982 (Health Insurance Association of America, 1987, 1988).

Recently, after 50 years of growth, the reach of private health insurance has begun to decline. As shown in Table 2-3, the percentage of the nonelderly population covered by employment-based plans dropped from 67.4 percent in 1979 to 64.8 percent in 1986 (Congressional Research Service, 1988). In the same period, the number of individuals with neither public nor private insurance expanded to an estimated 37 million in 1986

TABLE 2-3 Sources of Health Insurance Coverage for Nonelderly Population, 1979, 1983, and 1986

Coverage Source	Percentage of Nonelderly Population		
	1979	1983	1986
Employment-based plans			
Covered on own job	33.1	32.5	33.4
Covered through someone else	34.3	32.1	31.4
Total employment-based	67.4	64.6	64.8
Other plans[a]	17.9	18.5	17.7
Uninsured	14.6	16.9	17.5
Total	100.0	100.0	100.0

[a]Excludes persons covered by employment-based plans.

SOURCE: Congressional Research Service (1988, p. 181).

(Chollet, 1988; Congressional Research Service, 1988). Those people represent 17.5 percent of the civilian population, up from 14.6 percent in 1982. (A recent revised estimate puts the number of uninsured at 31.1 million in 1987 [Rich, 1989].) Some individuals move in and out of coverage as they take seasonal or other periodic employment, but many of the uninsured are full-time workers and their dependents. In 1986, 15 percent of workers reported no health insurance from any source (Monheit and Schur, 1988).

Although a variety of economic and social conditions lie behind the decline in insurance coverage, high costs for health care certainly contribute to it. In fact, the continuing escalation of health care costs is once again prompting questions about the insurability of medical care and the viability of private health benefit plans (Abramowitz, 1989; Freudenheim, 1989; National Health Policy Forum, 1988).

EARLY COST-MANAGEMENT EFFORTS BY THIRD PARTIES

The transfer of many health care costs from individuals to third parties has been accompanied both by a shift and a recasting of the cost problem. Insurance has added new complexities to the problem, along with new resources for managing it. Table 2-4, which shows changes in the general consumer price index and selected medical care items from 1929 to 1960, reveals a sharp postwar increase in hospital rates compared to physician fees.

Between 1920 and 1965, many of the basic elements of today's strategies for managing health benefit costs were identified, even if they were not persuasively articulated or successfully applied. These include

TABLE 2 4 Consumer Price Indexes for All Items, All Services, and Medical Care Items, Selected Years, 1929-1960 (Average Annual Index, 1947-1949 = 100.0)

Item or Service	1929	1935	1940	1950	1955	June 1960
All items	73.3	58.7	59.9	102.8	114.5	126.5
Medical care	73.5	71.4	72.7	106.0	128.0	156.1
General practitioners' fees	--	73.9	74.7	104.0	124.3	147.5
Surgeons' fees	--	73.8	74.0	104.5	116.4	129.3
Hospital rates	--	47.1	50.4	114.6	164.4	222.7
Hospitalization insurance[a]	--	--	--	--	115.5	174.3

NOTE: Values are annual averages, except for those in June 1960.

[a]Index for December 1952 is 100.

SOURCE: Adapted from Somers and Somers (1961, p. 545). Data from consumer price index, Bureau of Labor Statistics.

- management of the risk pool,
- design of the benefit plan,
- controls on payments to health care providers,
- constraints on the supply of health care resources, and
- review of the appropriateness of utilization.

Management of the Risk Pool

The founders of health insurance plans in the 1920s and 1930s had to abide by a fundamental principle of all insurance: The composition of the risk pool is critical to the cost and survival of a plan. If the people who buy health insurance are disproportionately those who expect high expenses for health care, then insurance will be, at best, a form of group budgeting for the ill minus the critical feature of risk-sharing with healthy individuals.

The choice of the employment group as the foundation for private health insurance was a key element in managing the risk pool. The employee group was attractive because it existed for reasons other than the purchase of insurance.

Many of the early nonprofit health insurance plans were also committed to "community rating." That is, they charged the same amount per individual based on the projected expenditures for all those covered in the community. However, "experience rating" soon emerged as a way for insurers to compete by segmenting risk. Insurers could attract business by offering lower premiums to groups with lower health cost experience or lower projected costs. This left smaller employers, groups with older and less healthy workers, and self-insuring individuals to pay higher premiums.

To make it feasible to sell insurance directly to individuals, most insurers have devised various controls. These include medical underwriting (that is, excluding those with conditions such as cancer or charging them higher rates) and waiting periods for coverage of preexisting medical problems. Such controls are designed to limit or compensate for the disproportionate selection of an insurance product by less healthy individuals.[3] Even so, individually purchased insurance was and is more expensive than comparable group insurance.

Recently, with many employers offering several health plans to their employees, the management of risk within and across these plans has become a major issue. The long-term impact of this new fragmentation of the risk pool on benefit costs and on the stability of health plans is the subject of spirited controversy (Scheffler and Rossiter, 1985). Efforts to create sound risk pools for small groups, the self-employed, the fragmented employer group, and others remain an elusive goal for those trying to extend health benefits to the nonpoor uninsured.

Design of the Benefit Plan

Like management of the risk pool, the centrality of benefit design was also quickly appreciated as a vehicle to control health plan costs. One way to limit expenses is to require patients to bear some of the cost of care themselves through deductibles, copayments (a flat payment per service), coinsurance (a percentage of a charge), and dollar maximums on benefits for all services or specific categories of service. Cost-sharing has two objectives—first, the simple transfer of some liability for costs to the patient and, second, the discouraging of patient demand for care.

Plan administrators also concluded that premiums could be held in check by excluding coverage for experimental and ineffective treatments, for treatments whose use was highly discretionary or difficult to monitor, for extended or custodial care for chronic conditions, and for relatively low-cost services that could be scheduled and budgeted. Early benefit plans often limited coverage to selected hospital services. These coverage limitations applied uniformly to the covered group and did not require patient-by-patient judgments of medical appropriateness. Later, as insurers

---

[3] The difference between individual and group coverage risk pools is illustrated by statistics from a recent report issued by Independence Blue Cross and Pennsylvania Blue Shield (1988). The Blue Cross plan offers individual coverage without medical underwriting on an open enrollment basis throughout the calendar year for residents of its five-county service area. In 1987, individual subscribers were 6 years older on average (44 versus 38 years), had a hospital admission rate that was 46 percent higher than that for all group subscribers, and incurred costs that were 60 percent higher. Fifty-five percent of the individual subscribers were age 50 or over compared with 35 percent of the group subscribers.

and employers became more comfortable with sponsoring health plans, coverage began to include nonhospital services.

Controls on Payments to Providers

During the financially uncertain years of the 1930s, contracting and risk-sharing with providers were important economic elements of prepaid group practice arrangements and some health insurance plans. One of the earliest prepaid group practices, the Ross-Loos Medical Group, was started in 1929 and later followed by the Group Health Association of Washington, D.C., the Kaiser Foundation Health Plan (as a community-based organization), and the Health Insurance Plan of Greater New York. Also in 1929, what is considered the first Blue Cross plan was established (for a public teachers group) and "underwritten" by Baylor University Hospital. Later Blue Cross plans also had provisions for some sharing of risk by their contracting hospitals or physicians, and negotiated limits on fees were elements in many plans (Donabedian, 1976; Hellinger, 1976).

Strong contractual relationships that included some risk-sharing or limits on payments to providers, however, were hard to establish and maintain (Werlin, 1973). The expansionary postwar decades stimulated hospital restiveness with the contractual relationship that guaranteed service to Blue Cross enrollees at a negotiated price (Anderson, 1975). Physicians continued to fight prepaid group practice plans and other forms of contracting and risk-sharing. However, some medical societies took a less negative approach, establishing Foundations for Medical Care (FMCs), beginning with the San Joaquin County (California) Foundation in 1954. Those FMCs that were based on contracts and physician acceptance of financial risk are the predecessors of today's independent practice associations (IPAs) (Egdahl, 1973).[4]

Constraints on Supply

Another approach to cost containment was developed under the rubric of health planning. Health planning had received much of its initial nationwide impetus as a tool for guiding the expansion in community hospital resources under the Hill-Burton program established after World War II. Beginning in the late 1950s, however, the growing supply of hospital resources came to be viewed as a source of rising health care costs (Roemer

---

[4]Egdahl (1973) distinguishes two types of FMCs. The comprehensive FMCs sponsored prepaid health insurance and performed peer review of health care quality. The other type provided peer review services to insurers and other organizations and became the model for government-mandated professional standards review organizations (PSROs) and peer review organizations established in the 1970s and 1980s.

and Shain, 1959), and health planning was seen as a way to limit excessive capital investment (Somers and Somers, 1961). By the 1970s, a full-blown federal, state, and local health planning program was attempting to regulate resource development (IOM, 1981; Yordy, 1972). Many insurance officials and employers were active supporters of these efforts (Ennes, 1974; Herod, 1974). Using a tactic pioneered by Blue Cross of Northeast Ohio as early as 1950 (U.S. Department of Health, Education, and Welfare, 1976), some insurers warned that unless hospitals cooperated with public or voluntary health planning, "we will not pay full reimbursement or continue our contract with a hospital" (Walter McNerney, quoted in Somers, 1969, p. 138). In the 1980s, faith waned that health planning could be effectively implemented as a cost-control tool (Schwartz, W., 1981), and much of the federal and state legal framework for health planning was dismantled.

Utilization Review

Historically, payers have concentrated their cost-containment energies on the unit price of medical services and have directed less attention to the volume of those services provided by institutions and practitioners. Although some hospitals used committees to monitor utilization in an effort to cope with the short supply of hospital beds during World War II, the first explicit use of retrospective utilization review to control fee-for-service payments for unnecessary and inappropriate hospital services seems to have begun in the 1950s (Payne, 1987, p. 724).[5] In 1954, Fred Carter, a physician, wrote in *The Modern Hospital*, "Why not appoint a standing hospital staff committee designated as the 'hospital utilization committee' to do in the field of hospital and medical economics what the tissue committee does . . . in the field of surgery. Abuses in the use of hospital services and facilities coming to the attention of this hospital utilization committee could be disciplined to the point of near deletion" (cited in London, 1965,

---

[5] To a considerable degree, this utilization review was built on earlier efforts to standardize medical care delivery and establish mechanisms for overseeing the quality of care (Payne, 1976; Starr, 1982). Before the turn of the century, Florence Nightingale had pioneered techniques for assessing and improving the quality of medical services and spurred advances in the training and use of nurses. In the early 1900s, the Flexner report (1910) stimulated reforms in medical education. Ernest Codman developed techniques to audit medical care and identify corrective strategies for treatment deficiencies. Studies by the American College of Surgeons (ACS) identifying problems in the quality of hospital care led in 1917 to the Hospital Standardization Program of the ACS, which was refashioned after World War II into the Joint Commission on the Accreditation of Hospitals (Roberts et al., 1987). The ACS also initiated the professional activities studies to develop abstracting techniques to help audit committees. Over time other professional societies, such as the American College of Physicians and the American Society of Anesthesiologists, have also worked to develop standards of care and guidelines for medical practice.

p. 77). Apparently, high optimism about the impact of utilization review was born with the idea itself.

The 1950s also appear to have seen the first attempt to establish provisions in health benefit plans to encourage or require second surgical opinions (Rutgow and Sieverts, 1989). The United Mine Workers Union tried to institute second opinion requirements but failed because of resistance from organized medicine. It was not until the 1970s that such provisions were successfully introduced by the Store Workers Health and Welfare Fund working with Eugene McCarthy and his colleagues at the Cornell University Medical College in New York City (McCarthy and Widmer, 1974).

The San Joaquin County Foundation for Medical Care (FMC), founded in 1954, not only served as a model for many IPAs but also helped inspire several medical societies to organize peer review of health care utilization and quality. FMCs pioneered many utilization review tools, including model treatment profiles to assess physician performance, protocols for reviewing ambulatory care, and computerized screening of claims. By 1973, there were 61 FMCs in 27 states (Egdahl, 1973).

Utilization review also spread in other settings (Werlin, 1973). In the early 1960s, more than 60 Blue Cross plans reported programs to review hospital claims for the appropriateness of admissions, and more than 50 looked at the length of stay.[6] Some required physicians to certify at admission that hospital care was necessary for cases such as diagnostic and dental admissions, and more than two dozen required physicians to certify the need for continued hospital care after a specified length of stay (Fitzpatrick, 1965; Young, 1965).

In an observation echoed many times over the next 25 years, one speaker at a 1964 conference on cost-containment programs observed that insurer staffs had varying opinions on the effectiveness of utilization review, lamenting that "specific data are lacking" (Fitzpatrick, 1965, p. 24). In a prescient comment, Odin Anderson noted in 1968 that as payers showed increasing interest in medical practice patterns, "the central concern of the medical profession today and in the years ahead might well be 'bureaucracy'" (Anderson, 1968, p. 161).

To summarize, as third-party payment for medical care services expanded from the 1930s into the 1960s, payers—primarily insurers and

---

[6] State insurance commissioners, who often have considerable power over Blue Cross plans by virtue of their power to approve rate increases, spurred some of the utilization review and other cost-containment initiatives of these plans. This was true, for example, in Michigan, Pennsylvania, and New York (Anderson, 1968; Law, 1974). However, these initiatives—at least their outward forms—seem to have spread rather quickly elsewhere without intervention by state officials (Fitzpatrick, 1965). In the late 1950s, many Blue Cross plans were in precarious financial condition (Anderson, 1975).

health maintenance organizations (HMOs)—tried various tools to control these costs. These tools may have had some impact, but they often were neither rigorously applied nor rigorously evaluated. In general, concerns about controlling costs were still overshadowed by society's desire to expand access and improve health outcomes through the development and implementation of advances in medical care.

GOVERNMENT AND EMPLOYER INVOLVEMENT

Two major developments differentiate third-party involvement in containing health care costs during the periods before and after 1965. The first is the entry of the federal government as a powerful force for both cost escalation and cost control. Second, and somewhat later, private employers began serious efforts to control their expenditures for employee health benefits.

Federal Government Initiatives

The federal government's interest in health care cost containment was prompted primarily by its creation in the 1960s of two major health benefit programs: the federal Medicare program for the elderly and the federal and state Medicaid program for some of the poor. (The latter program also gave states an increased stake in containing health care costs.) Both programs responded to inadequacies in private group insurance as a means for covering high-risk or low-income individuals. Government's stake in health costs consequently increased. State and federal spending for personal health care services rose from 22 percent of total spending on these services in 1960 to 40 percent by 1980 (Table 2-2).

When Congress established the Medicare and Medicaid programs in 1965 to increase access to health services, it also recognized the need for constraints against overuse of services. The initial strategy was to expand and strengthen provider-based utilization review. Hospitals and extended-care facilities were required, as a condition of participation in Medicare, to have operational utilization review committees to assure the medical necessity and quality of care "without involving government in day-to-day hospital operations" (Mills, 1967). This was consistent with the preamble to the Medicare legislation, with its famous prohibition against federal "supervision or control over the practice of medicine or the manner in which medical services are provided" (P.L. 89-97).

The costs of the Medicare program soon climbed at rates far above what was predicted when the program began. As one result, policymakers came to view the strategy of delegating utilization review as ineffective, "more form than substance" (U.S. Congress, Senate, 1970). In addition, the medical profession and some consumer groups were complaining about the claims reviews and payment denials instituted by the private contractors that processed Medicare claims. The U.S. Department of Health, Education, and Welfare had required these activities—which some contractors already used in their private business—when they saw that expenditures were quickly exceeding projections (Blum, et al., 1977; Law, 1974).

In the Social Security Amendments of 1972 (P.L. 92-603), Congress provided for the establishment of PSROs to control costs and improve the quality of care through independent peer review. Building on many of the concepts developed by the Foundations for Medical Care and the Experimental Medical Care Review Organizations (federal demonstration projects beginning in 1971), PSROs were to be physician-controlled community organizations that would develop and apply professional standards to the review of institutional health services (Blum et al., 1977; Ermann, 1988; Gosfield, 1975; Nelson, 1984). The law required PSROs to perform concurrent review, but preadmission and retrospective review were optional. In their decade or so of existence, the PSROs designed and refined many of the data collection and analysis techniques used by successor organizations to serve both public and private purchasers.

Congress also got interested in the mid-1970s in second surgical opinion programs as a means of reducing unnecessary surgery. A congressional subcommittee stated that there were more than 2 million unnecessary operations each year, a figure it reached by extrapolating from rates of nonconfirming second opinions found in early research (American College of Surgeons, 1982). Although researchers disavowed this kind of projection, the figures got a lot of attention and helped persuade Congress to authorize demonstration projects to test second-opinion programs for Medicare and Medicaid beneficiaries.

Despite some positive accomplishments, the PSROs—like hospital-based utilization review—disappointed policymakers (Berman and Gertman, 1981; Chassin, 1978; Congressional Budget Office, HCFA, 1979, 1981; Institute of Medicine, 1976; Nelson, 1984). Most PSROs delegated review to hospitals (Ermann, 1988), and the PSROs had little power to penalize physicians for inappropriate practices. Also, general problems in the economy of the United States—the combination of high inflation and low economic growth—complicated efforts to contain costs.

In 1982, Congress replaced PSROs with statewide "utilization and quality control peer review organizations," PROs for short (P.L. 97-248) (Gosfield, 1989). Three years later, Congress added a requirement for PROs to manage a focused second-opinion program, a provision not actually implemented until 1989. Appendix C of this report describes some ways in which PROs tend to differ from private review organizations. Many PROs also have review contracts with private employers.

Utilization review by PROs was intended to supplement and monitor another reform that most viewed as much more important—the introduction of the prospective payment system (PPS) for hospital services provided to Medicare beneficiaries. PPS itself was another response by government policymakers to the frustration with earlier cost-containment efforts, for example, the Economic Stabilization Program with its wage and price controls and the health planning program, which tried to limit major capital investments. The end result of the former, in one evaluator's assessment, was considerable effectiveness in "reducing rates of increase in hospital employees' wages but [little impact] . . . on hospital costs" (Ginsburg, 1978).

Private Purchasers Become a Force

In the private sector, purchasers more gradually came to understand that they too had to be aggressive and prudent buyers of health benefits for their employees. Indicative of employers' low profile in the 1960s was a National Conference on Medical Costs, convened at the request of President Johnson to consider the general problem of rising costs. This 1967 conference had no corporate members (outside the health industry) on its advisory committee, listed no business associations among the groups that were consulted, and included only one corporate representative on its agenda (U.S. Department of Health, Education, and Welfare, 1968). As one employee benefits manager put it later:

> In the past, many of us in the business community routinely paid bills for medical care with no questions asked. Unknowingly, we contributed to the continuation of many abuses in the medical care system by simply signing the check and looking the other way (Chinsky, 1986).

The oil embargo in 1973 and subsequent jumps in oil prices, rising interest rates, stiffer foreign competition, and other economic shocks combined with even sharper increases in health benefit costs finally overcame the employer passivity. By 1976 the Council on Wage and Price Stability was holding hearings, later published, on private sector concerns and initiatives to control costs (Council on Wage and Price Stability, 1976). The share of national spending for health services and supplies accounted for by business grew from 17 percent in 1965 to around 30 percent in 1987 (Levit et al., 1989).

One event that helped influence the thinking of the business community was the publication in 1978 of a 37-page report entitled, simply, "Labor-Management Group Position Paper on Health Care Costs" (Labor-Management Group, 1978). This labor-management group included former Secretary of Labor John Dunlop, the chairmen of eight major corporations, and presidents of seven influential labor unions. Their report, issued after 9 months of meetings and staff work, supported such utilization management precursors as retroactive utilization review (supported by explicit provisions in collectively bargained benefit plans) and coverage of alternatives to inpatient hospital treatment. It also promoted a variety of other initiatives, including prospective reimbursement, HMOs, health planning, technology assessment, medical malpractice reform, and health education.

In 1987, a new task force of the Labor-Management Group issued a statement that emphasized preadmission review, (high-cost) case management, and review of nonhospital care as key strategies for cost containment (Labor-Management Group, 1987). A related group, the so-called Dunlop Group of Six, has met on an ongoing basis to investigate and develop cost-containment proposals. The group consists of the American Hospital Association, American Medical Association, Health Insurance Association of America, Blue Cross and Blue Shield Association, Business Roundtable, and the AFL-CIO (Cronin, 1988).

Another early manifestation of greater business interest in health benefit costs was the move to self-insurance by employers large enough to bear the risk. In 1975, perhaps 3 percent of companies were self-insured (Gabel et al., 1986). Among companies surveyed in 1986, the proportion of those that were self-funded had jumped from 19 to 59 percent between 1980 and 1986 (The Wyatt Company, 1986). Many of the advantages of self-insurance lie not in reduced costs for health care but in reduced underwriting, tax, and other expenses associated with the insurance mechanism. Moreover, the Employment Retirement and Income Security Act allows self-insured employers to avoid paying benefits under state-mandated coverage for a variety of services and providers. These mandates raise both health care and administrative costs, particularly for multistate employers. Despite the apparent advantages of self-insurance, a recent study of Bureau of Labor Statistics data found that monthly costs for family coverage were higher for self-insured groups than for those with Blue Cross and Blue Shield or commercial insurance (Jensen and Gabel, 1988). It also reported that groups converting from insured to self-insured status showed higher cost increases (19 percent over 4 years) than did those remaining insured (10 percent) or those already self-insured (16 percent).

Once larger employers began to assume more active roles in managing their health benefit plans, their initiatives multiplied (Sullivan, 1984). These initiatives have included both individual and collective efforts and have often involved participation by other groups, such as labor representatives. A few examples can illustrate the wide variety of these activities.

- Beginning in 1979, General Motors started joint labor-management efforts to monitor the cost-containment activities of participating Blue Cross plans, implement pilot cost-containment projects, and undertake special studies. In 1984, management and labor agreed to a target 10 percent reduction in health benefit costs (in constant dollars) over 3 years (Labor-Management Group, 1987).

• The state of Pennsylvania and Council 14 of the American Federation of State, County, and Municipal Employees agreed in 1984 to institute a statewide plan for prior review of the medical necessity (not just site of care) of certain elective procedures. Other activities involve employee education, HMOs, preferred provider organizations, and program evaluation (Labor-Management Group, 1987).

• The Massachusetts Business Roundtable helped forge revisions in the state's regulation of hospital rates (Bergthold, 1988).

• The Greater Phoenix Affordable Health Care Foundation developed a software package for local physician offices (with monthly updates) that lists features of hundreds of employer-based benefit plans (Lockhart, 1988).

• Business coalitions, such as the Washington Business Group on Health and the Midwest Group on Health, have been formed to pursue a broad range of educational, data collection, and other activities.

More and more corporate benefits managers now talk about health benefits as a complicated instance of a familiar problem: the procurement of the supplies and services needed to produce the companies' products. A vivid illustration of this shift was described in 1986 by Patricia M. Nazemetz, Xerox's benefits development manager,

> We realize that the purchase of poorly defined products and services at undefined prices is not consistent with good business practice. It does not meet the standards of the quality improvement process that is applied to every other aspect of our business. While we have taken steps toward cost containment through plan redesign and expansion of alternative delivery options, we have continued to purchase off-the-shelf [health care] products that do not necessarily meet our customer requirements. A logical next step will be to define our customer requirements [and then] request proposals from providers and select those who can conform best to our specifications. . . .
>
> We realize the importance of developing measurement systems . . . that allow all the parties involved to determine if . . . service and quality standards are being met and if benefits are being delivered at the right level for the negotiated price. Conformance to service standards will be determined through employees' input. . . . Measuring quality will be much more difficult. The key will be to identify and agree upon those things that are appropriate quality indicators. For example, we may need to consider time lost from work, hospital readmissions, relapses, infections, etc. (Nazemetz, 1986).

Although many larger businesses can take advantage of these approaches, it should be noted that small businesses often lack the financial and managerial resources and the economic leverage necessary to implement many cost-management strategies. Many small employers see cutting or eliminating health benefits as their major option.

The ability of large purchasers to secure better terms for their purchase of medical care is attributable, in part, to shifts in the relative supply of providers versus users of care. The perceived shortage of health care resources following World War II enhanced the position of hospitals and physicians. More recently, the greatly increased ratios of hospital beds and physicians to population have turned the resource shortage into a surplus in most areas. What is in relatively shorter supply today is patients. Occupancy levels in community hospitals, for example, have dropped from a national average of 76 percent in 1980 to 65 percent in 1987 (American Hospital Association, 1988). Since ability to pay now depends largely on public or private insurance, one result is enhanced power for government and employers, at least large employers.

Many approaches now being used by payers to bring about modifications in patterns of care have been initiated by Medicare, the largest single payer. On the private side, the first use of utilization review requirements also appears to have occurred where certain purchasers were in a particularly powerful position vis-à-vis health care providers, for example, among manufacturers with large facilities in small or mid-sized cities (such as Caterpillar, Inc.) or among insurance plans with large local market shares (such as the Blue Cross and Blue Shield plans in Pennsylvania) (Richards, 1984). Although many individual employers in large cities lack leverage on their own, business coalitions in a number of communities are attempting to combine employer purchasing power. An estimated 200 to 250 business coalitions now operate; at least 72 have paid staff (Cronin, 1988).

OTHER FACTORS GIVING RISE TO UTILIZATION MANAGEMENT

The intensified involvement of government and private purchasers in efforts to contain health care costs has been a key element in the rise of more direct and assertive programs to influence patient care decisions. Purchasers have acted as both a stimulus and a lever for the development and application of new approaches to modifying medical practice patterns and limiting the unnecessary use of services (Webber and Goldbeck, 1984).

In addition, at least three other factors have played a role in the transition from the provider-based utilization review of the 1960s and 1970s to utilization management by third parties in the 1980s. These factors include

- a growing body of research suggesting that many medical services are unnecessary or inappropriate and could safely be eliminated;
- an increasing emphasis by purchasers on linking cost containment and quality assurance; and
- a proliferation of information resources, assessment tools, and organizations that make case-by-case review of proposed services feasible on a large scale.

More generally, the 1960s and 1970s saw the growth of doubts that greater expenditures on medical care were improving health status. As one sociologist has put it, this idea "hit with the force of a thunderclap" and added to pressure to constrain medical care expenditures (Starr, 1982).

Inappropriate Utilization as a Cost-Containment Target

The move by third-party payers to become more aggressive about detecting and eliminating the inappropriate use of medical services has been strongly influenced by research suggesting that some costly patient care is unnecessary or inappropriate and that less costly and more appropriate ways of providing care are possible. Support for these views comes from two directions: studies that document substantial variations in the use of medical services across different settings and studies that assess medical services by using explicit criteria of appropriateness.

Variations in Utilization

Some of the most influential research on medical care utilization has examined how the variations in the volume of medical services relate to variations in ways of organizing and financing medical care. For example, several studies suggest that the volume of physician services tends to increase when fee-for-service payment rates are frozen but levels off or decreases when prices are allowed to rise (Gabel and Rice, 1985; Mitchell, 1988; Rice, 1983; Rossiter and Wilensky, 1983; Schwartz, M., et al., 1981). Most widely known are the array of studies reporting that hospital use tends to be 5 to 35 percent lower in HMOs than in fee-for-service systems. Lower use rates in HMOs have been linked to (1) the financial incentives of capitated or salaried payment for services; (2) the advantages of group practice in providing peer pressure, feedback, and practice protocols; (3) the combination of organizational selection and self-selection that leads practitioners with different styles of practice into different practice settings; and (4) the tendency of healthier individuals to be more accepting of health benefit plans that limit their choice of physician (Epstein et al., 1986; Luft, 1987; Luft and Miller, 1988; Manning et al., 1984; Norbrega, 1982; Siu et al., 1986; Ware et al., 1986). The latter explanation is the only one in which differences in the clinical status of patients might play a significant role in explaining differences in utilization.

The view that medical practice patterns are not a precise and unvarying function of medical science is also supported by studies showing substantial and largely unexpected variations in patient care patterns across geographic areas. The studies date back to the late 1960s and early 1970s (Bunker, 1970; Lewis, 1969; Vayda, 1973). John Wennberg's 1973 article in *Science* on variations in small geographic areas attracted much attention, both for its findings and for its methodological innovations (Wennberg, 1973). Small-area studies frequently show two- to fourfold differences in the use of various procedures (Eisenberg, 1986; Lohr et al., 1985; Sandrick, 1984; Wennberg, 1984). They have led purchasers to ask increasingly pointed questions about the rationale for such variations.[7]

Small-area studies tend not to label any particular level of utilization as appropriate or inappropriate (Wennberg, 1986). Certainly, some variation in use is thought to be due to different population needs for care (Blumberg, 1987; Wennberg, 1987). For example, a small-area study sponsored by Blue Cross and Blue Shield of Minnesota found one rural county with unusually high rates of hospitalization for acute myocardial infarction (80 percent higher than the statewide average) and several other heart conditions or symptoms that are not thought to involve much discretion in hospital admission decisions (Thomas, 1989). The insurer asked academic epidemiologists to investigate, and they came up with evidence to suggest disproportionate rates of coronary heart disease in the county. (In response, the insurer joined with others to fund a $300,000 wellness program for the county.)

Inappropriate Utilization

Studies of variations in utilization levels have been complemented by research that attempts to distinguish clinically between appropriate and inappropriate care and to compare actual with correct use of services. These studies have examined hospital admissions, days of inpatient care, ancillary services, and surgical and other medical procedures.

This research has used a number of methods for identifying inappropriate use, including review of pathology specimens after surgery, second opinions on the need for recommended surgery, and audits of medical records. Some studies, for example, those employing second surgical opinions and early audits of medical records, have relied on clinical judgment without explicit written criteria. For other methods, such as certain kinds of medical record audits, explicit written criteria are central to the assessment process (Payne, 1987).

Taken together, research on appropriateness suggests that perhaps one-quarter to one-third of medical services may be of little or no benefit to patients (Brook and Lohr, 1986). For example, several studies have suggested that between 20 and 40 percent of ancillary services in hospitals

---

[7] To help PROs understand area utilization patterns and target potential problems, the federal government is funding a 12-state demonstration project to make small-area analyses available for use by PROs (Tokarski, 1989). In addition, small-area studies have been initiated by public and private organizations in such states as Maine, Minnesota, North Carolina, Iowa, California, and New York (Caper, 1987, Tokarski, 1989; Wennberg, 1984).

were unnecessary or inappropriate (Eisenberg, 1977; Hughes et al., 1984; Schroeder et al., 1984). Other studies have found similar rates of inappropriate hospital admissions and days of care (Restuccia, 1984). Recent work by the Rand Corporation suggests that one-third or more of coronary angiographies and coronary artery bypass surgeries may be performed for patients whose risk from the procedure equals or exceeds the expected benefit (Winslow et al., 1988b). Carotid endarterectomies (which remove clots in the arteries leading to the brain) were judged appropriate in only 35 percent of cases (Chassin et al., 1988; Winslow et al., 1988a).

Some inappropriate use of medical services is probably an inescapable consequence of the inexactitude of medical science, and geographic variations are not necessarily correlated with variations in appropriate use (Chassin et al., 1987). Nevertheless, the great variability in the use of medical services and the studies suggesting that many services are unnecessary have led purchasers to target such services for cost containment.

Linking Cost and Quality

Purchasers have also recognized that a single-minded concern with the costs of inappropriate utilization can be counterproductive. It can create suspicion, antagonism, and resistance rather than cooperation among payers, practitioners, and patients. By tying utilization management to quality of care as well as cost, purchasers do two things:

• they underscore the responsibilities of health care institutions and physicians for providing patients with safe, effective care, and
• they emphasize to policymakers and health plan beneficiaries that payment for poor-quality care and unneeded services is a bad use of limited resources.

Researchers have noted that where there is strong professional consensus on the appropriate use of particular services, such as surgery for cancer of the bowel or hospitalization for hip fracture, there tends to be less variation in levels of utilization. Where consensus is low, for example, on the need for hysterectomy and prostatectomy, utilization is more variable (Caper, 1984). Although differences among populations in the use of particular services can reflect differences in the incidence of the relevant medical problems, many variations appear to be due to differences in what Wennberg (1984) calls physician "practice styles." To strengthen consensus and reduce inappropriate care, the federal government, many medical societies, and other organizations are encouraging the development of practice guidelines or protocols for the appropriate and cost-effective use of specific medical services.

The value of linking cost and quality concerns is suggested by several developments over the past two decades. For example, the growing support for research on the effectiveness of medical services—support that cuts across purchaser, provider, and consumer interests—might not have materialized based on only cost *or* quality considerations. In addition, the legislative history of PROs and HMOs suggests that congressional support for these programs depends on their perception that quality of care as well as cost-containment goals are being served. When Congress banned hospitals from making incentive payments to physicians as an inducement to reduce services to Medicare beneficiaries, it also set restrictions on some financial incentives used by HMOs that were to take effect in 1989 (P.L. 99-509). The effective date has been shifted to 1990, and other changes may result from further study of these incentives, but the basic concern about the cost containment/quality link remains (Ready, 1989). The paper on utilization management in HMOs in Appendix B of this report discusses these concerns at greater length.

Improving the Tools and Structures for Utilization Management

Changing perceptions about the extent of unnecessary medical care and the impact of such care on both cost and quality have been intertwined with changes in information resources, analytical tools, and organizational structures. Although there is substantial need for improvement in each area, these technical and organizational developments have made it more feasible to move from problem identification to problem solving.

Information Resources

The past two decades have seen many advances in the quality and availability of data on the cost and use of health services. These advances include

- greater, though still incomplete, standardization of cost and utilization data from different provider and payer sources;
- more rationality and uniformity in the definition and coding of medical diagnoses and services;
- creation of more large utilization and cost data bases covering hospital, physician, and other services; and
- development of computer software to manage and analyze information.

Each of these developments has increased the ability of purchasers, researchers, and others to describe utilization and cost patterns, track changes across time, and identify anomalies. This kind of descriptive information has been a powerful stimulus for purchaser efforts to reduce inappropriate utilization.

The committee recognizes that, despite considerable progress, many problems with the availability and quality of data remain. Studies continue to document imprecise or inaccurate diagnosis and procedure coding, lack of diagnostic codes on most claims forms, only scattered documentation about entire episodes of treatment or illness, errors and ambiguities in preparation and processing of claims data, and limited information on patient and population characteristics (Larks, 1989; PPRC, 1988). However, the momentum for solving these problems is substantial and stems from multiple public and private interests and needs. These include the demands of purchasers for better documentation on claims for payment, the specter of malpractice, the interest of policymakers in data to develop and monitor changes in methods of paying providers, and technological advances in computer hardware and software.

Assessment and Education Strategies

Assessment and analytic tools that have helped the move toward utilization management include (1) explicit criteria for assessing the appropriateness of medical services, (2) statistical methods for setting utilization norms, and (3) methods for assessing the health status of different patients and population groups. On this analytic base are built feedback techniques for informing physicians about how their practice patterns compare with statistical norms and criteria for appropriate care (Eisenberg, 1986; Wennberg, 1984; Wennberg et al., 1977).

Explicit criteria for judging the appropriateness of medical services include methods that are diagnosis-specific and those that are not (Payne, 1987). The studies of carotid endarterectomies and cardiac pacemakers cited earlier rely on the former, whereas studies of the need for hospital admission or days of hospital care rely on the latter.

Statistical norms have been used most frequently to assess lengths of hospital stay and frequencies of diagnostic or treatment procedures. Average lengths of stay for patients in the western United States, which are lower than those for patients in other regions, are frequently used as a standard in continued-stay review.

Since one reason that health care use and costs may differ across groups is because the health status of group members differs, much effort has gone into methods to assess how severely ill individual patients are, whether they need to be hospitalized, and how institutions and practitioners vary in the overall severity of their mix of cases. These methods use various approaches, including patient resource consumption, organ system involvement, disease stage, and diagnosis (Aronow, 1988; Hornbrook,

1982). Some rely on claims data; others require abstracted information from medical records.

Two cautions should be offered about the current interest in developing medical practice guidelines to influence physician behavior. First, the quality of the relevant medical evidence and the quality of the guideline development process can have major impacts on the soundness and utility of the guidelines. A number of researchers have written persuasively about the limits of clinical research, the lack of fit between some guidelines and relevant clinical evidence, and the problems with methods for generating guidelines (Bunker, 1988; Chassin, 1989; Eddy and Billings, 1988; Schwartz, 1984; Wennberg, 1984). Moreover, empirical research itself can clarify but not fully resolve some questions, for example, whether it is an appropriate use of limited resources to perform cataract surgery to correct small visual deficits.

A second caution about the influence of guidelines is that the success of education programs in changing physician behavior is mixed (Donabedian, 1982; HCFA, 1979; Myers and Gleicher, 1988; Restuccia, 1982; Schroeder, et al., 1984; Wennberg et al., 1977; White et al., 1975). One thorough review of research in this area concluded that just presenting facts is not likely to accomplish much in the absence of other facilitating conditions (Eisenberg, 1986). These conditions include a supportive professional environment, a perceived need for the information, an active involvement by respected peers and professional leaders, and careful targeting of quality, utilization, and cost problems.

The growth of new contracting and payment techniques that put physicians at financial risk is increasing the perceived need for information feedback to practitioners. Analyses and comparisons of practice patterns may have a greater impact on practitioners when reenforced by the specter of future claims denials, exclusion from an HMO or PPO, or loss of a year-end bonus. Moreover, the skilled use of feedback techniques may avoid the tensions created when the more negative or punitive strategies are actually used.

New Organizations

The demand on the part of large public and private purchasers of care for ways to manage, rather than only review, health care utilization has been matched by the emergence of many "suppliers" wanting to take on this role (de Lissovoy et al., 1987; Freund, 1987; Gardner and Scheffler, 1988; InterStudy, 1989; Mayo Clinic, 1988). These suppliers fall into two broad categories: first, organizations that integrate utilization and cost control with service delivery and, second, organizations that offer specialized utilization management services to both health care providers and purchasers. One 1987 survey of over 700 employers found that about one-third of those covered by the employers' health plans were enrolled in "managed fee-for-service" programs and over a quarter more were enrolled in either HMOs or PPOs (Gabel et al., 1988).

The 1980s have seen substantial growth in the number and types of organizations that integrate, to some degree, cost-management and service delivery functions. The number of HMOs has grown from 175 in 1976 to over 600 in 1988, and membership has risen from 6 million to over 32 million (Group Health Association of America, 1988; Interstudy, 1989). A recent survey placed the number of PPOs at over 600 (American Medical Care and Review Association, 1988). Declining hospital occupancy rates and competition for the business of large purchasers has stimulated some of the country's largest multihospital systems and insurers to develop integrated service/insurance products. By 1986, all six of the largest multihospital systems, nine of the largest ten group insurance carriers plus the Blue Cross and Blue Shield system, and six of the eight largest HMO systems had developed some kind of integrated product or products (Patricelli, 1986).

These organizations differ in the weight they place on financial incentives, favorable unit prices, utilization management, and other means to control costs. Some, including many PPOs, develop and manage contractual arrangements with health care providers but do not underwrite the cost of services. Others, such as many HMOs, accept risk for the cost of services, although they typically share that risk with their participating hospitals and physicians.

The financial incentives used by many of these organizations, such as capitation and bonuses, target both elements of utilization risk, that is, the number of services per episode of care and the number of episodes. Although these arrangements may reassure payers that overuse of services is not being encouraged, that reassurance may be countered by concerns that some needed care will be discouraged (AFL-CIO, 1986; Halowell, 1989).[8] These worries are reflected in congressional requirements for PRO monitoring of the quality of care provided to Medicare beneficiaries in capitated HMOs and PPOs (P.L. 99-272) and in proposals that people be informed about financial arrangements for participating providers before they enroll in such health plans (Physician Payment Review Commission, 1989).

---

[8] One early critic of bonuses and withholds linked them pejoratively to such historic arrangements as "split fees, kickbacks, rebates, bribes, and so forth." However, these latter incentives have generally been regarded as unethical inducements to over- rather than underutilization (Geist, 1974, p. 1306).

Disappointing earnings, and perhaps increasing concern about regulatory restrictions, have led many sponsors and investors to drop their new products or move out of certain geographic markets. Still, the array of organizations offering integrated service delivery and cost management is larger and more diverse than it was a decade ago and gives employers more leverage than they had in the past.

Some of the vertically integrated organizations that remain are promoting and underwriting an integrated health benefit package, the so-called triple option. Such programs, which are not yet widespread, typically allow employees to enroll in an HMO, a PPO, or a traditional benefit plan based on their own weighing of coverage, premium, and freedom of choice of provider. Ideally, since all options are purchased from only one supplier, the employer gets a less complex program to manage plus an integrated premium that helps adjust for any tendency of sicker individuals to choose more generous and expensive plans while healthy individuals choose more restrictive and less expensive alternatives. A variant on this concept is the open-ended HMO that provides limited coverage for nonemergency use of providers outside the HMO panel.

A second market response to purchaser demands for cost containment has involved lower entry costs and lower risks than the product integration and triple-option strategies (McGraw-Hill, 1987). Many organizations have been established to offer freestanding utilization management services to providers, insurers, and employers. Although some purchasers, such as prepaid group practices, are well situated to undertake utilization management internally, others, such as many independent practice associations, have found it easier to obtain the services from an external agent. Also, some purchasers prefer not to buy an integrated product.

The utilization management industry, although growing fast and covering an increasing number of benefit plans and beneficiaries, has received little systematic study. This report is designed to help correct that deficiency.

CONCLUSION

Much of this century has been devoted, first, to improving the effectiveness of medical treatments, second, to increasing individual protection against the financial burdens of medical services, and, third, to trying to control the economic costs of expanding access to more sophisticated medical care. In each endeavor, various strategies or working hypotheses rise and wane in popularity as initial promising ideas or results are subjected to empirical evaluation, trials of administrative feasibility, or tests of political acceptability.

Most current approaches to controlling costs and improving the appropriateness of care have been tried and revised, with varying degrees of enthusiasm and sophistication, over several decades. Utilization management builds on the gradual accumulation of experience and data that suggest that externally applied assessments of the appropriateness of proposed medical services can constructively influence how care is provided and, as one consequence, help constrain health care costs. The next three chapters describe what we know about the varied ways in which utilization management works.

REFERENCES

Abramowitz, Michael, "Governments Pinched by Health Care," *The Washington Post*, May 28, 1989, p. C1.

American Federation of Labor and Congress of Industrial Organizations (AFL-CIO), Department of Occupational Safety, Health and Social Security, *Health Care Cost Containment Crisis: Bargaining for Improved Health Care Benefits*, Washington, DC, 1986.

American College of Surgeons, "Second Surgical Opinion Programs: A Review and Progress Report," Chicago, 1982.

American Hospital Association, *Hospital Statistics*, Chicago, 1988.

American Medical Care and Review Association, *Directory of Preferred Provider Organizations*, Bethesda, MD, 1988.

Anderson, Odin, *Blue Cross Since 1929: Accountability and the Public Trust*, Cambridge, MA: Ballinger, 1975.

Anderson, Odin, *Health Care: Can There Be Equity?* New York: Wiley, 1972.

Anderson, Odin, *The Uneasy Equilibrium*, New Haven, CT: College and University Press, 1968.

Aronow, David B., "Severity of Illness Measurement," *Medical Care Review*, Fall 1988, pp. 339-366.

Bergthold, Linda A., "Purchasing Power: Business and Health Policy Change in Massachusetts," *Journal of Health Politics, Policy and Law*, Fall 1988, pp. 425-451.

Berman, David E., and Gertman, Paul M., "Cost Containment and Quality Assurance," in *Federal Health Programs*, ed. by Altman, Stuart, and Sapolsky, Harvey, Lexington, MA: Lexington Books, 1981.

Blum, John D., Gertman, Paul M., and Rabinow, Jean, *PSROs and the Law*, Germantown, MD: Aspen Systems Corporation, 1977.

Blumberg, Mark S., "Inter-area Variations in Age-Adjusted Health Status," *Medical Care*, April 1987, pp. 340-353.

Brook, Robert H., and Lohr, Kathleen N., "Will We Need to Ration Effective Medical Care?" *Issues in Science and Technology*, Fall 1986, pp. 68-77.

Bunker, John P., "Is Efficiency the Gold Standard for Quality Assessment?" *Inquiry*, Spring 1988, pp. 51-58.

Bunker, John P., "Surgical Manpower: A Comparison of Operations and Surgeons in the United States and in England and Wales," *New England Journal of Medicine*, January 15, 1970, pp. 135-144.

Caper, Philip, "Variations in Medical Practice: Implications for Health Policy," *Health Policy*, Summer 1984, pp. 110-119.

Caper, Philip, Presentation to the Physician Payment Review Commission, Washington, DC, September 1987.

Chassin, Mark, "The Containment of Health Care Costs: A Strategic Assessment," *Medical Care*, October 1978 (Supplement), pp. 1-55.

Chassin, Mark, "Developing Good Medical Standards We All Can Live With," *The Internist*, May-June 1989, pp. 6-9.

Chassin, Mark R., Kosecoff, Jacqueline B., and Park, R. E., "Does Inappropriate Use Explain Geographic Variation in the Use of Health Services?" *Journal of the American Medical Association*, November 13, 1987, pp. 2533-2537.

Chassin, Mark, Kosecoff, Jacqueline, Brook, Robert H., and Solomon, David H., "How Coronary Angiography Is Used," *Journal of the American Medical Association*, November 13, 1988, pp. 2543-2547.

Chinsky, David, Employee Insurance Division, Ford Motor Company, Speech on February 19, 1986.

Chollet, Deborah, *Uninsured in the United States: The Nonelderly Population Without Health Insurance, 1986.* Washington, DC: Employee Benefit Research Institute, October 5, 1988.

Congressional Budget Office, *The Effects of PSROs on Health Care Costs: Current Findings and Future Evaluations*, Washington DC, 1979.

Congressional Budget Office, *The Impact of PSROs on Health Care Costs: Update of CBO's 1979 Evaluation*, Washington, DC, 1981.

Congressional Research Service, *Health Insurance and the Uninsured*, Report to Congress, Vol. 1, Washington, DC, June 9, 1988.

Cronin, Carol, "Business Wields Its Purchase Power," *Business and Health*, November 1988, pp. 4-8.

Council on Wage and Price Stability, Executive Office of the President, *The Complex Puzzle of Rising Health Care Costs: Can the Private Sector Fit It Together?* Washington, DC, December 1976.

de Lissovoy, Gregory, Rice, Thomas, Gabel, Jon, and Gelzer, Heidi J., "Preferred Provider Organizations One Year Later," *Inquiry*, Summer 1987, pp. 127-135.

Donabedian, Avedis, *Explorations in Quality Assessment and Monitoring*, Ann Arbor, MI: Health Administration Press, 1982.

Donabedian, Avedis, *Benefits in Medical Care Administration*, Cambridge, MA: Harvard University Press, 1976.

Eddy, David M., and Billings, John, "The Quality of Medical Evidence and Medical Practice," Paper prepared for the National Leadership Conference on Health Care, Washington, DC, 1988.

Egdahl, Richard, "Foundations for Medical Care," *New England Journal of Medicine*, March 8, 1973, pp. 491-498.

Eisenberg, John M., *Doctors' Decisions and the Cost of Medical Care*, Ann Arbor, MI: Health Administration Press, 1986.

Eisenberg, John M., et al., "Computer-Based Audit to Detect and Correct Overutilization of Laboratory Tests," *Medical Care*, 1977, pp. 915-921.

Ennes, Howard, Testimony in hearings on national health planning and resources development held by the Subcommittee on Public Health and Environment, Committee on Interstate and Foreign Commerce, U.S. House of Representatives, May 8, 1977, in Hearing Record, Serial No. 93-91, pp. 709-718.

Epstein, Arnold M., Begg, Colin B., and McNeil, Barbara J., "The Use of Ambulatory Testing in Prepaid and Fee-for-Service Group Practices," *New England Journal of Medicine*, April 24, 1986, pp. 1089-1094.

Ermann, Danny, "Hospital Utilization Review: Past Experience, Future Directions," *Journal of Health Politics, Policy and Law*, Winter 1988, pp. 683-704.

Fitzpatrick, Thomas B., "Utilization Review and Control Mechanisms: From the Blue Cross Perspective," *Inquiry*, September 1965, pp. 16-29.

Flexner, Abraham, *Medical Education in the United States and Canada*, New York: Carnegie Foundation for the Advancement of Teaching, 1910.

Freudenheim, Milt, "A Health Care Taboo Is Broken," *The New York Times*, May 8, 1989, p. D1.

Freund, Deborah A., "Competitive Health Plans and Alternative Payment Arrangements for Physicians in the United States: Public Sector Examples," *In Search of an Optimal Incentive Structure in Health Care*, special issue of *Health Policy*, 1987, pp. 163-173.

Gabel, Jon, Jajich-Toth, Cindy, and de Lissovoy, Gregory, "The Changing World of Group Health Insurance," *Health Affairs*, Summer 1988, pp. 48-65.

Gabel, Jon, et al., "The Emergence and Future of PPOs," *Journal of Health Politics, Policy and Law* Summer 1986, pp. 305-321.

Gabel, Jon R., and Rice, Thomas H., "Reducing Public Expenditures for Physician Services: The Price of Paying Less." *Journal of Health Politics, Policy and Law*, Winter 1985, pp. 505-609.

Gardner, Laura B., and Scheffler, Richard M., "Privatization in Health Care: Shifting the Risk," *Medical Care Review*, Fall 1988, pp. 215-254.

Geist, Robert W., "Incentive Bonuses in Prepayment Plans," *New England Journal of Medicine*, December 12, 1974, pp. 1306-1308.

Gibson, Robert, "National Health Expenditures, 1979," *Health Care Financing Review*, Summer 1980, pp. 1-36.

Ginsburg, Paul, "Impact of the Economic Stabilization Program on Hospitals," in *Hospital Cost Containment*, ed. by Zubkoff, Michael, Raskin, Ira E., and Hanft, Ruth S., New York: PRODIST for the Milbank Memorial Fund, 1978, pp. 293-323.

Gosfield, Alice, *PSROs: The Law and the Health Consumer*, Cambridge, MA: Ballinger Publishing Co., 1975.

Gosfield, Alice, "PROs: A Case Study in Utilization Management and Quality Assurance," *1989 Health Law Handbook*, New York: Clark Boardman Co., Ltd., 1989.

Group Health Association of America, *HMO Industry Profile*, Washington, DC, December 1988.

Hallowell, Elizabeth, "In Del., Challenging HMO Financial Incentives," *The Philadelphia Inquirer*, March 28, 1989, p. B1.

Health Care Financing Administration, *Professional Standards Review Organizations: 1978 Program Evaluation*, Washington, DC, U.S. Department of Health, Education, and Welfare, 1979, pp. 34-37.

Health Insurance Association of America, *1986-1987 Source Book of Health Insurance Data*, Washington, DC, 1987.

Health Insurance Association of America, *1988 Update, Source Book of Health Insurance Data*, Washington, DC, 1988.

Hellinger, Fred J. "An Empirical Analysis of Several Prospective Reimbursement Systems," in *Hospital Cost Containment*, ed. by Zubkoff, Michael, Raskin, Ira E., and Hanft, Ruth S., New York: PRODIST for the Milbank Memorial Fund, 1978, pp. 370-400.

Herod, James C., Testimony in hearings on national health planning and resources development held by the Subcommittee on Public Health and Environment, Committee on Interstate and Foreign Commerce, U.S. House of Representatives, May 8, 1974, in Hearings Record, Serial no. 93-91, p. 381.

Hornbrook, Mark C., "Hospital Case Mix," *Medical Care Review*, Spring 1982, pp. 1-43, and Summer 1982, pp. 73-123.

Hughes, Robert A., et al., "The Ancillary Services Review Program in Massachusetts: Experience of the 1982 Pilot Project," *New England Journal of Medicine*, October 5, 1984, pp. 1727-1732.

Independence Blue Cross and Pennsylvania Blue Shield, *Independence and Leadership in Health Care: Community Health Care Report 1988*, Philadelphia, 1988.

Institute of Medicine, *Assessing Quality in Health Care*, Washington, DC: National Academy of Sciences, November 1976.

Institute of Medicine, *Health Planning in the United States*, Washington, DC: National Academy Press, January 1981, two volumes.

InterStudy, *InterStudy Edge*, Excelsior, MN, 1989.

Jensen, Gail, and Gabel, Jon, "The Erosion of Purchased Health Insurance," *Inquiry*, Fall 1988, pp. 328-343.

Labor-Management Group, *Position Paper on Health Care Costs*, 1978.

Labor-Management Group, *Policy Issues in Health Care Costs and Six Case Studies*, Washington, DC, 1987.

Larks, Marlen, *Fostering Uniformity for Health Care Assessment Data Gathering*, Washington, DC, National Association of Health Data Organizations, May 4, 1989.

Law, Sylvia, *Blue Cross: What Went Wrong?* New Haven, CT: Yale University Press, 1974.

Letsch, Suzanne W., Levit, Katherine R., and Waldo, Daniel R., "National Health Expenditures, 1987," *Health Care Financing Review*, Winter 1988, pp. 109-129.

Levit, Katherine R., Freeland, Mark S., and Waldo, Daniel R., "Health Spending and Ability to Pay," *Health Care Financing Review*, Spring 1989, pp. 1-12.

Lewis, Charles, "Variations in the Incidence of Surgery," *New England Journal of Medicine*, October 16, 1969, pp. 880-884.

Lockhart, Carol Ann, "Physicians Operation Procedures: A Project for Enhancing Patient Flow Through a Competitive Health Care System," Phoenix, AZ: Greater Phoenix Affordable Health Care Foundation, 1988.

Lohr, Kathleen N., Lohr, William R., and Brook, Robert H., *Geographic Variations in the Use of Medical Services and Surgical Procedures: A Chartbook*, Washington, DC, George Washington University National Health Policy Forum, 1985.

London, Morris, "Medical Staff Utilization Committees," *Inquiry*, September 1965, pp. 77-95.

Luft, Harold S., *Health Maintenance Organizations: Dimensions of Performance*, New Brunswick, NJ: Transaction Books, 1987.

Luft, Harold S., and Miller, Robert H., "Patient Selection in a Comprehensive Health System," *Health Affairs*, Summer 1988, pp. 97-119.

Manning, Willard G., et al., "A Controlled Trial of the Effect of a Prepaid Group Practice on Use of Services," *New England Journal of Medicine*, 1984, pp. 1505-1510.

Mayo Clinic, "The 'Cost' of Effective Utilization Review Programs," Statement prepared for the Institute of Medicine Committee on Utilization Management by Third Parties, May 20, 1988.

McCarthy, E. G., and Widmer, Gor, "Effects of Screening by Consultants on Recommended Elective Surgical Procedures," *New England Journal of Medicine*, 1974, pp. 1331-1335.

McGraw-Hill, Inc., *Review Resources: Sourcebook of Private Independent UR Companies*, Washington, DC, 1987.

McIntyre, Duncan, *Voluntary Health Insurance and Rate Making*, Ithaca, NY: Cornell University Press, 1962.

Mills, Wilbur D., "Rising Health Costs: A View from Congress," in *Report of the National Conference on Medical Costs*, June 27-28, 1967, Washington, DC: U.S. Department of Health, Education, and Welfare, 1967.

Mitchell, Janet, Wedig, Gerard, and Cromwell, Jerry, "The Medicare Physician Fee Freeze," *Health Affairs*, Spring 1989, pp. 21-33.

Monheit, Alan C., and Schur, Claudia L., "The Dynamics of Health Insurance Loss," *Inquiry*, Fall 1988, pp. 315-327.

Myers, Stephen A., and Gleicher, Norbert, "A Successful Program to Lower Cesarian-Section Rates," *New England Journal of Medicine*, December 8, 1988, pp. 1511-1516.

National Health Policy Forum, Health Insurance Institute, Washington, DC, November 30-December 1, 1988.

Nazemetz, Patricia M., "Health Care Management Directions at Xerox," Speech at Government Research Corporation Health Leadership Conference, Washington, DC, April 1986.

Nelson, Alan, "Lessons from the Past," *The Internist*, January 1984, pp. 7-8.

Norbrega, F. T., "Hospital Use in a Fee-for-Service System," *Journal of the American Medical Association*, February 12, 1982, pp. 806-810.

Patricelli, Robert, "Musings of a Blind Man—Reflections on the Health Care Industry," *Health Affairs*, Summer 1986, 128-134.

Payne, B. C., et al., *The Quality of Medical Care: Evaluation and Improvement*, Chicago: Hospital Research and Educational Trust, 1976.

Payne, Susan M. C., "Identifying and Managing Inappropriate Hospital Utilization," *Health Services Research*, December 1987, pp. 709-769.

Physician Payment Review Commission, *Annual Report to Congress*, Washington, DC, 1988.

Physician Payment Review Commission, *Annual Report to Congress*, Washington, DC, 1989.

Ready, Tinker, "House Panel Modifies Physician-Incentives Law," *Managed HealthCare*, July 13, 1989, p. 5.

Restuccia, Joseph D., et al., "A Comparative Analysis of Appropriateness of Hospital Use," *Health Affairs*, Summer 1984, p. 130-138.

Restuccia, Joseph D., "The Effect of Concurrent Feedback in Reducing Inappropriate Hospital Utilization," *Medical Care*, January 1982, p. 46.

Richards, Glenn, "Business Spurs UR Growth," *Hospitals*, March 1, 1984, p. 96.

Rice, Thomas H., "The Impact of Changing Medicare Reimbursement Rates on Physician-Induced Demand," *Medical Care*, August 1983, pp. 803-815.

Rich, Spencer, "Health Plans May Cover More Than Was Estimated," *The Washington Post*, July 1, 1989, p. A-5.

Roberts, James S., Coale, Jack G., and Redman, Robert A., "A History of the Joint Commission on the Accreditation of Hospitals," *Journal of the American Medical Association*, August 21, 1987, pp. 936-940.

Rorem, C. Rufus, *A Quest for Certainty: Essays on Health Economics, 1930-1970*, Ann Arbor, MI: Health Administration Press, 1982.

Roemer, Milton I., and Shain, Max, *Hospital Utilization Under Insurance*, American Hospital Association Monograph Series No. 6, Chicago, 1959.

Rossiter, Louis F., and Wilensky, Gail R., "A Reexamination of the Use of Physician Services: The Role of Physician-Initiated Demand," *Inquiry*, Summer 1983, pp. 162-172.

Rutgow, Ira M., and Sieverts, Steven, "Surgical Second Opinion Programs," in *Socioeconomics of Surgery*, ed. by Rutgow, Ira M., St. Louis, MO: The C.V. Mosby Co., 1989.

Sandrick, Karen M., "Blue Cross and Blue Shield of Michigan's Efforts to Change Practice Patterns," *Quality Review Bulletin*, November 1984, pp. 349-352.

Scheffler, Richard M., and Rossiter, Louis F., *Biased Selection in Health Care Markets*, Advances in Health Economics and Health Services Research, Vol. 6, Greenwich, CT: JAI Press, Inc., 1985.

Schroeder, Steven A., Myers, L. P., and McPhee, S. J., "The Failure of Physician Education as a Cost Containment Strategy: Report of a Prospective Controlled Trial at a University Hospital," *Journal of the American Medical Association*, 1984, pp. 225-230.

Schwartz, J. Sanford, "The Role of Professional Medical Societies in Reducing Practice Variations," *Health Affairs*, Summer 1984, p.p 90-101.

Schwartz, Michael, et al., "The Effect of a Thirty Percent Reduction in Physician Fees on Medicaid Surgery Rates in Massachusetts," *American Journal of Public Health*, 1981, pp. 370-375.

Schwartz, William B., "The Regulation Strategy for Controlling Hospital Costs," *New England Journal of Medicine*, November 19, 1981, pp. 1249-1255.

Siu, Albert L., et al., "Inappropriate Use of Hospitals in a Randomized Trial of Health Insurance Plans," *New England Journal of Medicine*, November 13, 1986, pp. 1259-1266.

Somers, Anne R., *Hospital Regulation: The Dilemma of Public Policy*, Princeton, NJ: Industrial Relations Section, Princeton University, 1969.

Somers, Herman M., and Somers, Anne R., *Doctors, Patients, and Health Insurance*, Washington, DC: The Brookings Institution, 1961.

Starr, Paul, *The Social Transformation of American Medicine*, New York: Basic Books, Inc., 1982.

Sullivan, Sean, *Managing Health Care Costs: Private Sector Initiatives*, Washington, DC, American Enterprise Institute, 1984.

Thomas, M. Carroll, "Where Overutilization Does Not Mean Bad Doctoring," *Medical Economics*, May 1, 1989, pp. 65-68.

Tokarski, Cathy, "HCFA Conducting Market-by-Market Study of Physician Practice Patterns," *Modern Healthcare*, February 17, 1989, p. 30.

U.S. Congress, Senate, *Medicare and Medicaid: Problems, Issues and Alternatives*, Report of the Staff to the Committee on Finance, U.S. Senate, Washington, DC, February 9, 1970.

U.S. Department of Health, Education, and Welfare, *Trends Affecting U.S. Health Care System*, prepared by the Cambridge Research Institute, DHEW Pub. No. HRA 76-14503, Washington, DC, January 1976.

U.S. Department of Health, Education, and Welfare, *Report of the National Conference on Medical Costs*, June 27-28, 1968, Washington, DC.

Vayda, E., "A Comparison of Surgical Rates in Canada and in England and Wales," *New England Journal of Medicine*, 1973, pp. 1224-1229.

Ware, John E., Jr., et al., "Comparison of Health Outcomes at a Health Maintenance Organization with Those of Fee-for-Service Care," *Lancet*, May 31, 1986, pp. 1017-1022.

Webber, Andrew, and Goldbeck, Willis B., "Utilization Review," in *Health Care Cost Management: Private Sector Initiatives*, ed. by Fox, Peter B., Goldbeck, Willis B., and Spies, J. J., Ann Arbor, MI: Health Administration Press, 1984, pp. 69-81.

Wennberg, John E., Blowers, Lewis, Parker, Robert, and Gittelshon, Alan M., "Changes in Tonsillectomy Rates Associated with Feedback and Review," *Pediatrics*, June 1977, pp. 821-826.

Wennberg, John E., "Population Illness Rates Do Not Explain Population Hospitalization Rates," *Medical Care*, April 1987, pp. 354-359.

Wennberg, John E., and Gittelsohn, Alan M., "Variations in Medical Care Among Small Areas," *Science*, December 14, 1973, pp. 1102-1108.

Wennberg, John E., "Which Rate Is Right?" *New England Journal of Medicine*, January 30, 1986, pp. 310-311.

Wennberg, John E., "Dealing with Medical Practice Variations: A Proposal for Action," *Health Affairs*, Summer, 1984, pp. 6-32.

Werlin, Stanley, "Cost Control Methods in Health Care Delivery" in *PSRO: Organization for Regional Peer Review*, ed. by Decker, Barry, and Bonner, Paul, Cambridge, MA: Ballinger Publishing Co., 1973.

White, J. J., Satillana, M., and Haller, J.A., Jr., "Intensive In-Hospital Observation: A Safe Way to Decrease Unnecessary Appendectomy," *American Surgeon*, December 1975, p. 794.

Wilensky, Gail R., and Rossiter, Louis F., "The Relative Importance of Physician-Induced Demand for Medical Care," *Milbank Memorial Fund Quarterly*, Spring 1983, pp. 252-277.

Wilson, Florence A., and Neuhauser, Duncan, *Health Services in the United States*, Cambridge, MA: Ballinger, 1974.

Winslow, Constance M., Solomon, David H., Chassin, Mark R., Kosecoff, Jacqueline, and Brook, Robert H., "The Appropriateness of Carotid Endarterectomy," *New England Journal of Medicine*, March 24, 1988a, pp. 721-727.

Winslow, Constance M., Kosecoff, Jacqueline, Chassin, Mark R., Kanouse, David E., and Brook, Robert H., "The Appropriateness of Performing Coronary Angiography and Coronary Artery Bypass Surgery," *Journal of the American Medical Association*, July 22/29, 1988b, pp. 505-509.

The Wyatt Company, *1986 Group Benefits Survey*, New York, 1988, p. 18.

Yordy, Karl D., "National Planning for Health: An Emerging Reality," *Bulletin of the New York Academy of Medicine*, January 1972, pp. 32-38.

Young, Lee A., "Utilization Review and Control Mechanisms: From the Blue Shield Perspective," *Inquiry*, September 1965, pp. 5-15.

3
The Utilization Management Industry: Structure and Process

Analyzing the changes brought about by utilization management requires a basic understanding of how utilization management actually works. What decisions do utilization management organizations make and on what basis? To whom are they accountable and for what? How do they try to be effective in controlling costs without harming patients? How standardized are their methods and criteria?

To answer these questions, the committee set out to learn more about the workings of utilization management. What it found about prior review procedures is described in this chapter. Chapter 5 covers high-cost case management. Judgments and recommendations are reserved primarily for Chapter 6.

From the standpoint of the employers or governmental programs that purchase medical care, utilization management can be brought into play in one of three ways. The purchaser can

- engage in utilization management directly, as some Medicaid programs do;
- contract with another organization for utilization management services, as Medicare and many employers do; or
- shift some of the financial risk to another party, such as an insurer, an HMO, or a PPO, which is then faced with the same three choices of doing utilization management directly, contracting for the services, or shifting risk to still another party (for example, physicians or hospitals).

The committee did not focus on utilization management activities undertaken directly by employers. Rather, it looked at the broad and varied array of organizations that either contract directly with employers to provide utilization management services or, like some HMOs and insurers, provide utilization management as part of a larger package of services. The products, target markets, philosophies, and technologies of these organizations vary widely, but the industry is evolving so rapidly that summary is difficult. What follows is a snapshot of the field of utilization management.

INDUSTRY OVERVIEW

In 1980, there was no utilization management industry to speak of, although some of the building blocks existed in HMOs, professional standards review organizations (PSROs), insurance plans, and hospital utilization review programs. Now hundreds of organizations offer utilization management services to thousands of clients who employ perhaps half to two-thirds of all American workers (Foster Higgins, 1987; Gabel et al., 1988). A precise count of utilization management organizations is virtually impossible because the industry is changing constantly, and no single trade association or industry information source exists. A 1987 publication listed 158 private independent utilization review companies (McGraw-Hill, 1987). However, this list did not include the utilization management departments of those commercial insurers and Blue Cross and Blue Shield plans that do not have separate utilization management subsidiaries. Also not included were the internal utilization management departments of HMOs, independent practice associations (IPAs), and PPOs. A 1989 survey by Business Insurance reported 125 review organizations (Business Insurance, 1989). Again, utilization management departments of many insurers were not listed. The companies listed in this second survey covered from 10,000 to over 11 million individuals, and review services accounted for 2 to 100 percent of company revenues. The ten largest firms are listed in Table 3-1.

Figure 3-1 charts the industry's growth, a growth vividly illustrated by the experience of the Mayo Clinic (Mayo Clinic, 1988). In 1984, the Mayo Clinic was dealing with only one utilization management program—precertification for Medicare beneficiaries. Four years later it was working with approximately 1,000 utilization review plans. This does not equate to 1,000 review organizations, however, because many review companies alter some details of their programs to fit particular client preferences. (The Mayo Clinic, for example, reported dealing with over 200 Blue Cross and Blue Shield review programs, but there are fewer than 75 Blue Cross and Blue Shield organizations in existence.) The American Hospital Association (1989) reports that hospitals may deal with from 50 to 250 organizations doing prior and retrospective review.

TABLE 3.1 The 10 Largest General Service Utilization Review Firms

| Company (Ownership) | No. of Lives Serviced | No. of Full-Time Staff | | | Physicians on Retainer |
		Total	Physicians	Registered Nurses	
Intracorp (CIGNA Corp.)	11,500,000	600	NA	NA	NA
Corporate Health Strategies (Metropolitan Life Insurance Co.)	6,200,000	243	6	228	7
HealthCare COMPARE Corp. (independent)	5,000,000	433	27	300	NA
Peer Review Analysis, Inc. (privately held)	4,000,000	45	7	16	65
Corporate Health Care Management (EQUICOR, Inc.)	3,750,000	236	9	93	23
Cost Care, Inc. (independent)	2,900,000	268	19	136	6
Value Health, Inc. (privately held)	2,800,000	119	5	9	7
The Sunderbrunch Corp. (privately held)	2,683,000	293	2	89	0
Western Medical Review (nonprofit)	2,000,000	40	1	22	50
August International Corp. (privately held)	1,979,750	230	3	48	45

NOTE: NA, not available.

SOURCE: *Business Insurance* (1989).

Some utilization management organizations are spin-offs and descendants of the PSROs developed for Medicare after 1972. Many PSROs had private clients, as do many of the successor PROs. Over three-quarters of the PROs were listed in a 1987 compilation of private independent utilization review companies (McGraw-Hill, 1987), although only a handful appeared in a 1989 directory compiled by Business Insurance (Business Insurance, 1989).

Insurance companies, which are coping with the loss of business that resulted from employers' decisions to self-insure, offer utilization management services both to control costs for underwritten accounts and to provide new products for both insured and self-insured groups. From 1982 to 1986, the percentage of Blue Cross plans reporting prior review programs

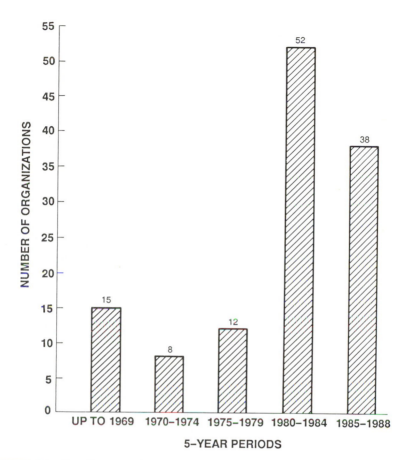

FIGURE 3-1 Founding years for utilization management organizations. All organizations founded before 1970 were founded to perform other functions such as insurance or claims administration. Some organizations founded later are subsidiaries of older insurance companies or other organizations. Regardless of founding data, most initiated utilization management services after 1982. SOURCE: *Business Insurance* (1988).

jumped from 28 to 95 percent (Scheffler et al., 1988). Third-party administrators, which began by specializing in processing claims for self-insured employers, have also diversified into prior review. In addition, a few community coalitions are administering utilization management programs for employers.

The strategies, lines of business, market niches, and sophistication of organizations in the utilization management field are quite varied. Some organizations specialize in a particular service, such as high-cost case management or review of mental health services, whereas others offer a broad range of services, including underwriting, claims administration, and provider contracting. Certain organizations concentrate on developing software packages for analyzing claims data and assessing the appropriateness of services but actually administer programs for relatively few clients.

The relative youth of utilization management organizations, their limited track records, and the inexperience of purchasers have created a small offshoot industry: firms that review the reviewers. These firms provide consulting services to employers and other purchasers. They also conduct independent audits of hospital medical records and compare their results with those of different review systems or organizations (Milstein et al., 1987).

The description of utilization management that follows is drawn largely from a series of site visits during the summer of 1988 to 12 organizations engaged in utilization management (see Appendix E for summaries of these visits). The organizations visited were selected for variability, not because they were believed to be exemplary. They included both industry leaders and organizations that are not as well known. Site visit teams were made up of two staff members and one or two members of the committee. The visits generally consumed a full day and focused heavily on the details of the operation of preadmission review and high-cost case management programs. The committee asked the utilization management organizations that it visited for examples of contracts with clients. Appendix F in this report presents a review of the agreements that were submitted.

The organizations visited included three independent utilization management companies, three insurance company subsidiaries, two third-party administrators, two PROs engaged in private review, and two HMOs (one staff model and one IPA). This mixture of organizations conveys something of the variety in the utilization management field but not the extent of cross-fertilization that is built into these organizations. The backgrounds of the organizations and their founders includes HMOs, PSROs, the insurance industry, claims administration, employee benefit management, disability management, and academic research. These differences in origins and backgrounds translate in complex and subtle ways into differences in corporate cultures, data systems, computerization, attitudes toward physicians and institutional providers, expectations about what utilization levels can be achieved, and sensitivity to the employee relations issues that utilization management can create for employers.

Although any simple categorizations inevitably oversimplify the situation, it is helpful to define several basic ways in which the utilization management function can relate to the functions of health care delivery, insurance, and benefit plan administration. The following four categories of utilization management are described below: (1) freestanding service,

(2) insurer-based service without provider contracts, (3) insurer- or broker-based service with provider contracts, and (4) provider-based service.

In the first category, utilization management is carried out by an organization that (1) does not have contracts or other formal relationships with providers and (2) is *not* at risk for the costs of medical care services. The party at risk may be an employer, an insurer, or even an HMO or PPO that contracts with the organization for utilization management services. Even though the review function may be freestanding, the organization itself may be a subsidiary or an affiliate of an insurance company or a subdivision of a third-party administrator rather than a completely independent organization. What distinguishes these programs from those that are integrated into the insurance or claims administration function is that they may be marketed as a freestanding product to purchasers that use other companies for insurance or claims administration or that perform those functions themselves.

The organizations that engage in utilization management as a freestanding service have gained so much attention that they are often thought of as constituting the utilization management industry. And, in fact, except for two HMOs, all of the organizations visited in this study—including the PROs—fit into the freestanding category.

In the category of an insurer-based service without provider contracts, utilization management is done by a party that is at risk for the costs of additional medical services but has no contractual relationship with the hospitals or physicians who are subject to its utilization management efforts. Many insurers, acting in their insurance capacity,[1] engage in utilization management as a way of controlling claims costs, with the administrative expense for the function built into their premiums. Alternatively, they may offer prior review as a separate option to their customers, but they do not market their service on a freestanding basis to clients whom they do not insure.

The third category of utilization management covers organizations that establish and manage explicit networks or panels of providers. These organizations include some HMOs, some PPOs, and some Blue Cross and Blue Shield plans. The specific arrangements vary from highly integrated group practice HMOs to PPOs and other models with weaker ties between the providers and the broker or other entity that organized the network. The entity that organizes and manages the network may act simply as a broker that does not accept economic risk for the cost of services delivered by network providers. Alternatively, the organization may accept risk, typically

---

[1] The implied distinction arises because insurance companies and Blue Cross and Blue Shield plans may either act as an insurer (accepting actuarial risk) *or* as an entity that provides only administrative services for self-insuring clients.

sharing it with the providers in the network. Generally, the provider agrees to initiate the prior review process and to not bill the patient for any claim denied for lack of medical necessity.

When an organization has the kinds of contractual relationships with physicians described above, it has at least three types of potential influence over physicians. The first lies in its control of continuing access to the network's patients, which can be effective with doctors who need the patients furnished by the network more than the network needs access to the services provided by that doctor. Second, because the organization generally has the provider's agreement not to bill patients when claims are denied for lack of medical necessity, the threat of a payment denial can be significant. The organization does not have to face unhappy patients whose bills are not being covered or unhappy clients whose employees are complaining about denied claims. Third, the organization can establish economizing or risk-sharing incentives, for example, capitation or bonuses, as part of its compensation arrangements. (The commissioned paper by Joan B. Trauner and Sybil Tilson in Appendix B describes utilization management in HMOSs in more details.)

Provider-based utilization management, the fourth category, is undertaken out of self-interest by hospitals or other health care organizations that have formal relationships with physicians, for example, employment or admitting privileges. One incentive for health care organizations to undertake utilization management is to reduce the potential for retrospective denial of payment for services judged medically unnecessary. In addition, hospitals paid on a prospective per-case basis have an incentive to minimize costs once a patient is admitted. Institutions may also undertake utilization management as an alternative to having the function performed by an external organization, as may happen with some HMOs or PPOs.

For provider-based utilization management, effectiveness may rest less on the threat of payment denial than on administrative pressure, a perceived mutuality of interest, and the risk that the institution might sever its relationship with the physician, for example, by not renewing an employment contract or by withdrawing admitting privileges. Although several payers (most importantly, Medicare) provide institutions with economic incentives to minimize unnecessary days of care, little documentation is available on the extent to which health care institutions actually use the methods of utilization management (Burda, 1989; Project HOPE, 1987).

The committee notes that those who consider the full research and policy questions raised by utilization management must recognize the existence of provider-based utilization management. The committee, however, has not focused on the utilization management activities of institutional providers of health care for several reasons. Most hospitals have been responsible for utilization review and discharge planning for many years, so hospital-based prior review is a less dramatic change from past practices than are programs undertaken by external organizations. Institutional providers also face comparatively small changes in their legal responsibilities for patient care, which exists independently of any prior review programs.

In theory, the differences among the various organizational contexts of utilization management described above could have important implications for an organization's efficiency and effectiveness, its sensitivity to the complexities and costs created for patients and physicians, its ability to assess the impact of its activities, and the extent to which it is exposed to legal risk. Unfortunately, as described in Chapter 4, virtually no research exists on the effects of these organizational differences. As Appendix B points out, this also holds true for many organizational differences among HMOs.

Even though the organizations visited do not represent the full range of organizations that carry out utilization management activities, the committee found many noteworthy variations in the ways that utilization management is designed and implemented. The description that follows covers several areas of variation in prior review processes. The short history and rapid evolution of the industry and the flux in employer-sponsored health benefits make it impossible to predict how long this description will hold.

THE REALITIES OF PRIOR REVIEW: HOW IS IT ACTUALLY DONE?

"We have the same things that everyone else has . . . a book, a WATS line, and nurses."[2]

Despite certain basic similarities implied by this quote and by the definitions offered in Chapter 1, each utilization management organization's programs are a mixture of invention, imitation, borrowing, and adaptation by an organization that has its own history, market niche, and strengths and weaknesses. Moreover, the industry is subject to little explicit regulation and has not developed any extensive form of self-regulation during its relatively brief existence. For these reasons, it is not surprising to find variations in how such "standard" methods as preadmission and continued-stay review are carried out by different organizations. Even the PROs that contract with Medicare, which are subject to very detailed oversight and performance specifications from the federal government, vary a great deal in their organization and activities (General Accounting Office, 1988).

---

[2] Robert E. Becker, M.D., founder of HealthCare COMPARE Corp., at the June 6, 1988, hearing of the Committee on Utilization Management by Third Parties. Dr. Becker followed this characterization with his views on why his company is, in fact, different.

Likewise, the means used by HMOs to influence patient care decisions vary widely, as described in Appendix B of this report.

To date, little or no documentation exists regarding the nature, extent, or consequences of such variations. This report attempts to correct some of that descriptive void, but the committee's charter did not and could not include empirical research on the impact of organizational differences.

Certain elements appear to be common to all or most programs in which prior authorization or certification must be obtained from an external organization regarding the necessity or appropriateness (different programs use different terms) of hospitalization or other services. First, all programs offer some or all of the prior review and high-cost case management activities described in Chapter 1.

Second, all rely on telephone rather than face-to-face contact with the patient or physician. The major exception is that some programs for continued-stay review programs use review nurses who are employed by the utilization management organization but who work on-site in the health care facilities that are subject to review. This arrangement was typical of PSROs and continues to be common in PROs. It is also used by HMOs, particularly those that have contractual relationships with a limited number of hospitals. In addition, for admissions planned weeks in advance, written forms may be used, with the telephone used for follow-up as needed.

Third, programs use a two-stage assessment process. In the first stage, the review organization obtains information about the patient and the proposed services; services that pass the screening criteria are certified as necessary or appropriate. This first stage is handled by nurses in most programs, although experienced medical secretaries perform this function in one program that the committee visited. Services that do not pass the screening criteria pass to the second stage, which involves physician review. Nurses may authorize services, but only physicians may deny authorization.

Fourth, the current focus of prior review is on the appropriateness of the site of care, the timing of an admission, or the duration of care. A few organizations examine the need for specific procedures, but most currently do not. During preadmission review, the cost of alternative care is not evaluated on a case-by-case basis. (As described in Chapter 5, high-cost case management includes such an assessment.)

The typical steps in the prior review process are described in Figure 3-2. Beyond these elements, organizations vary widely, as described below.

How Prior Review Is Integrated with Other Administrative Functions

Because utilization management is done by organizations with different purchaser and provider relationships, there are significant differences in the extent to which the prior review function is integrated with other

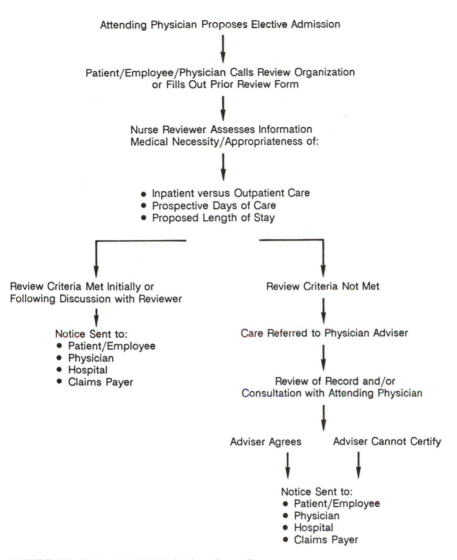

FIGURE 3-2 Typical basic steps in the prior review process.

aspects of benefit plan administration, such as determination of whether a proposed or alternative service falls in a category covered by a patient's benefit plan. Some organizations have no information about benefit plan provisions and thus can make judgments only about the appropriateness of proposed services, not whether a general category of care is covered for a particular patient. Such organizations typically tell the patient or the provider that they must find out from the employer, insurer, or claims administrator whether or not the benefit plan covers the particular services. Even organizations that have information about benefit plan provisions do not always have on-line information about whether a particular patient is still eligible for benefits or has left the employer, been dropped as a dependent, or joined another health plan.

Moreover, some review organizations have no connection with the claims payment function and possess little or no information about the actual use of services. Thus, they can report only on their activities (for example, the numbers of admissions requested and authorized), not on services actually used or paid for. They also cannot readily determine whether adherence to utilization management requirements is being checked during the claims payment process.

At the other extreme are organizations that do both utilization management and claims payment and that have fully integrated data systems. Such integration provides greater certainty that unauthorized services are not paid for inadvertently, a problem that may occur more often when one organization does utilization management and another pays claims. It also makes possible the generation of reports based on actual claims experience. Ready access to particular patients' claims histories, which some organizations possess, may permit more sophisticated judgments about the appropriateness of proposed treatment.

For example, a third-party administrator that the committee visited had a system in which the patient's claims history appeared automatically on the computer screen when the nurse reviewer began to enter data during a telephone request for prior authorization. The example that was demonstrated involved a child for whom a tonsillectomy was proposed—a procedure that was subject to a "focused second opinion" program under the insured's health benefits. The child's claims history showed that a series of office visits for tonsillitis had occurred over the previous year. Since this suggested a recurrent problem that was not responding to less intense treatment, the second-opinion requirement was waived because it was likely to concur. This saved the family some inconvenience and the purchaser the cost of the second opinion.

Systems that integrate utilization management with claims information also facilitate identification of potential cases for high-cost case management, for example, by flagging repeat hospitalizations. Integrated systems also make possible, at least in theory, a kind of outcome measurement, because future services will show up in additional claims. Although none of the organizations that were visited reported doing outcome studies, such assessments are not far beyond the capacity of several of them.

Another form of data integration takes place at some utilization management organizations whose activities are highly concentrated in a particular geographic area. PROs, Medicaid programs, Blue Cross and Blue Shield plans, HMOs, and PPOs operate largely in particular states or metropolitan areas, whereas the larger commercial insurance companies, third-party administrators, and independent review organizations often do business nationally and deal with a much more dispersed group of providers. The geographic concentration of a relatively high volume of business provides an opportunity, if data systems are properly organized, to accumulate considerable experience with particular hospitals and physicians and to better target review activities on problem services or providers.

None of the review organizations visited in this study confined their prior review or case management programs to providers who had been identified as problems. However, focusing on problem providers has been an important feature of the retrospective review activities of the PSRO, PRO, and carrier programs conducted for Medicare. One PRO visited by the committee reported that they had tried unsuccessfully to interest their private customers in a focused precertification program.

How Basic Logistical Matters Are Handled

For utilization management organizations, like most service companies, the ways in which basic operations are handled can have a major effect on relations with clients and suppliers. Purchasers often insist on visiting a review organization in an effort to assess how well the program is run, and many ask for periodic reports on service levels, for example, the percentage of telephone calls answered within five rings. Although the impact of logistical differences on benefit costs cannot now be documented empirically, the committee found a number of plan characteristics that are widely regarded as important.

Initiating Review

For organizations that do not have contracts with providers (and for some that do), the enrollee is usually responsible for initiating the review process. Otherwise, the enrollee may incur a financial penalty. One of the biggest challenges for purchasers and suppliers of utilization management services is to educate employees about this responsibility. Mere discussion in a benefits handbook is generally regarded as insufficient, and an array of additional information efforts are often attempted. These include highlighted notices on benefit plan identification cards, discussions during new employee orientation, and information letters that must be returned to the personnel office with a signed acknowledgment of receipt from the employee.[3]

As a practical matter, physician and hospital offices often make the initial calls to the utilization management organization since they generally end up discussing the case with the reviewer anyway and also want to reduce the risk of a denied claim or bad debt. For many years most hospitals have had standard routines to check a patient's insurance coverage before admission, and contact with review organizations can be incorporated into this process. Some utilization management firms say that they try to obtain all the information they need from the patient or the patient's family, but many make it a practice to talk to the physician's office to confirm the information, obtain additional information, and describe directly their review policies or guidelines.

Handling Telephone Calls

In some utilization management organizations, the calls from patients or providers are answered centrally and passed along to the first available review nurse. In other organizations, review nurses answer calls directly. Before the actual admission takes place, as many as three or four telephone conversations may take place, since review organizations may be notified of a pending admission by more than one party and may have to talk to the physician's office more than once, particularly if the proposed services do not pass the organization's screens for certification.

How quickly the caller gets through to the correct party will depend upon the organization's staffing levels, phone system, and other factors. Some firms with clients nationwide provide a single toll-free 800 number, but calls are automatically routed to different regional offices, depending on where the calls originate. Many but not all review organizations have computerized telephone systems that allow supervisors to monitor telephone waiting time and track how often callers encounter busy signals or hang up because the phone was not answered after several rings. Attention to these matters varies enormously from organization to organization. For example, some organizations lack the equipment for systematic telephone

---

[3]For example, the identification card for the indemnity health plan offered by the National Academy of Sciences includes one warning of special plan review requirements on the front of the card (in red capital letters) and two warnings (in boldface capital letters) at the top and the bottom of the card's reverse side. The reverse side also includes brief summaries of the plan requirements and relevant phone numbers.

monitoring, whereas others not only have the equipment but also have specific performance standards and incentives. In general, sophisticated phone systems are a high priority for major utilization management organizations.

Computerization

The degree of computerization also varies greatly across utilization management organizations. At one extreme there are organizations that use computers off-line only for recordkeeping purposes. Some organizations have gone to this approach after finding that their software was too slow to be efficient for data entry while the patient or provider was on the telephone. Since flexible and fast software can be very expensive to develop or license, some organizations have been slow to upgrade their systems. At the other extreme are organizations that use networked computers into which are built (1) questions for patients or providers, (2) decision protocols and criteria to assess the information and determine whether to certify care or refer it for further review, (3) details of client benefit plan limitations, (4) individual claims histories, (5) automatic diagnosis and procedure coding, (6) diagnosis or procedure-specific length-of-stay norms, and (7) addresses for practitioners and institutional providers. These systems may also allow the automatic preparation of letters to patients, physicians, and hospitals to confirm the results of the review. These aspects of computerization affect not only the comparative efficiencies of different utilization management programs but also the kinds of analyses and reports that can be generated.

Because multiple calls involving multiple parties may take place, logistics can be important for the patient or provider. In a highly computerized organization, any nurse reviewer or physician adviser can take up a case exactly where it was left on a previous call. Organizations that use pencil and paper or inflexible telephone and computer systems may require the person who took the initial call to take follow-up calls. Since nurse reviewers and physician advisers spend much of their time on the telephone, this means that the hospitals, doctors, or patients who deal with the latter type of organization may have to make many calls before they reach the right individual. Because this can be time-consuming, physicians often turn the function over to employees. Thus, the prior review process often becomes a discussion between a nurse reviewer at the utilization management organization and a secretary or nurse in the physician's office.

How Nurse Reviewers Work

Nurses play an integral role in most prior authorization programs. This role usually includes obtaining all requisite information about the patient and proposed treatment, entering the information into the computer, assigning diagnosis and procedure codes, reviewing the proposed treatment against the organization's criteria of appropriateness, and conveying approval for treatment that conforms to those criteria. Two organizations departed from this pattern. One uses experienced medical secretaries in this role. The other gives staff physicians—assisted by computerized screening criteria—the responsibility for reviewing treatment against approval criteria and conveying approval.

Several organizations report that nurse reviewers handle 40-50 calls per day, doing anywhere from 10 to 20 certifications (certification may require several calls to complete). In most organizations, nurse reviewers do other functions, such as high-cost case management and answering inquiries from beneficiaries. Some organizations assign those functions to a separate group or groups, and others rotate nurses through different functions.

Even in the organizations that use nurses for apparently similar functions, the nature of their authority varies substantially. No organization visited gives nurses the authority to refuse prior certification of care proposed by attending physicians, but most give nurses the authority to try to negotiate conformity with review criteria. However, two organizations instruct nurses *not* to negotiate with attending physicians or their employees; anything that does not fit the organization's criteria of appropriateness must be referred to a physician consultant. Even in these organizations, the nurse reviewer's questions may prompt the physician to modify a proposed plan of care.

Organizations also vary in whether they direct nurse reviewers *not* to coach attending physicians on how to gain approval of proposed care. In one organization that the committee visited, the attitude is that attending physicians do not always know the right language to be used to gain approval of an appropriate admission. If nurse reviewers' believe that a patient probably needs to be admitted, they can give the attending physician's office the cues needed to gain approval. Other organizations explicitly instruct nurse reviewers not to do this.

Another area in which nurse reviewers' authority varies from organization to organization is whether they are permitted to make exceptions to review criteria on the basis of their clinical judgment. At least two organizations visited permit review nurses to certify an admission that does not meet review criteria if, in their judgment, it is nevertheless appropriate. Many utilization management organizations do not permit this and require referral of all such cases for review by physicians.

Most organizations prefer to hire nurse reviewers who are registered nurses with at least 5 years of experience; however, one required only one year of experience. Most organizations also prefer reviewers with hospital experience. One mentioned experience in utilization review in hospitals as being important; another prefered nurse reviewers to have emergency room or intensive care unit experience.

The training of new nurse reviewers can be quite variable. Some are trained in one-to-one sessions with a supervisor; others go through formal training periods that last anywhere from 2 to 6 weeks. Most organizations report that after some initial loss of nurses who simply do not like the work, there is very little turnover. Recently, one national association implemented a training and monitoring program to instruct nurse reviewers how to analyze and listen to patient or provider requests and calls, explain insurance plan requirements, pose questions effectively, and manage difficult calls ("New Blues Program to Train Nurse Reviewers," 1989).

How nurse reviewers are monitored also varies. Supervisors in most organizations are responsible for anywhere from 6 to 12 nurse reviewers, but in a few organizations supervision is much less close. One PRO that was visited had 76 nurses and one supervisor. Monitoring ranges from informal oversight done by walking around and overhearing the nurse's end of conversations to very rigorous and systematic monitoring. Several organizations monitor telephone activity by using a computer (which can compute such things as the average length per call and number of calls per day) and by silently listening in on a sample of calls. Several organizations also systematically review a sample of cases handled by nurse reviewers by looking at the appropriateness and consistency of decisions made and the accuracy of coding. In a few organizations, the physicians who receive cases on referral from nurse reviewers play a role in monitoring their performance.

Several of the organizations visited provide incentives for accuracy and productivity. When asked, none reported attaching any rewards to such measures as days or dollars saved or utilization levels achieved.

What Role Do Physician Advisers Play?

All utilization management organizations that were visited refer cases that fail screens to physician advisers. These physician advisers are expected to use their clinical judgment and experience to determine whether the services should be certified as medically appropriate. One organization that was visited noted that under its state's law, this function could be construed to be the practice of medicine and thus must be carried out by a physician who is licensed to practice in the state. All organizations visited said that their physician advisers are *not* bound by the organization's criteria or rules about what services are appropriate. This is quite consistent with the logic of the entire process—otherwise, decisions not to certify services could be made by computers. Thus, the physician adviser's role is crucial.

However, responsibilities and work arrangements vary in some important ways across organizations.

One important source of variation involves the nature and sources of the information on which the physician advisers base their decisions. In most of the organizations visited, the physician advisers call the attending physician to discuss cases that the nurse reviewers cannot certify. Companies say that physician advisers have excellent success in establishing direct contact with attending physicians. One reason for this is that, in at least some companies, the physician adviser calls the patient's physician's office directly, announces himself as Dr. X without disclosing the purpose of the call, and asks to speak with the attending physician. (The committee's site visitors were unable to ascertain physicians' reactions to receiving a call from another physician and finding out when they come on the line that the calling physician was from a review company.) Companies also say that by approaching attending physicians as colleagues, physician advisers, are often able to obtain important additional information that was not provided to the nurse reviewer, and they can work out a satisfactory agreement with the attending physicians about the services that will be certified as appropriate.

Some utilization management organizations, however, use their physician advisers in quite a different way. In a pattern that may be particularly characteristic of PROs, some physician advisers have no contact with attending physicians. Ordinarily, they make their decisions based only on the information obtained by the nurse reviewers and then convey their results to these nurse reviewers, who carry on from there.

The relationship between physician advisers and utilization management organizations varies. Four arrangements were seen during the site visits:

- The medical director and physician advisers are full-time employees of the utilization management organization.
- The medical director and physician advisers are part-time employees and part-time practitioners.
- The medical director is employed by the utilization management organization, and physician advisers are outside consultants.
- The medical director and physician advisers are outside consultants.

In the first arrangement, the medical director and physician advisers are full-time employees who work from the utilization management organization's offices. This requires a certain volume of business to be practical, but it provides advantages in standardizing operations such as recordkeeping, monitoring performance, and developing a corporate culture. A potential danger is that the corporate culture will include a significant degree of cynicism about the abilities and motivations of practicing physicians. Also, this type of arrangement is inconsistent with a strongly held, though non-validated, belief of practicing physicians (and some people in the utilization management business) that physicians who leave practice to work as reviewers lose touch with important realities of medical practice. The opposing argument, also unverified, is that physicians who work for a large review firm deal with thousands of clinical situations each year and therefore not only keep current but have a broader and deeper understanding of what goes on in medical practice (such as variations among practitioners).

The second arrangement, the use of reviewers who are part-time employees and part-time practitioners, appears to combine the advantages of the first arrangement while avoiding the criticism about the loss of touch with the realities of medical practice. Of course, the use of part-time physician advisers is a less stable situation, since their practices may grow or they may assume full-time responsibilities elsewhere. However, with the growing physician supply nationally, review organizations in many areas of the country are able to find practitioners who can commit a certain number of hours per week to review. By law, physician advisers for PROs must be in active practice.

The third arrangement involves the use of an in-house medical director who is responsible for the organization's medical decision-making and consults, as needed, with a panel of practicing physicians in particular specialties, most of whom work from their own offices. The medical director may seek advice from these advisers or may refer to them an occasional case that they need to deal with fully, including discussion with the attending physician. Because most decisions and most feedback from practicing physicians pass through a single individual, this arrangement may provide for a comparatively high degree of consistency in the organization's decisions. However, the arrangement also has dangers if the medical director's judgment is idiosyncratic and not balanced by other on-site physicians.

The final arrangement, which was observed in several organizations and may be the most common of all, particularly in small organizations, involves the use of physician advisers (and even medical directors) who do their work for the utilization management firm from their own offices. Although this is probably the least expensive way to organize the function, it has several potential weaknesses. It can be difficult to monitor reviewers' performance, maintain consistency, and develop a corporate culture. Some organizations say that it can be difficult to reach a physician adviser who has a busy practice, to get him or her to attend to cases in a timely fashion, and to produce the necessary documentation. Some organizations have found that physicians who agree to be on their panel are reluctant to call the attending physicians or to raise the necessary questions with them. This reluctance may be a source of the delays in the review process complained of by some attending physicians.

Variations among utilization management organizations in the use of local versus nonlocal medical advisers also have important implications. Again, several arrangements exist. First, there are organizations that operate in a relatively confined geographic area, like PROs, and that use local physicians as reviewers. These reviewers may be more reluctant to challenge their peers because of social or professional contacts.

A second variation is for an organization to do prior review on a national basis but draw physician advisers from the areas where the firm's offices are located. (An unusual version of this model involves a large insurance company that uses its own nurse reviewers but contracts with organizations located elsewhere for the services of physician advisers.) During the site visits, such organizations did not complain of having difficulty in getting their physician advisers to make the necessary phone calls. On the other hand, this arrangement can lead to problems when practice standards that are commonplace where the reviewers are located differ from the standards where the attending physician is located. For instance, several organizations reported substantial regional differences in whether surgeons will admit patients on the morning of rather than the day before surgery or whether they will perform tonsillectomies on an outpatient basis.

Probably the least common situation is for a company to do business over a large geographic area with little or no use of local physician advisers. In part, this approach may reflect the logistical difficulties that a review organization can face in developing and monitoring physician advisers scattered around a larger region. In one state that the committee visited, an entrepreneurial group of physicians put together a statewide network of physicians who were willing to do reviews on a contract basis. It can ensure that the physician reviewer who is assigned to a case is from a different part of the state than the attending physician.

There are also major differences among utilization management organizations in how much physicians are involved in prior review. On the low side, the proportion of cases that go to physician advisers for review runs about 1 or 2 percent in two organizations visited and about 10 to 15 percent in five organizations visited. In contrast, 40 percent of cases go to physician advisers in one of the oldest and best established firms, and another firm advertises 100 percent physician review.

Given these differences, it is not surprising that caseloads for physician advisers vary enormously from organization to organization. The physician advisers who work on-site at one organization handle about 10 cases per full-time reviewer per day, whereas those at another organization do 200-250 certifications per day. Note that for a hypothetical 6-hour "review day" the latter rate appears to allow a physician, on average, less than 2 minutes per review. This suggests that many cases may be just scanned and signed in such organizations.

Except for the organizations in which the physicians' determinations are based purely upon a written or computerized record, all organizations report that the process of physician review is collegial. Rarely do the attending physician and the reviewing physician fail to reach agreement about a case. Most organizations report that denials of certification are issued in fewer than 1 or 2 percent of all cases, but a much larger proportion of cases involve some modification of proposed services at some stage in the review process. By way of comparison, based on both prospective and retrospective review, PROs deny payment for about 2 percent of all Medicare admissions (PPRC, 1989).

In hiring physician advisers, most organizations that the committee visited state that the main credentials they seek are board certification and experience in practice. Some organizations mention additional factors, such as professional reputation or experience in utilization review. Investigations of qualifications do not appear to be extensive. One organization recruits some reviewers from among the physicians with whom they have contact as subjects of review.

The training of physician advisers is minimal—from 1 day to several days—and performance monitoring varies greatly. In some organizations, up to 10 percent of each reviewer's cases are reviewed either by the medical director or a quality assurance committee. Alternatively, a sample of cases may be exchanged among reviewers for mutual review. One organization uses an outside panel to review a sample of its reviewers' decisions. In contrast, some organizations do not engage in such systematic oversight. They may only review cases in which an attending physician appeals the physician adviser's decision. One organization states that its main review of its physician advisers' performance was by the nurse reviewers to whom the decisions are conveyed.

Physician advisers are paid in several different ways, reflecting the diversity of their arrangements with the review organizations. The basis of payment seen in the site visits included payment per call made, per case, per hour, per month, and by an annual salary. Although explicit or implicit productivity incentives are common, none of the organizations that were visited indicated that they tie payments to physician advisers to such measures as denial rates or the amount of money that they save the purchaser. Virtually all of the organizations visited report little turnover among their physician advisers.

To summarize, the utilization management physicians in whose hands rest decisions about the necessity or appropriateness of services

- may be full-time or part-time employees of either the utilization management organization or a subcontractor;
- may or may not have an active medical practice;

- may work from their own offices or from the review organization's office;
- may review only local cases, only cases from other regions of the country, or both;
- may deal directly with attending physicians or may rely completely upon information assembled by nurse reviewers; and
- may review as few as 10 or as many as 200 cases per day.

These differences may well affect such matters as the reviewers' toughness in trying to eliminate inappropriate services, their sympathy with the position of the attending physician, the efficiency of the program, and the consistency of the organization's decisions.

What Style Is Used with Attending Physicians?

Utilization management organizations generally state a preference for negotiating agreement rather than attempting to impose decisions on attending physicians. This preference stems, in part, from reluctance among review organizations to risk legal liability for patient care decisions, but it also may reflect client wishes. In addition, employers who purchase utilization management services vary in their desire to maximize the economizing effects of these activities and in their willingness to risk employee relations problems by backing up negative review decisions. Numerous factors may contribute to these variations, including corporate culture, the composition of the labor force, and competitive pressures. Companies that have an expanding market and a highly educated labor force may put quite different demands on a review organization than may a company whose profits are threatened by health care costs and whose labor force is poorly educated and decentralized.

One organization, most of whose clients had unionized labor forces, particularly stresses its practice of trying hard to convince attending physicians to accept its determinations of appropriateness or agree to a negotiated alternative. They say they want to avoid putting patients in the middle between the provider and the payer. Several organizations stated that some clients want to be contacted before denial letters are issued, presumably so they can make case-by-case decisions about whether to risk employee relations problems.

However, other organizations take pride in backing their reviewers' determinations and believe that their clients expect them to refuse payment authorization for inappropriate services. The impact of such a policy has not been empirically compared with more lenient policies.

What Criteria Are Used to Assess Care?

The results of prior review of medical services by utilization management organizations are shaped by *criteria*—an imprecise term employed here to refer to the written policies, decision rules, or guides used to evaluate what services are appropriate or necessary for patients in different clinical circumstances (Donabedian, 1981). Organizations refer to several different types of criteria, although the boundaries between categories are not necessarily well-defined.

Lists of Procedures

Most utilization management organizations have lists of procedures that are used to target services for assessment. The most common lists involve (1) surgical or diagnostic procedures for which payment is ordinarily authorized only if the procedure is done on an outpatient basis without an overnight stay in the hospital and (2) surgical procedures or other services for which a second opinion may be required. These lists may be included in the benefit plan information provided to patients to alert them to the general policies of the utilization management program. The utilization management organization then uses the lists in evaluating proposed inpatient services, a step that relieves the patient of keeping track of a long procedure list. (Depending on whether the benefit plan includes preprocedure review, the patient may still need to be aware of outpatient procedures for which second opinions are required.) To consider whether an admission might be warranted for a target procedure, the reviewer relies on exceptions criteria.

Exceptions Criteria

Exceptions criteria specify the circumstances under which certain utilization management policies or requirements might be waived. For procedures that are ordinarily certified only as outpatient procedures, exceptions might include patients with a history of bleeding disorders or heart disease. Also common are defined exceptions to the general rule against authorizing a patient's admission to the hospital prior to the day of surgery. Both of these types of exceptions criteria tend to be generic, and they are applied without reference to the particular diagnosis or procedure for which an admission is proposed.

Hospitalization Criteria

Utilization management organizations use a variety of criteria to determine whether an individual needs inpatient care. Most are based on criteria that were originally developed for retrospective review in the PSRO program or for research on unnecessary use of the hospital (Payne, 1987). These criteria have been refined and are marketed in hard copy or computer disk versions by a handful of major vendors for use in both prospective and retrospective reviews.

Most of the review organizations the committee visited base their hospitalization criteria either on the appropriateness evaluation protocol (AEP) or on the ISD-A criteria set (intensity of services, severity of illness, discharge, and appropriateness screens). These tools, which were originally developed for retrospective research on the extent of inappropriate hospital use, have been adapted for prospective use to discourage inappropriate hospitalization (Restuccia, 1986). A 1987 study of PROs indicated that the AEP and ISD-A criteria are also widely used by PROs (Project HOPE, 1987).

The AEP criteria for adult medical/surgical services and for pediatric and elective surgery, which were initially prepared with federal financial support in the late 1970s, are in the public domain and have been the subject of several studies that have indicated that they are reliable and valid (Gertman and Restuccia, 1981; Strumwasser et al., 1987). More recent work on the AEP has been proprietary, although it is readily available and relatively inexpensive. The ISD-A criteria are proprietary (InterQual, Inc., 1987), and no specific reports on their reliability appear to have been published.

The AEP, which has been revised and expanded since it was developed in the mid-1970s, is comprised of lists of symptoms (such as sudden acute loss of vision) or services (such as the need for vital signs monitoring every 2 hours or more often). The lists are specific to major clinical services (for example, surgery and pediatrics) and are designed so that any one symptom or service suffices to justify a day in the hospital. Table 3-2 includes an excerpt from a recent training manual describing criteria for determining when inpatient surgery is warranted based on respiratory status. The ISD-A criteria operate by a logic similar to that of the AEP but are specific to different body systems.

Most organizations purport to use a modified version of whichever criteria set they have adopted. The committee cannot judge whether these modifications are designed to make the criteria tougher, more appropriate locally, or easier for reviewers to use.

To explore variations in two specific areas, site visitors inquired about the circumstances that would warrant certification of admission to the hospital for combined tonsillectomy and adenoidectomy and for nonsurgical back pain. Some organizations consider their criteria and guidelines to be proprietary, but all responded to these specific questions. As summarized in Table 3-3, the responses varied considerably in content and specificity. It should be noted, however, that tonsillectomy and adenoidectomy and lower

TABLE 3-2 Excerpt from the *Surgery Appropriateness Evaluation Protocol Reviewer's Manual*

V. CRITERIA OF ADMISSION--LOCATION OF SURGERY/RISK FACTOR ASSESSMENT
    This section includes those factors felt to identify patients and procedures requiring that surgery be performed on an inpatient basis rather than on an ambulatory or day of surgery admission basis. These criteria for determining location fall into three categories: (1) comorbidity (the presence of concurrent medical problems which place the patient at special risk, no matter what kind of surgery is to be done), (2) potential for complications post-operatively, and (3) the need for intensive post-operative care. If any one of these criteria is met, inpatient admission for the surgical procedure is deemed appropriate. Conversely, if none of the criteria are satisfied, inpatient admission is not justified. The reviewer, however, does have the option to override the criteria in either direction (see pages 9-10).

Comorbidity

    The diagnoses or measurements in this section must be documented as being present and the data (whether test results or clinical observations) should be from within the past four months prior to admission. Do not use "suspected" diagnoses.

A. Respiratory Status
    1. Significantly abnormal pulmonary function measurements
        Independent of what particular respiratory disease is present any one of the following four measures of pulmonary function will suffice:
        a. Functional Vital Capacity (FVC) of < 1.0 liters
        b. Forced Expiratory Volume in the First Second (FEV_1) of < 50% x FVC
        c. Arterial pCO_2 > mmHg
            This test must have been done while the patient was breathing room air, not an atmosphere higher in oxygen concentration.
        d. Arterial pO_2 < 50 mmHg
            This test must have been done while the patient was breathing room air, not an atmosphere higher in oxygen concentration.
    2. Sleep apnea
        Documented as present regardless of how severe or frequent.

SOURCE: Reprinted with permission from Restuccia (1986). Copyright © 1986 by Restuccia.

back pain were picked deliberately because the committee knew they were particularly likely to show variation.

Length-of-Stay Norms

To assess proposed hospital lengths of stays, most utilization management organizations use statistical norms based either on data published by the Commission on Professional and Hospital Activities (CPHA) or on data compiled by the review organization itself. These statistics are generally disaggregated by geographic region and diagnosis. Most of the organizations visited base their continued-stay review on the CPHA's average length of stay for the CPHA Western region, where lengths of stay are shortest. Many review organizations do continued-stay review either on the

TABLE 3-3 Circumstances Warranting Hospital Admission as Identified by Various Organizations Visited by the Committee

Site	Tonsillectomy and Adenoidectomy
1	Distance from home to facility; complications
2	Physician insistence on admission
3	Complications
4	Age; comorbidities
5	Physician insistence; high risk; 2 hours or more of travel time
6	Bleeding disorders; distance
7	Physician request for admission
8	Patient's history
9	None specified
10	One-night stay permitted
11	Physician request for admission
12	No special conditions required
Site	Lower Back Pain
1	Patient requires intramuscular injections for pain control; inability to move
2	Need for intramuscular injections for pain control; motor defects
3	Pain; complications
4	Severe pain; need for traction
5	Three days of traction allowed for pain
6	ISD-A criteria
7	Failure of outpatient treatment
8	Neurological deficit
9	If physician requests, having tried outpatient treatment first
10	Physician insistence on admission
11	Physician request for admission
12	Rare, only for intensity of service

day by which 50 percent of patients with a given diagnosis are discharged in the Western CPHA region or on the day before that. However, one HMO visited initiates continued-stay review on the day when, on average, the first 10 percent of patients are or have been discharged. Most of the organizations visited do not use the length-of-stay norms to certify a specific length of stay as appropriate but, instead, use them as guides for scheduling continued-stay reviews. They then assess whether a patient is ready for discharge based on AEP, ISD-A, or similar criteria. Some organizations do not employ statistical norms for scheduling continued-stay review but rather check back on a regular basis, for example, every third day after admission.

Thus, although some organizations still tell providers and patients how many days of stay they can certify at the outset, others simply state when they will check back to see how the patient is doing. Two reasons have been cited for this practice. First, when a particular length of stay is certified, physicians and patients may interpret it as a fixed limit, not a guide. Patients who do not understand the process may get anxious when they know that 3 days of stay have been authorized and then their physician tells them on the third day that they are not ready for discharge. Second, some physicians may regard a statistical norm as a minimum length of stay or may focus on the length-of-stay numbers rather than on the justification for continued hospitalization.

Necessity of a Procedure

The least commonly used criteria at this time are those designed to assess whether a specific procedure (usually surgical, but sometimes diagnostic) is appropriate for a particular patient. Although considerable research evidence has accumulated to suggest that certain procedures—insertion of pacemakers, carotid endarterectomies, and others—are used much more commonly than is medically justifiable, utilization management organizations have moved cautiously to require prior review of procedures based on medical necessity grounds. PROs are now required to review the need for care on a prospective basis for several procedures (see Appendix C). Fear of legal liability undoubtedly contributes to the reluctance of other organizations to accept the responsibility that such determinations would entail. Nevertheless, a growing number of programs are expanding or planning to expand in that direction.

The most commonly mentioned criteria for this kind of review involve the medical review system developed by former Rand Corporation researchers (Value Health Sciences, Inc., 1989). In this system, the review protocols for procedures like tympanotomy tube insertion or knee arthroscopy involve a series of questions on such matters as the chronicity of the patient's problem, prior treatment by drugs or specified nonsurgical options, and physical findings. The answers are evaluated through scaling and other techniques to determine whether the proposed care is indicated (Value Health Sciences, Inc., 1989).

At present, it appears that most organizations that make medical necessity judgments combine prior review with provisions for a nonbinding second-opinion in cases in which the clinical indications for a procedure are dubious. In certain cases in which clinical indications for a specific procedure are nonexistent (based on information provided to the reviewer), some review organizations say they now refuse to certify the necessity of the services.

How Criteria Are Adopted and Modified

Many approaches are used to adopt or modify criteria, but virtually all involve the organization's medical director and physician advisers (or a committee thereof), who are supplemented in some cases by an external advisory group. Some organizations describe a fairly formal and extensive internal process for developing criteria that includes using systematic review of the clinical literature on a topic and consensus panels. However, criteria are often borrowed, licensed, or adapted from outside sources or are developed less formally through discussions among physician advisers.

Utilization management organizations generally report that their criteria are in a continuous process of modification, although some also schedule periodic reviews for particular sets of criteria. The process of modification can be rather informal in smaller organizations. In large organizations in which many different nurses and physicians use the criteria, the process is necessarily more formal.

The decision to revise a criterion may be prompted in several ways. Members of the medical staff may raise an issue because of differences among themselves over how certain situations are being handled, because they are encountering a great deal of resistance from attending physicians, or because new information has come to light in medical literature or conferences. In addition, pressure from customers to reduce medical care utilization may prompt a new examination of criteria to search for areas in which additional savings are possible.

Several organizations mentioned that they revise criteria based on their own utilization data. They may find, for example, that although they are still authorizing hospitalization for a particular procedure, the majority of the patients covered by their program undergo the procedure on an outpatient basis. Length-of-stay criteria may be revised when data show that many patients are being discharged before the scheduled concurrent review. Examples like these suggest that utilization management organizations tend not to be the pioneers in the move to more parsimonious forms of care but are, instead, consolidators of movement in that direction.

How Organizations Use Criteria

Utilization management organizations most commonly use written or explicit criteria to differentiate patient conditions that warrant certification in a first level of review (usually by a nurse reviewer) from those that require more detailed review, usually by a physician based on implicit professional standards. The written criteria are, as a result, often described as *screens*, although that term is sometimes reserved for computerized edits of claims that flag certain types of claims for more detailed examination by nurse reviewers.

The main users of criteria are the nurse reviewers who are empowered by most (but not all) programs to certify services that conform to the criteria or to negotiate changes in proposed services so that they conform to the criteria. Criteria for outpatient surgery, presurgical days, or appropriate hospital days may be applied more or less strictly, depending on the utilization management organization's philosophy and the purchaser's requirements. In most instances, physician advisers make little direct use of such formal screening criteria. They are expected to make decisions based upon their own clinical judgment. However, physician advisers are expected to be familiar with the formal criteria and not contradict them without sound clinical justification. It does not ordinarily suffice for a physician adviser to certify services on the grounds that he or she does not agree with the criteria.

In some cases, medical directors and physician advisers cannot agree on how particular circumstances should be handled, and it is left to the discretion of the physician adviser who receives the case.[4] In some organizations, the nurse reviewers have the power to select the physician adviser to whom a case will be referred. With the passage of time, the nurses can learn a great deal about different physician advisers' tendencies and can make referrals based on their own assessment of what decision should be made and their knowledge of which physician adviser is most likely to make that decision.

Appeals Processes

The appeals process used by organizations that engage in utilization management are quite diverse, although it appears that all organizations have some mechanism for appeals. Among the organizations visited, variations in these mechanisms appear particularly significant along two dimensions. One dimension is the elaborateness of the process. The other is whether parties external to the organization are involved.

PROs have a very formal and extensive appeals process. (For a brief overview of some general differences between the PRO program and private programs, see Appendix C.) This is a function of the requirements that PROs accept as part of their contracts with the federal government to review care for Medicare beneficiaries.

In most of the organizations the committee visited, an appeal involves a review of the case by a new physician adviser, the medical director, or a

---

[4] A particularly interesting situation was described in one review organization visited in which the two specialists to whom a particular type of case was referred had different preferences regarding the two treatment options that were available. Depending upon which physician adviser received the case, either treatment A or treatment B would be authorized. For the organization to send all such cases to either of the physicians would have involved a policy decision that the organization was not prepared to make. The organization decided to alternate cases, without regard for the fit between the therapeutic preferences of the attending physician and the physician adviser. So the luck of the draw determined whether an attending physician received authorization with no difficulty or might not be able to obtain authorization at all.

committee. Additional discussion with the attending physician may or may not be a part of the process.

Several organizations indicated that their clients, usually an employer, may get drawn into the appeals process when the issue is whether the proposed service will be covered by the patient's benefit plan. In at least one organization, appeals are shifted directly to the clients.

Reporting and Feedback Mechanisms

In inquiring about the impact of the programs operated by the organizations the committee visited, it became apparent that interpretation of results and comparisons across organizations are extremely difficult. What can be made of information from one organization that the number of hospital days per 1,000 covered individuals ranges from 300 days for one client to 600 days for another and from a second organization that reports a range from 200 to 1,300 days per 1,000? For a third organization, the range is 487 to 1,583 days, but the review organization at least knows that the second number applies to a group of retirees. Despite the well-recognized differences in medical care cost and use experience for different age, sex, and other groups and the considerable variation across employee groups, there are no standard adjustments or reporting conventions used by utilization management organizations to account for these differences.

Organizations that provide review services under contract generally provide their clients with periodic reports on their activities. These reports vary considerably in usefulness. At one extreme are organizations that calculate savings based on the difference between services requested and services authorized. At the other extreme are organizations that can provide detailed analyses of inpatient and outpatient utilization for the covered group. Some firms have clients that demand relatively sophisticated, or at least extensive, data, and they risk losing these clients if they cannot respond to those demands. (Problems with different measures of program results are discussed in Chapter 4.)

Discussions of reporting requirements during the site visits conveyed a clear sense that clients evaluate utilization management organizations based on their apparent success in reducing hospital utilization or holding hospital utilization to comparatively low levels. Client reaction to reports of cost and use experience are, thus, an important feedback mechanism to review organizations.

Review organizations also receive several other kinds of feedback. One source is appeals and objections from physicians and patients regarding the organization's decisions. Criteria that produce too much negative reaction and consume too much of the physician advisers' time may be revised.

None of the organizations that provide utilization management services under contract report any routine mechanism to evaluate the impact that their decisions have on the quality of patient care. For example, no systematic mechanisms are in place to track the experience of patients whose care is shifted from an inpatient to an outpatient basis. Similarly, no organization has any systematic process to assess the burden that their procedures place on providers of care. Some organizations, however, report that they survey patients who have gone through prior review. Also, clients may have (or may be planning) programs to monitor quality of care based, for example, on retrospective reviews of certain types of claims such as those showing rehospitalization within a specified number of days after discharge.

SECOND-OPINION REQUIREMENTS

Second-opinion programs were not the subject of much systematic inquiry during the site visits because few of the organizations regard second opinions as a major element in their package of services. Second-opinion programs, which are generally confined to a list of 15-30 surgical procedures, have two major objectives. First, they are intended to save money by reducing the likelihood that unnecessary procedures will be recommended and performed. Second, they are an educational device designed to increase the amount of information available to the patient who is contemplating elective surgery.

There are several types of second-opinion programs. Some employers and insurers have voluntary programs that pay for a second opinion if the patient wants it. Other programs are mandatory, that is, they make obtaining a second opinion a requirement for full payment of benefits, but they do not condition payment on the receipt of a confirming opinion. Some benefit plans require a third opinion if the second opinion does not confirm the first. Most programs, like those for preadmission review, require that the patient initiate the process with a call to the utilization management organization.

Several permutations were encountered in the site visits. For example, organizations vary in whether they refer patients to particular physicians for second opinions. Some have panels of physicians who have agreed to provide second opinions, and these organizations generally offer patients the names of three participating physicians whom they can call for an appointment. Other organizations leave the selection to the patient. With regard to procedures about which there may be differences of opinion across medical specialties (for example, between cardiac surgeons and a cardiologists), some programs require that the second opinion be obtained from the nonsurgical specialist. One organization has a second-opinion program that consists of record reviews and telephone consultations by their regular panel of physician advisers. No face-to-face consultation is required.

Although older second-opinion programs required (with few exceptions) a second opinion for any targeted procedure, several organizations now waive the requirement when preadmission or preservice review determines that the clinical indications for the procedure are clear. A typical example would be a patient with uterine cancer recommended for a hysterectomy. The screening of cases during preadmission or preservice review is intended to reduce the cost and inconvenience of the program. However, by retaining the provision for second opinions for cases in which indications are in doubt, the review organization has a means of dispute resolution that can supplement the usual appeals process.

LEGAL ISSUES

In Appendix A of this report is a commissioned paper by William A. Helvestine that discusses the legal implications of utilization review, primarily prior review, and continued-stay review techniques. It describes the general lack of explicit legislative, administrative, or judicial rules involving prior review. It also describes standards of behavior that have been applied by the courts to other aspects of health plan administration that are, in many respects, similar to prior review.

In one well-known case, *Wickline* v. *California*, a state court has held that a review organization (in this case the state Medicaid program) could be held liable for "defects in the design and implementation of cost containment mechanisms" that result in the denial of medically necessary services. In this particular instance, the organization was not held liable because the harm to the patient was attributed to the negligence of the attending physician. A later case, *Sarchett* v. *Blue Shield of California*, explicitly upheld the right of an insurer to challenge an attending physician's decisions about medically necessary care.

A few states have passed laws regulating private review organizations (American Hospital Association, 1989). Maryland and Arkansas have established (but have not implemented at the time of this writing) a certification process that requires submission by organizations of information about review standards, appeals provisions, personnel, confidentiality policies, information for patients and providers, and accessibility to patients and providers (for example, business hours). The laws do not require detailed disclosure of review criteria. Other states have considered, but not passed, legislation that would require that review physicians be licensed within the state, that no penalties (for example, reductions in benefit payments) be imposed on patients or providers for failing to follow review procedures, and that all reviews (including those now performed by nurses) be done by licensed physicians. The efforts to impose state regulation have been attributed, in part, to concern about controlling a few "bad apples" and getting accountability, especially from the smaller organizations. However, physician resistance to outside review and unwillingness to change challenged practice patterns is also cited (Page, 1989). Some proposed regulations could make operations much more difficult for organizations operating on a nationwide basis, and some might make reviews prohibitively expensive.

Despite the lack of much explicit regulation, the committee found that review organizations are aware of the legal risks inherent in efforts to influence patient care decisions and to operationalize the terms of health benefit contracts. There also appears to be a general appreciation of the conventional—but not infaliible—protections offered against liability by good management, good judgment, good faith, and good documentation. The contract provisions analyzed in Appendix F reflect the sensitivity of utilization management firms to these legal issues.

CONCLUSION

As might be expected for a new and evolving activity, prior review programs are not standardized. Aside from a few common elements—the absence of face-to-face contact with patients, the focus on site, timing, and duration of care, and the requirement that negative determinations be made by a physician—all aspects of the process vary markedly from organization to organization. This variation includes the roles and responsibilities of the nurses and physicians who are involved in the review process, the logistics of the process, the nature and availability of the criteria used in prior review, the types of decisions that are made, the appeals process, and reports of impact.

Although review organizations vary in their inventiveness and willingness to tackle new issues of appropriate use, they generally follow the lead of researchers or medical groups in selecting targets for attention. The evolving focus on assessing the clinical indications for selected procedures is a case in point.

Some variation among review organizations is prompted by clients, some by the origins or roots of the organization. Variations in state regulation, which affect many aspects of insurance company operations, do not account for differences among review organizations since little regulation of these programs exists. One exception involves PROs, which face many requirements for their federal business that also govern their private contracts. However, PROs still vary considerably. It might be expected that the outside consulting firms that assess review programs for employers would have a certain standardizing influence over time, but the committee has seen no obvious evidence of this to date.

Through its site visits, the committee developed a clear sense that some organizations have better designed programs or more effectively implemented programs than others. However, as the next chapter reports, the limited evidence on the impact of prior review programs does not include any assessment of the link between differences in program characteristics and differences in program results.

REFERENCES

American Hospital Association, *Private Utilization Review*, State Issues Forum Monograph Series, August 1989.

Burda, David, "Changing Physician Practice Patterns," *Modern Healthcare*, February 17, 1989, pp. 18-26.

Business Insurance Survey, "Directory of Utilization Review Companies," *Business Insurance*, February 20, 1989, pp. 33-68.

Donabedian, Avedis, "Criteria, Norms and Standards of Quality: What Do They Mean?" *American Journal of Public Health*, April 1981, pp. 409-412.

Foster Higgins, *Health Care Benefits Survey*, New York, 1987.

Gabel, Jon, Jajich-Toth, Cindy, de Lissovoy, Gregory, and Cohen, Howard, "The Changing World of Group Health Insurance," *Health Affairs*, Summer 1988, pp. 48-65.

General Accounting Office, *Medicare PROs: Extreme Variation in Organizational Structure and Activities*, GAO/PEMD-89-7FS, Washington, DC, November 1988.

Gertman, Paul M., and Restuccia, Joseph D., "The Appropriateness Evaluation Protocol," *Medical Care*, August 1981, pp. 855-871.

InterQual, Inc., *The ISD-A Review System*, Chicago, 1987.

Mayo Clinic, "The Cost of Effective Utilization Review Programs," Statement for the Institute of Medicine Committee on Utilization Management by Third Parties, Washington, DC, May 20, 1988.

McGraw-Hill, Inc., *Review Resources: Sourcebook of Private Independent UR Companies*, Washington, DC, 1987.

Meyer, Harris, "Two States Lead Move to Regulate Utilization Review," *American Medical News*, April 21, 1989, pp. 1, 45.

Milstein, Arnold, Oehm, Marvis, and Alpert, Geraldine, "Gauging the Performance of Utilization Review," *Business and Health*, February 1987, pp. 10-12.

"New Blues Program to Train Nurse Reviewers," *American Medical News*, April 14, 1989, p. 49.

Page, Leigh, "AMA, Insurers Agree on Guidelines for Hospital Admission Review," *American Medical News*, July 21, 1989, pp. 3, 34-35.

Payne, Susan M. C., "Identifying and Managing Inappropriate Hospital Use," *Health Services Research*, December 1987, pp. 706-769.

Physician Payment Review Commission, *Annual Report to Congress*, Washington, DC, 1989.

Project HOPE, *A Study of the Preadmission Review Process*, Prepared for the Prospective Payment Assessment Commission, Washington, DC, November 1987.

Restuccia, Joseph, *Appropriateness Evaluation Protocol Reviewer's Manual*, Boston: Boston University, 1986.

Scheffler, Richard M., Gibbs, James O., and Gurnick, Deborah, *The Impact of Medicare's Prospective Payment System and Private Sector Initiatives: Blue Cross Experience 1980-1986*, HCFA Grant No. 15-C-98757-50-1, Research Program in Health Economics, University of California, Berkeley, July 1988.

Strumwasser, Ira S., et al., *Estimates of Non-Acute Hospitalization*, Final Report, HCFA Grant No. 18-C98582/5-01 and 2, Washington, DC: Health Care Financing Administration, 1987.

Value Health Sciences, Inc., *Medical Review System*, Santa Monica, CA, 1989.

4
Impact of Prior Review Programs

The explosive growth of utilization management activities, organizations, and expenditures raises an obvious question: Does utilization management work? More specifically, does it do what it is intended to do at a reasonable cost without unacceptable effects on quality or access to care? And under what circumstances do programs have better results? How have patients, physicians, and other involved parties fared?

Unfortunately, in its search of the literature, the committee found that relatively little rigorous empirical evidence is publicly available on the effects of these programs. What is available only covers those elements of utilization management that have been in place long enough for assessment data to have been accumulated. Prior review of the actual medical need for specific procedures is mostly too new to have been evaluated.

This chapter summarizes the evidence available to the committee, describes weaknesses in the evidence, and considers the positive and negative aspects of prior service for patients, providers, and purchasers. Most of the evaluations cited here focus on preadmission review and continued-stay review. A review of evidence specific to the effects of high-cost case management is presented in Chapter 5. Appendix B of this report discusses the limited information about the effects of different methods used by HMOs to influence patient care decisions.

The committee has not attempted a global assessment of the broad societal effects of utilization management. At this point, the base is simply too weak to estimate how utilization management has specifically affected total health care expenditures, overall use of health services, and attitudes toward medical care.

DIRECTION OF AVAILABLE EVIDENCE: IMPACT ON UTILIZATION AND COST

Although reports of the impact of prior review programs on utilization and cost suffer individually from an array of methodological weaknesses, they present a reasonably consistent pattern of positive results. Taken together, the studies show:

- a substantial initial drop in inpatient hospital utilization following introduction of prior review, with use rates tending to decline at a lesser rate or to level off thereafter;
- an increase in the use of outpatient facilities and physician office services following the introduction of prior review;
- a greater decline in inpatient utilization for reviewed groups than for nonreviewed groups during a period of generally declining hospital use;
- among groups covered by prior review, a more sizable drop in inpatient utilization for groups that started with higher than average initial utilization rates compared with those with lower than average initial utilization rates; and
- a lower rate of increase in the short-term in per-employee medical care costs for groups covered by prior review compared with those that were not, but no long-term reduction in the rate of growth in total medical care spending.

Evidence discussed in this chapter about the effects of prior review programs was discovered through site visits by the committee, computerized literature searches, presentations to the committee, and less formal efforts. The majority of reports take the form of marketing materials, press releases, and client reports prepared by review organizations. Much scarcer are more sophisticated assessments prepared by review organizations or academic researchers.

The earliest studies typically were simple one-group before-and-after studies with no comparison groups. Several recent studies are more methodologically sophisticated, although they too are imperfect. Limitations of available research are described at the end of this section and in the appendix to this chapter.

Before-and-After Studies

Most of the early and influential attempts to demonstrate the effects of prior review programs were based on simple before-and-after comparisons.

These comparisons are typical of the promotional materials, conference presentations, and materials that most utilization management companies release to the public to show changes in utilization for client groups.

The trend data presented in summary form by one utilization management company that the committee visited are illustrative. For a large food and chemical company, the number of hospital days per 1,000 covered individuals dropped from 579 days before initiation of prior review management to 486 and then 389 days in the subsequent 2 years. For an aerospace company, the comparable figures were 627 for the preprogram year and 514 and 416 for the next 2 years. And for a large consumer products company, the number of inpatient days per 1,000 covered individuals went from 1,065 days before to 889 to 703 days after the program. Many other companies report similar drops in inpatient use after the introduction of prior review.

In 1984, the journal *Hospitals* included some typical press release information in a story on preadmission review programs ("Preadmission Review Cuts Hospital Use," 1984). The story noted that Blue Cross and Blue Shield of North Carolina reported that a pilot preadmission review program helped cut hospital days by 37 percent and that Blue Cross of Northeast Ohio reported a 23 percent decrease in hospital days and savings of $30 million during the first 5 months of a preadmission review program.

More fully described is the experience of Deere & Company of Moline, Illinois, as presented in a case study prepared by the Health Systems Management Center at Case Western Reserve University (Kauer, 1983). Deere initiated a utilization management program in 1977 by using PSROs to perform preadmission and concurrent review. Over 36 months, inpatient days dropped 21 percent, and the company estimated savings of $11 for every program dollar spent. The case study noted that one PSRO performed its own reviews, whereas another PSRO delegated the review responsibility to each area hospital. The nondelegated program showed greater initial results, with the delegated program catching up somewhat in later months.

The Deere study mentions that company staff accompanied PSRO officials to discuss utilization problems with individual hospitals, and the company added HMO options to its benefit offerings in 1980. These activities point to a major problem with before-and-after studies. While prior review programs were being introduced, other changes were also occurring that affected utilization patterns within particular companies and across society more generally.

Comparative Studies

Over the past decade, several factors, including the growing safety and acceptance of procedures done on an outpatient basis, the increasing supply of outpatient resources, and restrictions on inpatient payments, have

TABLE 4-1 Some Factors That May Affect the Impact or
Assessment of Prior Review

Benefit Plan Characteristics
        Coverage of noninpatient benefits
        Levels and types of beneficiary cost-sharing
        Choice among alternative benefit plans

Other Initiatives
        Quality of care monitoring
        Selective contracting
        Hospital payment method and financial incentives
        Physician payment method and financial incentives
        Retrospective utilization review
        Provider audit, feedback, and education
        Consumer education and health promotion

Government Regulation
        Medicare prospective payment system, PRO programs
        State rate setting and other hospital regulation
        Mandated benefits and other insurance regulation
        Medicaid program features
        Health planning

Individual, Group, and Community Characteristics
        Age, income, education, race, and sex
        Union membership
        Marital and family status
        Other health insurance coverage
        Health status
        Occupation and industry
        Geographic region
        Urban or rural location

Health Care Delivery System
        Supply of hospital and other institutional resources
        Supply and distribution of physicians and other practitioners
        Medicare and Medicaid market shares
        HMO and PPO market shares
        Blue Cross and Blue Shield market shares
        Proportion of self-paying and uninsured patients

changed the balance of incentives for using inpatient versus outpatient care
and have contributed to substantial general reductions in hospital use (Table
4-1). Data from the American Hospital Association, the Hospital Discharge
Survey, the Health Interview Survey, and the Blue Cross and Blue Shield
Association indicate that hospital days per 1,000 people under age 65 were
beginning to level off and then drop in the latter part of the 1970s (Lerner
et al., 1983b). The drop accelerated in the 1980s, before it appeared to
level off again recently. Simple before-and-after studies are not capable
of distinguishing the impact of utilization management from the impact of
other factors and, thus, may wrongly credit those programs with changes
that would have occurred anyway.

Some studies have attempted to control for the impact of systemwide influences by comparing the utilization and cost experience of groups covered by prior review programs with groups that were not. The RCA organization tried this approach within its own organization. In 1985, it instituted an array of utilization management programs (called Plan for Health) for about half of its employees, early retirees, and dependents while continuing the old plan for the other half. Although inpatient hospital utilization dropped for both groups, it dropped more for the utilization management group. Inpatient days for medical care patients showed the same general pattern. However, surgical days unexpectedly increased for both groups, although more for the nonmanaged group. Nevertheless, net benefit costs for employees under utilization management dropped by 4 percent, whereas they rose by 6 percent for the nonmanaged group. The company estimated a 4:1 return on its investment in the utilization management program (O'Donnell, 1987).

In 1984, Blue Cross and Blue Shield of Massachusetts added a comprehensive utilization management option for its fee-for-service business and then compared what happened to hospital utilization for its subscribers who were covered by the option, those who were not covered by the option, and those who were covered under an HMO. In 1983, the number of hospital days per 1,000 covered individuals was 680 for the traditional plan and 409 for the organization's HMOs. By 1985, traditional plan days had dropped to 600 (a 12 percent drop), "managed" fee-for-service days were 520 (down 24 percent), and HMO days dropped to 374 (a 9 percent drop) (Getson, 1987).

An analysis prepared for the Service Employees International Union and the State of Michigan took a somewhat different approach. The evaluation of the group's precertification program attempted to measure "the difference between what experience was expected to occur if no intervention took place, and what actual experience was given implementation of the program" (SEIU, 1988). The decline in hospital use for the program group was higher than that for a statewide comparison group for the first year of the program but not for the second year. However, in both years the program had lower hospital utilization than predicted on the basis of preprogram trends for the union group. The analysis estimated a gross savings/cost ratio for the program of 2.27 to 1. The savings were not reduced by the cost of alternative services but did exclude the estimated fixed costs of avoided admissions (Service Employees International Union, 1988).

Yet another approach was used by Blue Cross of Greater Philadelphia, which established a utilization management program as part of its 1985 contractual agreement with area hospitals. Because this agreement covered all enrollees unless a client explicitly rejected application of the utilization management features (which was rare), the company did not have an adequate base to compare enrollees with and without prior review. Instead, the company compared inpatient days per 1,000 covered individuals for contracting hospitals, which dropped 23 percent from 1984 to 1986, with inpatient days for noncontracting hospitals (mostly specialized mental health, rehabilitation, and similar facilities), which saw inpatient days increase by 28 percent. One consequence was that the share of inpatient days accounted for by noncontracting hospitals went from 17 to 27 percent of the total inpatient days. Total inpatient days per 1,000 covered individuals for all hospitals decreased by 20 percent from 1984 to 1987. Combined inpatient and outpatient surgical rates (excluding physician office surgery), which had increased from 48.2 procedures per 1,000 in 1980 to 53.1 in 1983, declined to 47.9 in 1986 (Blue Cross of Greater Philadelphia and Pennsylvania Blue Shield, 1986, 1987).

Multivariate Studies

A potential contaminant in simple comparative studies is the fact that the introduction of utilization management may have been accompanied by other changes that could affect utilization and costs. For example, other cost-containment methods such as increased cost-sharing by beneficiaries have often been implemented along with prior review, and sales and acquisitions can change the work force composition, which in turn can affect health care use. Also, the purchasers that self-select utilization management could differ in various ways from those that do not. Although not all such factors can be controlled, some multivariate studies have attempted to rule out alternative explanations for changes in cost and use after the introduction of prior review.

One utilization management company structures its comparisons by trying to match review and nonreview groups by industry, geographic region, and other characteristics. In an analysis for one insurance company client, the firm reported that hospital days per 1,000 covered individuals dropped 14 percent for review groups, whereas for nonreview groups they dropped 7 percent. The percentage increase in expenditures for groups with prior review was lower than the rate of medical inflation, whereas the opposite was true for comparison groups (Health Data Institute, 1988).

An analysis of early state programs to contain Medicaid costs reported that prior authorization for elective surgery and specific services appeared to reduce growth in real hospital expenditures by controlling growth in the number of beneficiaries receiving hospital care. For the period 1977-1984, states with prior authorization showed a 1.4 percent average annual increase in real total inpatient expenditures, whereas states without this policy experienced a 6.5 percent increase. The number of beneficiaries receiving inpatient care dropped, on average, by 1.2 percent a year for prior authorization states but rose 1.9 percent a year for the other states. A multivariate statistical analysis linked prior authorization with a 2.7 percent annual reduction in beneficiaries who received inpatient care after several other changes in Medicaid policy and state environments were controlled (Zuckerman, 1987).

Feldstein et al. (1988) and Wickizer et al. (1989) analyzed claims data for one insurer to compare utilization and costs for clients with and without utilization management. Using a combination of cross-sectional and longitudinal analyses that included controls for some differences in case mix, employee characteristics, market factors, and benefit plan features, the authors concluded that for the period 1984-1986 prior review reduced admissions by 13 percent, inpatient days by 11 percent, and total medical expenditures by 6 percent. (Because some groups included in this part of the analysis had a utilization management program in place *before* the first year for which data were analyzed, these results do not reflect straightforward preprogram-postprogram utilization.) From their statistical analysis, the authors concluded that the review programs produced a "one-time" reduction in use and costs but had little impact on growth in use and costs over time. In another analysis, the researchers compared groups with high utilization prior to adoption of utilization review to groups with low prior utilization. The former were found to have significant decreases in use and costs, but the latter did not (Feldstein et al., 1988).

After introduction of a utilization management product called HEALTHLINE, Aetna Life and Casualty compared postimplementation utilization and cost experience for employee groups with (122,299 employees) and without (296,519 employees) the program. The time period for the study was a six-quarter period ending December 31, 1987. The study controlled for some claimant, group, and benefit plan differences across the two samples (for example, claimant age, total covered employees, and coinsurance rates). The multivariate analysis also included a time trend variable. The researchers found that hospital admission rates dropped nearly 8 percent for the program sample but only 1 percent for the nonprogram sample; overall hospital days per 1,000 covered individuals dropped about 4 percent for the former and about 2 percent for the latter. Surgical outpatient costs per employee increased at about the same rate for both samples (15.5 and 16.1 percent, respectively), but inpatient medical and surgical costs rose about 5 percent for the sample with utilization management and 9 percent for the sample without.[1] Combined inpatient costs and outpatient surgical costs rose 6 and 10 percent, respectively. The study estimated gross savings from utilization management to be around 12 percent

---

[1] Inpatient costs included room and board, ancillary services, and physician services. Surgical outpatient costs included physician but not facility charges.

during the six-quarter period. The researchers emphasize that the results apply only to the study period and should not be used to predict program performance in other periods or for other employer groups. Further analyses will include preprogram data, data on nonsurgical outpatient use and costs, and other control variables (Allen and Khandker, 1988; Harris Allen, Aetna Casualty and Life, personal communication, November 3, 1988).

Scheffler et al. (1988) studied the impact of the Medicare prospective payment system (PPS) and Blue Cross benefits cost-management programs using quarterly claims data (1980-1986) on Blue Cross inpatient admissions and lengths of stay, hospital outpatient visits, total inpatient and total outpatient benefit payments, and total payments per member (adjusted for inflation). When controlled for the effects of the Medicare PPS, several other Blue Cross cost-management programs, and an array of environmental variables (for example, state regulation, state average income, and state age composition), the study found that (1) preadmission review was associated with lower hospital admission and outpatient visit rates but did not affect payments per 1,000 members for inpatient services or outpatient visits; (2) concurrent review was linked to lower inpatient and higher outpatient payments per 1,000 members and had a negative but not statistically significant impact on total payments per member; and (3) retrospective denial of payment to hospitals for inappropriate utilization was correlated with lower values for all utilization and payment measures.[2] In addition, the study attributed significant declines in utilization rates and rates of payment increase to the spillover effects of Medicare PPS and Blue Cross hospital payment policies (Scheffler et al., 1988).

Impact of Second-Opinion Programs

The committee did not closely examine the impact of second-opinion programs. In part, this choice reflects the fact that second-opinion programs have a longer history of application and assessment than do the other utilization management techniques investigated by the committee. (For an up-to-date review of the evidence on the impact of second-opinion programs, see Rutgow and Sieverts [1989]).

---

[2]This statistical analysis is complicated by characteristics of some of the independent variables. In all but 2 years between 1980 and 1986, over 95 percent of the Blue Cross plans reported that they had (and had used) policies to deny reimbursement for inappropriate use. In all years, over 95 percent had retrospective utilization review. The percentage of plans with concurrent review went from 52 percent in 1980 to 90 percent in 1986. No information was available on preadmission review in 1980 or 1981, but between 1982 and 1986 the percentage of plans with this program went from 28 to 95 percent. The analysis was not able to consider variations in the scope of programs nor what percentage of enrollees were covered by review requirements. Thus, a plan with 1 percent of its enrollees covered would rank the same as one with 90 percent.

The research on private sector second-opinion programs is even less likely than the research on other prior review techniques to include comparisons with groups not subject to second-opinion requirements. Moreover, refinements in the use of second opinions, particularly prior screening of cases for medical necessity before referral, are too new for much data to have accumulated on their effects; and it is not clear from discussions with those involved in such programs that the second opinions themselves are expected to have a major cost-containing effect. The major expectation is that referred patients will have more information on which to base their decisions about whether or not to have the recommended surgery.

During its site visits and other discussions of utilization management, the committee found relatively little interest in second-opinion programs and very mixed opinions about their cost-effectiveness. To some degree, this may reflect the inclination of purchasers and vendors to pay more attention to newer rather than older programs. Discussions with purchasers, however, suggest that programs that include no screening prior to mandatory referral for a second opinion are increasingly seen as wasteful.

In sum, the committee felt that a thorough, independent investigation of traditional second-opinion programs was not a high priority. The following reflects its assessment of such programs:

• Both voluntary and mandatory second-opinion programs may enhance consumer knowledge and affect some patient decisions about whether to have surgery. The effect may be to encourage surgery in certain cases (for the reluctant patient who gets a confirming opinion) and discourage it in others (for the patient who gets a strong nonconfirming opinion).

• Compared with voluntary programs, mandatory programs tend to show much higher rates of confirmation; that is, the second opinion confirms the first opinion or, more specifically, does not reject some form of surgical intervention.

• Voluntary second-opinion programs generally have much lower rates of participation by patients than do mandatory programs that include penalties if a patient does not seek a second opinion.

• Evidence on the net impact of second-opinion programs on utilization and costs is less supportive of the conclusion that it contains costs than is the (also imperfect) evidence about other utilization management techniques.

WEAKNESSES IN THE EVIDENCE ON EFFECTS OF PRIOR REVIEW

Because prior review programs have been developed and implemented in an operational rather than a research context, rigorous evaluation has not been a high priority for most organizations, and studies by outside researchers have been limited. One consequence is that much of the evidence about the impact of programs is of marginal value in answering the major questions that are asked by clients, policymakers, and other interested parties. All available studies suffer one or more of the following deficiencies in research design and measurement:

- absence of comparisons between groups with and without prior review that use such methodologies as random selection of study participants and random assignment of participants to program and nonprogram groups;
- use of short time series (for example, 1 year of preprogram data and 1 or 2 years of postimplementation data) that do not allow confident identification and assessment of preexisting trends, cyclical patterns characteristic of the health insurance industry, and long-term effects of utilization management;
- heavy reliance on inpatient utilization data with little or no evidence about (1) potentially offsetting changes in inpatient prices, (2) shifts in noninpatient prices, utilization, and overall costs, (3) changes in net benefit costs, and (4) savings relative to program costs;
- failure to control statistically or otherwise for nonprogram variables (for example, other cost-containment activities, scope of benefits, shifts in group composition, and market area characteristics) that may affect utilization and costs;
- knowledge by evaluators of whether data are from groups with or without utilization management;
- absence of comparisons of the relative impact of different program elements (for example, preadmission review versus continued-stay review) or alternative program designs (for example, greater emphasis on physician rather than nurse judgment); and
- failure to specify conditions associated with better or worse program results (for example, type of client and the supply of local health care resources).

Most importantly, all of the studies reviewed above confine their focus to utilization patterns and costs to the purchaser. The committee found no empirical research on the possible effects of private sector prior review programs on quality of care, patient out-of-pocket costs, patient convenience, patient-physician relationships, and attitudes and administrative costs of health care practitioners. (Four reports on the effects of Medicare payment and review programs are cited later in this chapter.) The appendix at the end of this chapter discusses methodological issues in more detail.

The committee did not study actuarial estimates of the impact of prior review that insurers and others employ in setting premiums or projecting benefit expenditures. Informal conversations suggest that actuaries may initially have estimated a 5-10 percent lower premium for companies that adopted prior review. Rate reductions of 1-5 percent are said to be more common for groups that have only recently adopted prior review. One explanation for the changes in estimates is that actuaries initially underestimated how much of the reduction on inpatient use would be offset by higher inpatient prices and higher outpatient use and prices and thus set premiums too low. This is consistent with the recent report of the Prospective Payment Assessment Commission (1989) which concluded that Medicare prospective payment and other public and private cost-containment efforts have reallocated health expenditures but not slowed their growth.

Another explanation for changes in actuarial estimates of prior review savings is that late-adopting groups have already gained some benefit from changes in physician behavior produced by the prior review (and other) programs implemented earlier by other purchasers. Also proposed is an analog of "herd immunity," in which coverage of one-half to three-quarters of the insured population by prior review may produce "spillover" protection for the rest. There has been no systematic test of this proposition. However, one study of an insurer's program to promote inhospital ambulatory surgery in the late 1970s and early 1980s suggested spillover effects for other payers whose inpatient surgery rates also began to drop. Nonetheless, the decrease for the sponsoring insurer started earlier and the gap in rates persisted over several years (Lerner et al., 1983a).

The committee notes that many reports on the impact of prior review come from those with an interest in positive results. This is most obvious for the organizations that provide prior review services. However, even union and corporate benefits managers may incline evaluations toward favorable results—unions may do this because utilization management can be seen as an alternative to benefit cutbacks and benefits managers may do this because good results can make them look effective to higher levels of management. Some purchasers of prior review services, recognizing that utilization management firms may be biased or may lack expertise in evaluation, ask that data be turned over for analysis by outside consultants. The study committee did not have access to the reports of these outside consultants.

EFFECTS OF PRIOR REVIEW ON SPECIFIC PARTIES

Although empirical data are very limited, it is important to consider how private sector prior review programs may positively or negatively affect different parties—enrollees of benefit plans, health care practitioners and institutions, and purchasers. The following discussion is based on committee members' experiences, testimony at the committee's June 1988 hearings, site visits of the committee members, a roundtable discussion among benefits managers of several major companies with prior review programs, and discussions among committee members over the course of several meetings.

The committee is aware that efforts to tease out the impact of prior review are complicated by the multiple cost-containment programs to which individuals and organizations are exposed. It may be impossible to isolate the effects of utilization management from the effects of prospective payment, benefit redesign, or provider and consumer education. And private review programs may be confused with those involving Medicare and Medicaid patients. Also, changes in clinical and management technologies would inevitably have spurred some shifts in clinical and administrative practices in the absence of utilization management.

Effects on Enrollees and Patients

Quality of Care

The foremost question about the effects of prior review on enrollees and patients is whether and how it affects the quality of care. Does prior review, which is explicitly aimed at unnecessary care, discourage necessary care as well?

The evidence on these points, which is very limited and pertains primarily to Medicare beneficiaries, does not suggest that prior review, as implemented thus far, has threatened the quality of care. The Prospective Payment Assessment Commission, prompted by concerns similar to those of this committee, contracted for a qualitative assessment of the impact of preadmission review on Medicare beneficiaries that found no evidence of harm (Project HOPE, 1987). Another study followed patients whose proposed hospitalizations had failed to receive certification by a PRO and also found no evidence of appreciable harm (Imperiale et al., 1988). In contrast, a more general study of what happened in one city to Medicare patients with hip fractures following the introduction of prospective payment indicated that patients were being discharged with significantly less functional capacity after the initiation of PPS and were more likely to remain in nursing homes 1 year later (Fitzgerald et al., 1988). Another study of PPS (not prior review) documented a shift in the location of death for elderly patients from the hospital to nursing homes but included no assessment of medical appropriateness (Sager et al., 1989).

On the other hand, a recent American Medical Association survey found that almost one-third of the responding physicians said they believed their patients had suffered an aggravation of illness or injury resulting from delayed or denied prior authorization for coverage (American Medical Association, 1989b). The response rate to this survey was only 30 percent, and it seems likely that physicians who had clinical, practical, or philosophical problems with prior review were most likely to have responded.

Prior review could be improving the quality of care, although this also is not documented. Unnecessary care can expose patients to needless risks from anesthesia, blood transfusions, hospital errors and infections, adverse drug reactions, and other hazards. It may also cause people to miss excess time from work and other customary activities. Still, unnecessary is not always harmful, and it may sometimes add to a patient's psychological or physical comfort (for example, the extra hospital day for the overburdened mother).

The absence of documented cases of quality problems linked to prior review might be seen as indirect evidence that these programs are, in fact, not harming patients. This is obviously a tenuous inference, and better monitoring and study of prior review's relationship to quality of care is needed.

Navigating Health Care and Health Benefits

Most employers and utilization management firms make some effort to educate employees about prior review requirements, although the level of effort appears to vary considerably. Many have added notices to insurance identification cards and taken other steps to help remind patients and providers about prior review requirements. Nevertheless, health plan requirements tend to be more complicated today than they were before, and some lapses in patient compliance seem inevitable. Even when a review organization or employer waives a penalty for employee failure to comply with requirements, the extra procedural responsibilities can cause anxiety or resentment.

Anxiety may also arise on the relatively uncommon occasions when a physician recommends a preoperative day of care that the review organization will not certify or when the patient receives a second opinion that disagrees with the attending physician's recommendation. To some extent, these anxieties are analogous to the stresses of trying to be an informed consumer in a complex medical care system. Utilization management requirements, like some patient education materials, may bring to patients or prospective patients an unwelcome awareness of the subjectivity and variability of many medical decisions.

Although prior review is one more bureaucratic hurdle in an increasingly complex health care system, it may also help patients deal with this complexity. Many employers and review companies report that benefit plan members often use nurse reviewers as a source of descriptive information about medical conditions, treatment options, alternative sites of care, and other issues related to a planned course of care. Some review companies have recognized this as a public relations opportunity and a job-enrichment vehicle for reviewers, and they have added training for reviewers in handling questions and providing descriptive information. (The companies emphasize that reviewers do not attempt to diagnose problems or recommend treatment.)

Patient Costs, Comfort, and Convenience

If prior review does help control benefit costs and deflect more onerous cost-containment strategies, then the aggregate economic impact on employees should be positive. That is, employees collectively may avoid higher deductibles, coinsurance, or other forms of reduced benefits.

In an individual case, depending on the structure of an individual's coverage, out-of-pocket costs may be lower or higher if utilization management changes the course of treatment. For example, out-of-pocket costs could be higher for patients in health plans that have higher coinsurance rates for outpatient care and do not cover outpatient prescription drugs. Patients' costs may be lower when health plans have equivalent coverage for inpatient and outpatient care or impose steep per-admission deductibles on hospital care. In some programs, patient failure to comply with review requirements may prompt a financial penalty.

When inpatient care is avoided, outpatient care may be either more or less convenient and comfortable for patients and patients' families. This depends on home conditions, income, distance from sites of outpatient treatment, and the complexity of alternative care needed. Some review organizations appear to be more willing than others to consider these sorts of circumstances in making decisions, as indicated in the presentation in Chapter 3 of circumstances considered to warrant hospitalization for lower back pain and tonsillectomy and adenoidectomy (see Table 3-3).

Some review organizations survey a sample of those who have been subject to utilization management to determine their views of the process. This information may be used in reporting to clients and refining programs. It has not, to the committee's knowledge, been published in any systematic way.

To summarize, prior review has both potential positive and negative implications for patients, depending on the specifics of their coverage and their understanding of it, the nature of the alternatives available to them, and the design and implementation of the review program affecting them. Physician and hospital reactions to utilization management may also affect patients.

Effects on Health Care Practitioners and Institutions

Most clinicians and hospital administrators now see prior review as a fact of life (Weinstein, 1988). In a recent American Medical Association (1989b) survey, for example, physician respondents reported that over one-third of their cases required prior review as a condition of payment. The growth of the utilization management industry, which depends on cooperation from hospitals and physicians, is itself an indicator of acceptance. Most physicians understand that complete prohibitions against payer "supervision or control . . . over the manner in which medical services are provided" (as stated in P.L. 89-97, the original Medicare legislation) are no longer realistic.

This recognition, however, has not come without some resistance. At a minimum, complaints about prior review requirements continue, and instances of noncooperation are still reported by review organizations. This physician's response in a focus group discussion of Medicare is illustrative of the resistor's stance: "I don't think that at this point in my life I have changed what I would do based on the fact that someone is pushing me. It just adds time to my day because I have to take telephone calls from so-and-so. And I resist the urge to be nasty on the phone saying, 'what do you think I'm going to treat this case with? I'm going to treat them with whatever I see fit, thank you' " (cited in Walker, 1989).

Physician-Patient Relationship

For those cases subject to prior review, third parties have a role in decisions on patient care that alters the context of the physician-patient relationship. However, the potential ramifications are easier to enumerate than to document systematically and almost certainly affect some specialties, such as surgery, more than others. The testimony provided by medical organizations at a hearing sponsored by this committee (summarized in Appendix D of this report) reflects both positive and negative views of utilization management.

Some physicians feel that prior review compromises their professional autonomy and increases their vulnerability to malpractice suits. Some are resentful when they must soothe patients worried about prior review requirements or act as advocates for their patients when review organizations promote a course of care that they see as less safe, comfortable, or convenient. This resentment could spill over into their relations with their patients. Some observers worry that certain physicians may acquiesce to a reviewer's judgments because they would rather avoid hassles than challenge a questionable review determination. On the other hand, some physicians note that utilization management may be contributing to improved patient relations—that they are explaining proposed services more carefully, jointly exploring more options, and documenting treatment rationales and details more carefully (Carroll, 1988; London and Anderson, 1988).

Physician-Hospital Relations

Utilization management, in combination with prospective hospital payment and other purchaser strategies to contain health care costs, has also affected relationships between physicians and hospitals. With hospital occupancy at or near record lows in most areas, physicians are more important than ever as the source of patients. However, physicians who are profligate orderers of resources once patients are admitted may make hospitals vulnerable to retrospective denials of payment or losses under a per-case payment system.

Hospitals clearly have increased their monitoring of physician behavior. Many have initiated their own preadmission review processes and have strengthened efforts to ensure that physicians adequately document their actions and decisions (Anderson, 1988). The objectives are to see that payer requirements have been met and to protect the hospital against after-the-fact payment denials for care judged to be medically unnecessary. More generally, utilization management reinforces other trends that are increasing the severity of hospital case mix and encouraging hospitals to diversify, sometimes successfully and sometimes not, into areas such as home health, health promotion, health insurance, and administrative services for physicians and other institutions.

Overall, utilization management appears to be one of many factors contributing to tighter integration of hospital medical staffs and more physician involvement in hospital management. Most physicians recognize their stake in the fiscal soundness of the hospitals in which they practice, although hospital-based review and related actions may nonetheless provoke irritation. For example, this reaction to hospital pressure came in a focus group discussion: "You see, what's happening is you're putting the doctor in a vice between what he feels he wants to do for the patient and what the hospital administrator wants to tell the doctor about how he should take care of the patient. There are a lot of MBAs between us and the patient telling us what care we can administer, for how many days, what they will pay for and what they won't pay for" (cited in Walker, 1989).

Provider-Purchaser Relations

Physician and hospital relationships with employers, insurers, and other third-party payers have also changed dramatically. More time and money are being invested by hospitals and physicians to keep up with a broad array of payer requirements, including utilization management. And it is not only the number of requirements but also the number of organizations involved that makes demands on institutions and practitioners. Much of the organized response to prior review, as reflected in the committee's June 1988 hearing, shows provider interest in greater standardization of utilization management processes across organizations, as well as better communication of requirements, criteria, and results. Timely handling of review requests and appeals is another major issue.

The American Hospital Association says that hospitals may deal with 50 to 250 organizations doing prior and retrospective review (American Hospital Association, 1989). The Mayo Clinic, which employs over 800 physicians and scientists, estimates that it deals with hundreds of review programs and would spend at least $0.5 million in 1988 to meet the requirements of utilization management programs (Mayo Clinic, 1988). The American Medical Association survey referred to earlier (American Medical Association, 1989b) showed that while "complex administrative services" related to patient health benefit plans took 1 hour of office time (physician and staff) for about one-quarter of responding physicians and 2 hours for another quarter, one-fifth of the respondents reported spending more than 6 hours a day on such activities. These results were not categorized by type or size of physician practice.

Payer questions about the appropriateness of physician decisions—and physicians' concerns about the appropriateness of payer judgments of appropriateness—have prompted physician organizations to become more involved in the development of guidelines and standards of care (Meyer and Page, 1988; Physician Payment Review Commission, 1988, 1989). The American College of Physicians is notable for its work in this area for more than a decade (American College of Physicians, 1986; Schwartz, 1984). Recently, the American Medical Association has discussed work with the Rand Corporation to develop practice guidelines, and there is a complementary effort with the Blue Cross and Blue Shield Association and the Health Insurance Association of America to incorporate the guidelines into insurers' utilization management programs (McIlrath, 1988; Meyer and Page, 1988).[3] And, to name one other initiative, physician organizations have been cooperating with the efforts of the Physician Payment Review Commission to improve the definition and coding of medical services and to suggest methodological standards for developing practice guidelines (Physician Payment Review Commission, 1988).

On the administrative side, the American Hospital Assocation is working with the American Medical Association, the Blue Cross and Blue Shield Association, and the Health Insurance Association of America to develop

---

[3] In addition, some former Rand Corporation researchers are now working independently with a for-profit organization, Value Health Sciences, to develop better criteria and supporting software for use in both prospective and retrospective reviews (Findlay, 1989; Michaelson, 1988).

voluntary guidelines for private review (American Hospital Association, 1989). The last three organizations already have cooperated on guidelines for the conduct of utilization management programs (American Medical Association, 1989a). There are eight guidelines specific to prior review.

• The medical protocols as well as other relevant medical issues used in prior authorization programs should be established with input from physician advisers selected by the health benefit plan.

• Prior authorization programs may be conducted on a targeted review basis rather than attempting to prereview all services eligible for coverage.

• All preadmission review programs should provide for immediate hospitalization of any patient for whom the treating physician determines the admission to be of an emergency nature, so long as medical necessity is subsequently documented.

• In the absence of any contractual agreement between physician and health benefit plan, the responsibility for obtaining prior authorization required by a claims administrator should be that of the enrollee.

• The claims administrator and employee benefits manager should work together to alert enrollees to the need to be aware of and to inform the physician of any prior authorization requirements applying to their insurance coverage.

• In cases where a claims administrator requires prior authorization, the claims administrator should respond promptly and efficiently to requests for authorization. A physician or a patient should receive a response within 2 business days.

• In any instance where authorization is questioned on the basis of medical necessity, the attending physician should be able to review medical necessity with the physician adviser representing the claims administrator.

• To the extent that prior authorization programs are administered efficiently with minimal disruption to the provision of medical care, additional payment to physicians for complying with prior authorization requirements should not be necessary.

Effects of Prior Review on Purchasers

Employers are the principal purchasers of private sector review programs and are affected by its application in a variety of ways. Initial employer reaction to prior review has been positive (Jennings, 1987; Vibbert, 1989). They feel it has had some impact on benefit costs and has improved the value they receive for their expenditures.

On the other hand, the fact that prior review programs seem not to have shifted the basic slope of the cost curve intensifies employers' frustration with rising expenditures. This frustration over basic trends repeats employers' experiences with other cost-containment tools, including increased employee cost-sharing and alternative delivery systems (such as HMOs).

In general, the adoption of prior review programs by private purchasers has reinforced their long-standing dissatisfaction with data about the health services they are buying and has strengthened their efforts to obtain better information. Most utilization management firms are under heavy pressure to report more utilization and cost data and present more credible analyses of program impact.

Some employers are concerned that prior review exposes them to a new risk of liability, particularly if they administer the programs directly. The case of *Wickline* v. *California* held that third-party payers "can be held legally accountable when medically inappropriate decisions result from *defects in the design or implementation* of cost containment mechanisms . . ." (emphasis added) (see the paper by William A. Helvestine in Appendix A of this report for further discussion). Employers often seek protection from such liability in their contracts with review organizations, but the latter are understandably reluctant to promise to indemnify their clients against damages.

As purchasers move from retrospective to prospective review of care, relationships with employees may change. Many employers recognize the need to enlist the employee in their efforts to hold down costs. Some have developed programs that teach employees about making informed health care decisions and assist them with decisions about the course and place of treatment. At a minimum, most prior review programs increase the administrative responsibilities of employees.

Purchasers of prior review services also may find themselves in a different relationship with providers. Until recently, purchasers generally paid for whatever treatment the doctor ordered. Now, in their new role as managers of utilization and armed with data on the prices and practices of community providers, they are using their purchasing power to influence community practice standards.

The committee noted that purchaser decisions are shaped by many factors. For example, although the committee is unaware of any systematic research on this point, different industries and different firms within industries appear to have different norms governing their decisions on employee benefits. For example, in a roundtable discussion with benefits managers from several large companies that the Institute of Medicine held in December 1988, some firms were portrayed as slow to adopt prior review out of concern that they would antagonize their white-collar employees. In areas where workers are in short supply, less restrictive health benefits may help in recruiting new workers but may be of little significance where unemployment is high. Employers that have multiple locations and small work sites may find it difficult to locate and coordinate effective utilization management services.

Overall, employer reaction to prior review has been positive, but the long-term picture is uncertain. This uncertainty has two aspects, neither empirically documented. First, to the extent that prior review and other programs influence provider practices throughout the community regardless of a particular benefit plan's provisions, some employers may consider dropping programs in the hope that the spillover benefit from other employers' programs will suffice. Others may feel that prior review has had all the impact it is going to have, that changes in practice patterns are now entrenched, and that they do not need to be reinforced by continued application of these techniques.

Second, employer discontent with the reemergence of sharply rising benefit expenditures may lead some to make drastic changes in their funding of employee benefits. For example, if employers switch from a defined benefit to a defined contribution program that limits their yearly increase for health benefits to a level they can control, regardless of what happens to health care costs, then their interest in various cost-control programs may diminish. Defined contribution programs have become common for employee pension plans but are not widespread for health benefit plans.

CONCLUSION

Although the evidence on prior review is generally not rigorous, it does tend to be consistently positive about the short-term effects of prior review on hospital use and expenditures. It focuses almost entirely on reviews of the site, timing, and duration of care rather than on the medical necessity of specific procedures, because the latter emphasis is too new to have produced adequate data for evaluation.

The impact of prior review techniques on access and quality of care has not been assessed systematically, but no serious suggestion of negative consequences has come to the committee's attention. Qualitative assessments of the impact of utilization management on patients, providers, and purchasers suggest the potential for both positive and negative effects.

The committee recognizes that rigorous evaluations are expensive and difficult. In the clinical arena itself, rigorous evaluations of the impact of specific medical services are the exception, not the rule. Furthermore, the committee recognizes that many health benefit programs are adopted, maintained, or discontinued by private and public decision-makers on the basis of evidence as weak as or weaker than that available for utilization management. Nevertheless, the committee is concerned about the limited commitment to systematic evaluation of utilization management. Its recommendations on this point are contained in Chapter 6.

APPENDIX
SOME METHODOLOGICAL ISSUES IN ASSESSING THE EFFECTS
OF UTILIZATION MANAGEMENT PROGRAMS

An exhaustive review of methodological problems in evaluating the effects of utilization management is beyond the scope of this report. However, a brief overview of key issues illustrates the array of difficulties faced by purchasers, program managers, policymakers, and others interested in the consequences of utilization management. This overview includes a table describing typical measures of program impact and their limitations (Table 4-2).

Claims Data

Health care cost and utilization data based on claims submitted by providers or patients may suffer from a variety of defects (Wennberg, 1987). The claim form itself may be improperly designed to capture the needed information about the site of care, type of care, or diagnosis in an unambiguous form. Information submitted on the claim form may be inaccurate because of errors in medical records, transcription mistakes, imprecise diagnosis or procedure codes, and deliberate provision of false information (for example, recording a medical problem for an examination undertaken purely for screening purposes). Claims information from different companies may be difficult to merge for multigroup studies. Claims data alone are not sufficient to establish the severity of illness for purposes of comparison over time or across groups.

Even when data are accurate, they may not be available until months or even years after care has been provided. This limits the efforts of program managers to identify problems and adjust programs in a timely fashion. Also, individual claims data may be accurate but limited in scope, often not reflecting an entire episode of care for a patient, particularly if the patient uses some care for which claims are not recorded (for example, care covered by a spouse's plan or care from a noncovered provider). This means that actual utilization and costs per episode of care may be underestimated for alternative modes of treatment. Information that tracks multiple episodes of care for an individual is even more limited, and the patient-level links between prior review decisions and subsequent care are typically not examined.

Group Data

Important characteristics of employee groups and individuals covered by utilization management may be unmeasured or measured inadequately.

TABLE 4-2   Measures of Prior Review Impact

ACTIVITY DATA
      Number of admissions or days requested
      Number of requests approved, negotiated, or denied
      Number of requests referred to physician reviewers
      Number of denials appealed and upheld or not upheld
      Number of admissions or days averted (requested minus approved)
      Number of second opinions obtained and confirmed or not confirmed
      Number of nonconfirming opinions not followed by surgery
      Source
            Review organization
      Comments
      •   Do not measure health services use or costs
      •   Are helpful in assessing workload and checking some administrative practices
      •   Are relatively simple to collect
      •   Can be manipulated by utilization management organizations to project unrealistically
            favorable results
      •   Can be manipulated by providers who request more days than are really wanted
      •   Cannot tap "sentinel effect" (that is, admissions discouraged with no prior
            authorization approval sought)
      •   May not be matched to actual utilization (that is, may ignore days or admissions
            approved but not used; days or admissions denied but approved upon appeal or after
            an emergency admission; for second opinion, may ignore individuals encouraged by
            second opinion to get surgery when they otherwise would not have)

INPATIENT AND OUTPATIENT UTILIZATION
      Inpatient hospital days per 1,000 covered individuals
      Inpatient admissions per 1,000 covered individuals
      Average length of stay
      Outpatient medical claims per 1,000 covered individuals
      Inpatient and outpatient surgical claims per 1,000 covered individuals
      Total outpatient claims per 1,000 covered individuals
      Physician office visits per 1,000 covered individuals
      Source
            Claims data
            Benefit plan enrollment statistics
      Comments
      •   Can correct some limitations of activity data
      •   Are needed to help interpret changes in site of care, plan costs, and other variables
      •   May involve questionable denominators for rates if the number of covered dependents
            is unknown or is estimated by using outdated multipliers for family size and if
            additional coverage for working spouses is not accounted for
      •   May count only hospital outpatient facility services and not visits to physician offices
            or other sites
      •   Are generally not aggregated to show entire episodes of care

TABLE 4.2 (continued)

INPATIENT AND OUTPATIENT COSTS

Inpatient payments per admission or day of care
Inpatient payments per 1,000 covered individuals
Outpatient payments (medical, surgical, or total) per claim
Outpatient payments per 1,000 covered individuals
Payments for inpatient or outpatient physician services per 1,000 covered individuals

Source

Claims data
Hospital cost reports

Comments

- Are useful for assessing changes in hospital payments, which have traditionally accounted for the largest share of total outlays
- May not adjust for differences in costs for days of care averted earlier versus later in a hospital stay
- May not adjust for fixed costs that are eventually absorbed by most retrospective cost- or charge-based payment systems
- Do not adjust for severity of remaining admissions and days of care
- May have same problems with denominators of rates as utilization statistics

PROGRAM SAVINGS AND COSTS

Benefit payments per 1,000 covered individuals
Premium per covered individual
Administrative charge per contract (or other basis)
Ratio of review program costs to program savings
Benefit payments less program costs per 1,000 covered individuals
Number of hospital days averted and savings
Number of surgeries averted and savings

Source

Claims data
Plan contract, enrollment, and premium data
Review organization

Comments

- Are needed to assess trends in overall benefit costs and to assess net savings
- May not measure true costs to the supplier, depending on market strategy of utilization management company (importance of this issue depends on evaluator's objectives)
- May not reflect costs of alternatives to admissions or surgeries or costs from care only temporarily averted
- May exclude noncontractual costs to client for explaining program to employees, etc.
- Do not include any costs or savings or other effects for providers or patients

If different employee groups or subgroups vary in their exposure to benefit claims in unmeasured ways, then per-employee or per-covered-individual use and cost comparisons may be misleading (see also Table 4-1). The scope of health plan benefits for a group can have an important impact on the use of services but is often unmeasured. Age, geographic location, and many other factors can also have an impact.

A fundamental inadequacy of many data bases is imprecise specification of the size of the groups covered by a health plan. Although the number of covered employees (contracts) is generally known, the number of covered dependents may only be estimated by "family" factors that ignore drops in average family size and increases in alternate primary coverage for spouses. This imprecision makes the denominators for utilization and expenditure rates problematic. Plans such as HMOs that require explicit enrollment information are in a stronger position to calculate use and payment rates. In addition, although plan managers are making strenuous efforts to coordinate benefits (that is, see that care for dependents with primary coverage from another source is not improperly reimbursed under their employee's contract), the extent of such duplicate coverage is often not known in the aggregate (Lerner et al., 1983b; Luft, 1981)).

Important information about the health status of group members is often tapped in only the most rudimentary way, if at all. This has been a major controversy in comparisons of HMOs and fee-for-service groups. Some claim that HMOs are getting healthier enrollees, and thus price and use comparisons are misleading (Luft, 1987; Scheffler and Rossiter, 1985).

Program Data

Information about the prior review program often is limited. Programs may theoretically go into effect on a specified date, but actual implementation may lag considerably. Differences in program quality, scope, techniques, and other characteristics may not be described, much less assessed, in reports on prior review program effects.

Savings Calculations

Many utilization management organizations estimate savings by taking the number of hospital days requested by a physician or hospital, subtracting the number of hospital days not authorized, and multiplying the result by the average cost of a hospital day. This approach has many flaws—the days requested may be overstated by providers who are trying to game the program, the number of days approved may be exceeded without subsequent adjustment, and the average cost of a hospital day may overstate the cost of days avoided at the end of a hospital stay when care is normally less intense than it is earlier in the stay.

Other Interventions

Prior review programs are often one of many efforts to deal with escalating benefit costs. Their implementation frequently coincides or overlaps with initiatives to collect more detailed and accurate information about use, costs, and covered individuals. Although such initiatives typically improve subsequent data, earlier data generally cannot be supplemented to provide a comparable time series for analysis. In addition, retrieval of preprogram data is often time-consuming and expensive, particularly when data are being aggregated for several groups and must be obtained from a separate claims payer.

Utilization management also may be introduced simultaneously with a major redesign of benefits (for example, increased cost sharing) and the addition of a choice among multiple health plans. This complicates efforts to distinguish any effects due independently to, or interactively with, utilization management. The study by Scheffler et al. (1988) attempts to distinguish the effects of Blue Cross cost-containment programs from each other and from the Medicare prospective payment system. Any such effort is inevitably plagued with problems in combining data from multiple sources, evaluating the accuracy of these data, measuring the intensity and quality of programs, and adjusting for statistical characteristics and quirks of the data.

Medical Care Prices

Costs are a function of both utilization and unit prices of services. If inpatient prices are better controlled than outpatient prices, then savings from shifting care may be illusory. Likewise, if hospitals increase their prices to cover fixed costs in the face of reduced occupancy and if payers cannot limit their exposure to these increases because they pay uncontrolled hospital charges or costs, the reduced inpatient use may not bring a net savings for purchasers of care. If some payers can limit their exposure to these increases, as Medicare and some other payers do, then costs for payers without such protection may increase even more.

Noneconomic effects

Sometimes claims data can be explored in an effort to assess possible effects of prior review programs on quality of care. For example, emergency admissions, readmissions, admissions following outpatient surgery, length of home or nursing home care, and other events can—with varying degrees of difficulty—be identified and links with prior review decisions can be attempted. PROs track some of these events in an effort to monitor the effects of prospective hospital payment. Some utilization management organizations are trying to build data systems that allow patient histories to be easily retrieved and analyzed.

More direct information on health status and health outcomes is more expensive and difficult to obtain. Medicare, other purchasers, and other organizations, such as the Joint Commission on the Accreditation of Health Care Organizations, are actively working on quality assurance programs to identify potential quality problems at various sites of care. Much remains to be done. The Institute of Medicine is engaged in a major project to help design a quality assurance program for Medicare (Institute of Medicine, 1989).

Some employers and utilization management organizations survey employees to assess their reactions to utilization management programs. This is more the exception than the rule. Possibly, the absence of volunteered complaints from employees is taken as evidence that employees are not unhappy with the program. They are not adverse to complaining about other aspects of benefit plan administration, for example, retrospective claims denials, slow payment of claims, and confusing explanations of coverage.

Systematic assessments of provider problems and attitudes are even less common than checks on beneficiary attitudes.

REFERENCES

Allen, Harris, and Khandker, Rexaul, "Aetna's HEALTHLINE Program: Fourth Quarter, 1987 Update," Unpublished paper, September 30, 1988.

American College of Physicians, *Clinical Efficacy Assessment Project*, Philadelphia, PA, October 1986.

American Hospital Association, *Private Utilization Review*, State Issues Forum Monograph Series, Washington, DC, August 1989.

American Medical Association, *Guidelines for the Conduct of Prior Authorization Programs*, Chicago, 1989a.

American Medical Association, *Summary Report: 1988 Payer Accountability Monitoring Survey*, Chicago, May 1989b.

Anderson, Suzanne, "Hospitals Can Improve Cash Flow by Managing Preauthorizations," *Healthcare Financial Management*, December 1988, pp. 56-59.

Blue Cross of Greater Philadelphia and Pennsylvania Blue Shield, *Extending the Influence Beyond the Source: Community Data Report 1987*, Philadelphia, June 1987.

Blue Cross of Greater Philadelphia and Pennsylvania Blue Shield, *State of the Art Health Care Management: Community Data Report 1986*, Philadelphia, July 1986.

Carroll, Robert P., "The Problem with PROs Is Hard Heads Like Me," *Medical Economics*, December 19, 1988, pp. 103-115.

Feldstein, Paul J., Wickizer, Thomas M., and Wheeler, John R. C., "The Effects of Utilization Review Programs on Health Care Use and Expenditures," *New England Journal of Medicine*, May 19, 1988, pp. 1310-1314. (See also Zwarenstein, M. B., et al., letter to the editor and P. J. Feldstein response, *New England Journal of Medicine*, October 17, 1988, p. 1158.)

Findlay, Stevan, "Looking over the Doctor's Shoulder," *U.S. News & World Report*, January 30, 1989, pp. 70-73.

Fitzgerald, John F., Moore, Patricia S., and Dittus, Robert S., "The Care of Elderly Patients with Hip Fracture," *New England Journal of Medicine*, November 24, 1988, pp. 1392-1397.

Getson, Jacob, "Reforming Health Care Delivery: The Massachusetts Blues' Role," *Business and Health*, February 1987, pp. 30-35.

Health Data Institute, Inc., "OPTIMED Managed Care Program," Lexington, MA, April 1988.

Imperiale, Thomas, et al., "Preadmission Screening of Medicare Patients," *Journal of the American Medical Association*, June 17, 1988, pp. 3418-3421.

Institute of Medicine, "Designing a Strategy for Quality Review and Assurance in Medicare: Twelve Month Update," Washington, DC, February 1989.

Jennings, Susan, "Survey of PEW Corporate Fellows in Health Policy," Unpublished paper, Boston University, December 1987.

Kauer, Robert, "Evaluating a Corporate Health Care Utilization Review Program: The Case of Deere & Company," Working Paper No. 013, Cleveland, OH, Health Systems Management Center, Case Western Reserve University, December 1983.

Lerner, Monroe, Salkever, David S., and Davis, Leonard, "Evaluation of Program to Move Care for Certain Surgical Procedures to an Ambulatory Care Setting," Paper presented at the annual meeting of the American Public Health Association, Dallas, November 14-17, 1983a.

Lerner, Monroe, Salkever, David S., and Newman, John F., "The Decline in Blue Cross Plan Admission Rates: Four Explanations," *Inquiry*, Summer 1983b, pp. 103-113.

London, Alan E., and Anderson, Richard A., "Provider and Reviewer Speak Out on Utilization Management," *Federation of American Health Systems Review*, July/August 1988, pp. 36-40.

Luft, Harold, "Divergent Trends in Hospitalization: Fact or Artifact?" *Medical Care*, October 1981, pp. 979-994.

Luft, Harold, *Health Maintenance Organizations*, New Brunswick, NJ: Transaction Books, 1987.

Mayo Clinic, "The 'Cost' of Effective Utilization Review Programs," Statement submitted to the Institute of Medicine Committee on Utilization Management, May 1988.

McIlrath, Sharon, "AMA, Rand Corp. Plan Joint Development of Practice Guidelines," *American Medical News*, October 28, 1988, pp. 2, 27.

Meyer, Harris, and Page, Leigh, "New Era in Utilization Review," *American Medical News*, December 9, 1988, pp. 1, 42-45.

Michaelson, Leslie, *Medical Review System*, Santa Monica, CA: Value Health Sciences, Inc., 1988.

O'Donnell, Peter S., "Controlling Costs Under a Fee-for-Service Plan," *Business and Health*, March 1987, pp. 38-41.

Physician Payment Review Commission, *Annual Report to Congress*, Washington, DC, March 1988.

Physician Payment Review Commission, *Annual Report to Congress*, Washington, DC, 1989.

"Preadmission Review Cuts Hospital Use," *Hospitals*, August 1, 1984, pp. 54-55.

Project HOPE, *A Study of the Preadmission Review Process*, Prepared for the Prospective Payment Assessment Commission, Washington, DC, November 1987.

Prospective Payment Assessment Commission, *Medicare Prospective Payment and the American Health Care System: Report to Congress*, Washington, DC, June 1989.

Rutgow, Ira M., and Sieverts, Steven, "Surgical Second Opinion Programs," in *Socioeconomics of Surgery*, Ira Rtugow, ed., St. Louis: C. V. Mosby Company, 1989.

Sager, Mark A., et al., "Changes in the Location of Death After Passage of Medicare's Prospective Payment System," *New England Journal of Medicine*, February 16, 1989, pp. 433-439.

Scheffler, Richard M., and Rossiter, Louis F., eds., *Biased Selection in Health Care Markets, Advances in Health Economics and Health Services Research*, Vol. 6, Greenwich, CT: JAI Press, Inc., 1985.

Scheffler, Richard M., Gibbs, James O., and Gurnick, Deborah, *The Impact of Medicare's Prospective Payment System and Private Sector Initiatives: Blue Cross Experience, 1980-1986*, HCFA Grant No. 15-C-98757-5-01, Berkeley, University of California, July 1988.

Schwartz, J. S. "The Role of Professional Medical Societies in Reducing Variations," *Health Affairs*, Summer 1984, pp. 90-101.

Service Employees International Union, "Utilization Review and Case Management in Employee Benefit Plans," Washington, DC, July 1988.

Vibbert, Spencer, "Is Utilization Review Paying Off?" *Business and Health*, February 1989, pp. 20-26.

Walker, Allison, "Findings of Physician Focus Groups," Unpublished paper prepared for the Institute of Medicine Committee to Design a Strategy for Quality Review and Assurance in Medicare, Washington, DC, January 1989.

Wennberg, John, "Use of Claims Data Systems to Evaluate Health Care Outcomes," *Journal of the American Medical Association*, February 20, 1987, pp. 933-936.

Wickizer, Thomas M., Wheeler, John R. C., and Feldstein, Paul J., "Does Utilization Review Reduce Unnecessary Hospital Care and Contain Costs?" *Medical Care*, June 1989, pp. 632-647.

Zuckerman, Stephen, "Medicaid Hospital Spending: Effects of Reimbursement and Utilization Control Policies," *Health Care Financing Review*, Winter 1987, pp. 65-77.

5
High-Cost Case Management

High-cost case management is a set of techniques to promote more cost-effective and appropriate modes of care for patients with expensive illnesses. Even more than prior review, these techniques have gained acceptance in a very short period. As recently as 1983, a survey of employer cost-containment programs conducted for Equitable included no questions about high-cost case management (Equitable Life Assurance Society of the United States, 1983). At that time, formal programs to manage expenditures for very expensive medical cases were uncommon, except for the programs of private firms and state agencies working with recipients of worker's compensation benefits.

The situation is different now. A 1988 survey of benefits managers for large companies found that 83 percent said they used high-cost case management (called "medical case management" in the survey) (Corporate Health Strategies, 1988). Although the surveyed group is not a representative sample, clearly this approach to utilization management has become common. Virtually all major commercial insurers and Blue Cross and Blue Shield plans offer the service either directly or through subsidiaries (Henderson and Wallack, 1987), as do most of the larger utilization management firms and third-party administrators. Some review firms are actually outgrowths of organizations originally established to manage worker's compensation cases. For health care institutions and other organizations trying to cope with the multiple and complex needs of patients with acquired immune deficiency syndrome (AIDS), high-cost case management

119

is one prominent strategy (Health Insurance Association of America, 1988; Taravella, 1987).

Because the case manager is not managing care as a physician does but rather is trying to see that health plan benefits are used wisely, some organizations prefer to call their programs "individual benefits management." Other organizations, reluctant to highlight cost objectives, use the term "medical case management."

FOCUS OF HIGH-COST CASE MANAGEMENT

What distinguishes high-cost case management from other utilization management or managed care programs is its intensive and specialized focus on high-cost medical cases. Preadmission and continued stay review, in contrast, cover a broader array of cases in a much less intense fashion.

The generic label "case management" seems to have arisen in the 1970s with government projects to encourage the integration of services for clients of social welfare programs (Monroe County Long Term Care Program, Inc., 1986). These include the Services Interaction Targets for Opportunities program in the 1970s and the channeling and Social/Health Maintenance Organization demonstration projects for the elderly in the 1980s (Merrill, 1985). High-cost case management shares with other case management approaches an emphasis on assessing individual needs and circumstances and then planning, arranging, and monitoring needed services. However, because it focuses on a relatively small number of expensive cases, high-cost case management can be distinguished from so-called primary-care case management approaches often used in HMOs and Medicaid programs. In these programs, all individuals are assigned to a case manager who ordinarily must authorize or provide most services. And because health care cost containment is a central goal, high-cost case management can be distinguished from social welfare case management that is aimed at helping clients get the services they need from the complex labyrinth of welfare programs and agencies.

In focusing on very expensive patients, high-cost case management responds to an important characteristic of medical care: a small group of individuals with very costly illnesses or injuries account for a large share of the total expenditure. The experience of one company is typical: 2 percent of plan members with yearly expenses of $10,000 or more accounted for 38 percent of plan medical expenses (Rosenbloom and Gertman, 1984). In another company, 6 percent of those making benefit claims (and not all employees submit claims) accounted for more than 55 percent of health plan expenditures (Alexandre, 1988). National data suggest that 1 percent of the U.S. population (all age groups) accounts for 29 percent of total health expenditures (Berk et al., 1988). High-cost case management focuses on these expensive patients.

Two basic types of high-cost patients can be identified (Rosenbloom and Gertman, 1984). The first are those who suffer a sudden, catastrophic event, such as a heart attack, stroke, accident, or complicated birth, that may require a long period of hospitalization. Recovery to normal or near normal functioning is often possible, and even those with a less complete recovery may need little special medical care. The second category of patients is those with serious, often fatal, chronic conditions, such as muscular dystrophy, certain cancers, AIDS, and amyotrophic lateral sclerosis (ALS), who may be hospitalized repeatedly and become more severely ill over time.

Not all high-cost cases are appropriate for case management. Sometimes no less costly modes or sites of care are suitable or the patient's plan of treatment already includes these alternatives.

The opportunities for savings through high-cost case management by third parties arise from the complexity and fragmentation of the medical care system and the limits built into health benefit plans. It is not easy to chart the most cost-effective path of service for patients with catastrophic medical problems. Certainly, most patients and families with high-cost medical problems start out with relatively little knowledge of what lies ahead of them, and they may not always learn from their physician about the subsequent care alternatives that are possible or available. Specialized high-cost case managers can help patients and families to understand what these options are and what they mean in terms of cost, quality, convenience, and comfort.

Although physicians and hospital staff typically are more informed than patients and families, they too may lack detailed knowledge about the range of options that might benefit specific patients, particularly during the recovery or long-term-treatment stages. The care of catastrophically ill patients often involves several specialists, each tending to focus on specific problems, not the whole situation. An individual with severe burns, for example, may receive services from an internist, nephrologist, pulmonary specialist, burn surgeon, infectious disease specialist, orthopedist, neurologist, gastroenterologist, and psychiatrist (Mazoway, 1987). Hospital discharge planners often aid in arranging posthospital services, but identifying the most cost-effective option is generally not their charge.[1] A case

---

[1] The prospective per case method of paying hospitals used by Medicare encourages hospitals to discharge Medicare patients as soon as it is medically appropriate. PROs, intermediaries, or carriers are not authorized to undertake case management. The Health Care Financing Administration (HCFA), however, is planning demonstration projects to assess the role it might play, given Medicare's special characteristics. For payers whose method of paying hospitals does not, in itself, stimulate hospital discharge planning, continued-stay review may be used to prompt its

manager who is accountable to a purchaser of services, on the other hand, does have that responsibility.

Case managers can also deal with limitations of benefit plans. Some coverage limits, such as restrictions on frequency of home nursing care, may keep down overall expenditures in a benefit plan but nevertheless increase outlays for specific patients. Many employers who shy away from across-the-board expansions in coverage have welcomed high-cost case management because it looks at cost-effectiveness on a patient-specific basis.

ROLE OF THE PURCHASER

As is true of other types of utilization management, purchasers can bring high-cost case management into play in at least three different ways. First, the purchaser may actually employ case managers, as, for example, Ciba-Geigy and Zenith have (Henderson and Collard, 1988). Second, and more typical, purchasers may contract with an outside organization—an insurer, a utilization management firm, a PRO, or other entity—for high cost case management services. Third, they may rely on an HMO, insurer, or other entity that bears the financial risk for benefit costs to undertake the function as part of their regular cost-containment activities. For purchasers who offer multiple benefit plans to employees, both the second and third strategies may be in place for different employees, depending on which kind of health plan they select.

For those employers who contract for or agree to case management services, some become closely involved with the function. They look for cases to refer, demand detailed reports, analyze data and estimate savings independently, and insist on controlling all exceptions to coverage limitations. Other employers want only general reports and refuse any role in decisions to waive coverage limitations.[2]

Employers also vary in their objectives of high-cost case management. Some are concerned almost exclusively with avoiding unnecessary costs. Others have multiple objectives: lower costs, higher quality of care, more humane care, and assistance to patients and families in negotiating the complexities of the health care system during a stressful and difficult period.

---

initiation. For uncomplicated cases, discharge planning may be quite modest, involving no need to identify or help in arranging posthospital services.

[2] The federal Office of Personal Management (OPM), for example, has been relatively uninvolved with case management. Although OPM has agreed to allow some plans serving federal employees to make coverage exceptions and to provide other case management services, they originally did not allow the program to be mentioned in brochures distributed to employees. In addition, OPM does not ask for reports on costs or savings achieved through high-cost case management (Eileen Thomas, Blue Cross and Blue Shield Federal Employees Program, personal communication, November 22, 1988).

The latter group of employers may accept the possibility that high-cost case management might increase the cost of care for some patients. For example, a patient near death from cancer might be allowed, through case management, to receive short-term but expensive support through 24-hour-a-day nursing services so as to be able to die at home—even though palliative care in a hospital might be less expensive.

HOW HIGH-COST CASE MANAGEMENT WORKS

Permutations are numerous, but the basic approach of high-cost case management is fairly straightforward: to bring a knowledgeable party who is concerned with cost containment into the process by which patient care decisions are made for patients with expensive medical problems. The most common elements of high-cost case management programs are

• efforts to find less costly alternatives to the care (usually hospital care) that would be provided for specific patients in the absence of case management;

• willingness to approve payment for services not covered by the patient's benefit plan, if doing so will help reduce overall costs; and

• concurrence from all relevant parties—patient, family, and physician—in implementing cost-saving alternatives for meeting the patient's needs.

Although the first two of the above elements appear to be virtually universal in high cost case management programs, the third element is not, even though it is often described as part of a standardized model.

Figure 5-1 charts in more detail the steps that are often involved in high-cost case management. The process starts with case identification, proceeds through assessment of the patient's suitability for high-cost case management and the availability of alternative courses of treatment, and continues with the development of a specific plan that is agreed to by all involved parties and then implemented and monitored. The final step is closure of the case. This may occur when the patient's condition changes or when coverage under a benefit plan is exhausted or otherwise lost. Table 5-1 provides two hypothetical case summaries.

The four categories of utilization management described in Chapter 3 generally apply to high-cost case management. The distinction between those organizations with and without provider contracts is probably less important for high-cost case management because cooperation rather than contractual compliance tends to be stressed in either situation. However, because case identification, as described in the next section, is such an important step in high-cost case management, freestanding programs may face more difficulties than case management undertaken by the insurer

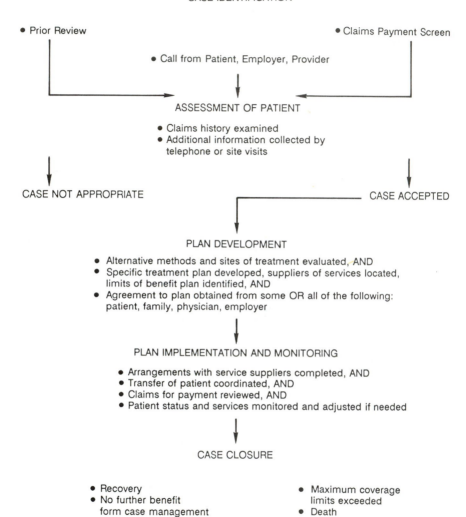

FIGURE 5-1 Examples of steps and variations in case management.

or claims administrator. There is no systematic evidence on this point, however.

Operational Variations

The committee learned during its site visits that high-cost case management programs are highly variable in ways that are not always easy to describe. The narrowest programs are, in essence, hospital discharge planning programs that operate by means of telephone and confine themselves

TABLE 5-1 Typical Case Management Summary and Analysis

<u>CONFIDENTIAL CASE REPORT 1</u>

Patient:	YYYY	Client: XXXX				

Patient: YYYY   Client: XXXX
Referred by: VVVV
Prepared by: WWWW
Diagnosis: Lymphoma   Date Opened: 2/14/88   Date closed: 3/9/88

INITIAL CASE SUMMARY

Patient is a 56-year-old woman with terminal breast cancer. Chemotherapy has been ineffective, and death is expected within a month of this referral. Patient requires pain management and skilled nursing and personal care. Family can provide some care but not 24 hours a day. Physician will continue hospitalization unless adequate home support can be arranged.

OUTCOME

Patient was transferred home with support from registered nurse and home health aide. Death occurred 14 days later.

COST ANALYSIS ASSUMPTIONS

Patient would have required continued hospital care.
Case management permitted discharge and maintenance at home.
Hospital days averted: 14 days
Dollars per hospital day averted: $600 (average billed this admission to date)
Actual home health expenses: (within contract) $2,000
                               (outside contract) $1,200
Case management fee: $700

SAVINGS

Hospital costs averted (14 days x $600)	$8,400
Home health expenses	($3,200)
Case management fee	($700)
Net savings	$4,500

TABLE 5-1 (continued)

CONFIDENTIAL CASE REPORT 2

Patient: RRRR   Client: XXXX
Referred by: SSSS
Prepared by: WWWW   Date Opened: 4/15/88   Date closed: 10/88

INITIAL CASE SUMMARY

Patient is a 15-year-old boy with head injury suffered in football game. After surgery, patient was comatose and was in intensive care unit (ICU) for 1 week before mother's employer contacted case manager. Attending physician estimates hospital care will be needed for at least an additional 3 months followed by transfer to a rehabilitation facility for several weeks.

OUTCOME

Patient spent 3 more weeks in ICU and was then transferred to a rehabilitation unit for an additional 4 weeks. Home care was provided for 3 months. Family has taken over therapy and the state is providing a tutor to prepare the boy to return to classes.

COST ANALYSIS ASSUMPTIONS

Patient would have been hospitalized for 3.5 months and would have spent another 3 months in a rehabilitation facility.
Case management permitted earlier transfer to rehabilitation facility and then substitution of home care.
Hospital days averted: 75 at $1,200/day
Rehabilitation hospital days averted: 21 at $900/day
Actual home care expenses: $8,000
Case management fee: $6,200

SAVINGS

Hospital costs averted:	$80,000
Rehabilitation costs averted:	$18,900
Home health expenses:	($8,000)
Fee:	($6,200)
Net savings	$64,700

---

to arranging out-of-hospital services that will allow earlier discharge of patients. In broader programs, case managers may be involved with patients and their families for many months and may visit them in the hospital, home, or elsewhere. The activities of these case managers are not confined to facilitating discharge from the hospital but extend to identifying and coordinating a broad range of services.

High-cost case management programs also vary in how they identify cases, who acts as case manager, who the case manager works with, and how directly case managers are involved with patients and providers. The differences among case management programs undoubtedly have important implications for the impact and effectiveness of high-cost case management.

However, these differences have received virtually no empirical study, and studies of one particular program are often generalized and assumed to apply to quite different strategies.

How Cases Are Identified and Screened

The case management process may be activated in several different ways. In many instances, the case manager is notified of a potential case by an employer, family member, or provider who is aware of the program and knows a patient who may benefit from it. In such situations, the case manager is likely to become involved early when the opportunities are greater for influencing the course of treatment to avoid needless expense. For these reasons, case management organizations may work with the purchaser to increase employees' awareness of the program and encourage early contact. Organizations with a significant presence in a local area may also work with community hospitals and physicians to bring them into the case identification process. In addition, an employer's disability insurance plan may refer cases for high-cost case management.

If the organization providing high-cost case management also provides other utilization management services, it may use its preadmission, admission, and continued-stay review programs to identify patients that are candidates for preadmission review. Generally, this involves specifying a set of target diagnoses such as stroke, ALS, or muscular dystrophy that are flagged by reviewers or their computer software. The lists of target diagnoses overlap but are not identical across different companies. Repeated admissions or multiple extensions of length of stay may also serve as flags. Overall, preadmission review and admission review may be of limited use, because many patients with catastrophic illnesses or injuries are admitted on an emergency basis and the prognosis may be highly uncertain for several days. Also, high-cost case management is generally handled by a separate staff that may not routinely communicate with the prior review nurses.

Potential high-cost cases may also be identified through the claims administration process. Claims may be screened for target diagnoses; for cumulative payments beyond a certain threshold, for example, $25,000; or for certain patterns of care, such as repeat admissions. However, by the time a high-cost case is identified from claims for payment, several months of care may already have been provided and chances to initiate less costly care missed. Nevertheless, retrospective analysis of claims caught and missed by a case management program may be useful in improving the program by suggesting where opportunities are being overlooked.

To avoid inefficient use of expensive case management resources, the first step is a review of basic demographic, clinical, and claims information.

Cases with a reasonable potential for case management may then be subject to a more intensive review, including direct communication with the patient and family.

Although all case managers make judgments about what cases to accept, they vary in how they make their decisions. These variations relate either to client objectives and concerns or to vendor capacities and strategies. Some organizations, based on their own and their client's objectives, reject cases with no or little potential for short-term savings. Other organizations reject cases with complications they feel they are unable to handle (for example, psychosis). Some clients want intensive case management efforts for AIDS and psychiatric cases but are less concerned about other problems. If high-cost case management operates in tandem with per-case payment to hospitals, third-party case managers may get involved only when hospital staff face an unusual case, perhaps one that requires exceptions to benefit plan limitations to make more cost-effective care feasible.[3] These sorts of decision rules may or may not be codified in internal procedure manuals and contracts with clients.

Who Serves as Case Manager?

One of the largest national companies offering high-cost case management services uses physicians as case managers. In all other programs known to the committee, nurses are used. The nurse managers always have access to physicians for consultation but manage most assessment, planning, coordinating, and monitoring activities themselves. Organizations differ in whether their nurses handle a wide array of cases or specialize. The most frequent area of specialization is in psychiatric case management. Some organizations use psychologists, social workers, and other professionals to assist case managers or handle certain types of patients or specific problems. They often speak of a "team approach" to case management in which several types of professionals contribute to patient assessment and recommendations.

How Case Managers Relate to Patients and Providers

Most high-cost case management programs report that they seek to work with all interested parties—the patient and family, the doctor, the

---

[3]Blue Cross and Blue Shield plans that pay hospitals on a diagnosis-related group (DRG) or other per-case basis report some difficulties in serving national employers who want a uniform program at all company locations—even if it is not cost-effective at some sites (Michael Cologero, Blue Cross and Blue Shield Association, November 21, 1988).

discharge planners at the hospital, home care agencies, and others. Their initial contact may be with any of these parties. However, some organizations work primarily with the patient and family, whereas at least one major national company works only with the patient's physician.

The emphasis placed on patient and family concurrence with high-cost case management recommendations varies. HMOs appear to be more directive, perhaps insisting on a choice between termination of coverage for services outside the treatment plan or agreement to follow the plan. However, not a lot is documented about HMO management of high-cost cases. Much of that management may be invisible to the patient because it occurs when the physician calls for approval for hospitalization or use of out-of-plan facilities or services. High-cost case management appears to be integrated into HMO administration (group, staff, and independent practice associations [IPAs]) more than in fee-for-service administration.

To date, most utilization management organizations and insurers working with fee-for-service health plans appear to use a voluntary approach. There are no statistics on patients who refuse case management, but some patients are reported to regard coordination with the case managers as a hassle rather than a help. The committee heard suggestions that some purchasers could become more insistent on high-cost case management when the likely cost of a patient's rejecting case management is significant. Some case management organizations do follow-up surveys of patients and families who have been involved in the process; others do not.

Case managers generally seek the cooperation of attending physicians. The attending physicians have essential information about the patient and the course of treatment, can influence patients' and families' acceptance of case management recommendations, and can assist in implementing recommendations by approving hospital discharges, ordering or providing necessary medical services, or supervising the care provided by others.

Face-to-face work with patients and physicians is most characteristic of HMOs and utilization management programs that operate in a relatively confined geographic area. However, at least one national company the committee visited attempts to do on-site case management through a national network of offices and employees. Blue Cross and Blue Shield plans in different states sometimes contract with each other to provide on-site case management services for patients located outside of their service area. Over 25 Blue Cross and Blue Shield plans are involved in a program for national employers that includes a utilization management component and involves a certification process using written application forms, site reviews, and ongoing guidance groups. Since on-site work is more expensive, particularly if it involves travel or subcontracting, most organizations target its use carefully.

Some case management firms establish contractual relations with home health care agencies, nursing homes, rehabilitation centers, durable medical equipment suppliers, and other institutions. These contracts may specify that clients of the firm have priority when the health care organization is operating near capacity. Contracts may also provide for discounts or negotiations on charges. However, even without such contracts, case managers may negotiate with provider organizations on charges for particular patients. Centralized firms without a local presence may be at some disadvantage in developing these kinds of relationships with providers.

How Much Case Management Costs

Another variable factor with high-cost case management programs is their cost, whether cost is defined as the price the purchaser of the service pays or the resources the utilization management organization requires to operate (Henderson and Wallack, 1987; Cologero, personal communication, 1988). Some insurers have not explicitly charged for case management services but have incorporated the cost as part of their premium or administrative services charge. Other insurers and some independent firms set a flat charge per covered employee, particularly if high-cost case management is part of a larger package of utilization management services. Most commonly, programs bill on a flat-fee or hourly basis for assessment, coordination, and other services. Hourly charges of $25 to $100 or more have been reported, with charges tending to fall toward the higher end of this range. For a case involving 40 hours of management services, the difference in administrative fee could be $3,000 for companies at the low versus the high end of the range.

IMPACT OF HIGH-COST CASE MANAGEMENT

There seems to be general acceptance that high-cost case management can save money and improve the quality of care and the quality of life for patients and families. Results probably vary depending on a large number of factors—the nature of the patient's problem, the family circumstances, physician and hospital cooperation, community health resources, employer objectives, and sophistication of the case management program. However, very little systematic evidence is available to support any specific conclusions about the effects of high-cost case management. Illustrative reports on case management program results suggest the kind of information and analysis typically available.

In Oregon, for example, the Bargaining Unit Benefits Board for the Service Employees International Union (SEIU) decided in 1985 to replace concurrent review with high-cost case management. The case management services were provided by the Oregon PRO that also administers pread-mission review and second surgical opinion programs for SEIU. Program savings from case management were calculated by projecting charges that were averted by the use of case management (such as additional days of hospital care) and subtracting the cost of alternative services and the PRO administrative fee. In the first year, the union reported that more than $13 was saved for each program dollar spent, but the savings-to-cost ratio subsequently dropped to 4:1 (Service Employees International Union, 1988; Jo Anne Browne, Service Employees International Union, personal communication, January 19, 1989).

The Bank of America adopted a case management program for patients with catastrophic illnesses as one outgrowth of its efforts to deal with its growing number of employees with AIDS. In the program's first year, the bank reported savings of $1.2 million compared with costs of $155,000, a savings-to-cost ratio of more than 7.5:1 (Ricklefs, 1988).

Independence Blue Cross of Philadelphia (formerly Blue Cross of Greater Philadelphia) began individual case management in 1987. For the 30 cases actively managed in that year, it reported savings of nearly $2 million, over $65,000 per case on average (Independence Blue Cross and Pennsylvania Blue Shield, 1988).

Intracorp, a firm with a history in case management in the workers compensation arena, has reported savings as high as $75 for every dollar spent on case management. It reports a savings ratio of 17:1 for a recent review of 14 typical cases (Tonsfelt, 1986).

In a study of an unnamed insurer (and an unnamed separate utilization management firm), Brandeis University researchers tried to project what would have happened without high-cost case management. They asked consultant physicians to examine a sample of the study and project how much hospital care would likely have occurred without the intervention of the case manager. Among the small numbers of cases examined initially, savings to cost ratios ranged from 1.18:1 to 0.42:1. The researchers identi-fied spinal injury cases as likely to have higher rather than lower costs under case management because of improved identification and use of rehabilita-tion options and institutions. In general, the consultants were considerably more conservative in their projections of savings than the case managers (Henderson et al., 1987; Mary Henderson, Brandeis University, personal communication, November 21, 1988). One purchaser of case management services, Caterpillar, Inc., attempts to compensate for exaggerated esti-mates of cost savings by making its own projections of what use and costs would be in the absence of intervention and then cutting those estimates by one-quarter. Caterpillar uses a PRO to provide the case management services (Richard Wright, personal communication, November 22, 1988).

EFFECTS OF HIGH-COST CASE MANAGEMENT ON
SPECIFIC PARTIES

For the most part, high-cost case management appears to have been favorably received by patients, families, and health care providers. The committee heard few complaints but numerous anecdotes of positive responses. The following discussion is based on the committee members' experience, testimony at the committee's June 1988 hearings, the 12 site visits, the roundtable discussion among corporate benefits managers in January 1989, and the six meetings of the committee.

Effects on Enrollees

In discussions with those offering and purchasing high-cost case management services, most recounted—with some feeling—stories of individuals who have been assisted by case management in confronting devastating medical problems. Even in the less dramatic cases, the picture conveyed is of people who are grateful for additional information, guidance, and support in dealing with stressful and complex situations. The major concern expressed to the committee involved questions of confidentiality for patients with AIDS, cancer, or other conditions that might provoke negative reactions at their place of work.

Three characteristics of case management, as currently practiced, appear to be responsible for its generally positive reception. First, case management tends to be quite individualized and cognizant of the special problems created for the patient and family by the particular nature of the patient's medical problem, the quality of the home environment, and the limitations of the community's health care resources. To some degree, then, high-cost case management escapes the impersonality and rule-bound image that tends to accompany programs dealing less intensively generally with more patients. Second, most organizations emphasize cooperative work with patients, families, and physicians and consensus on the design and implementation of the treatment plan. They do not put patients in the position of going along or losing benefits. Third, high-cost case management is often a vehicle for providing a patient and family with more services and options than would normally be available under the patient's benefit plan. The patient and family ordinarily are quite aware of these extra benefits.

To the extent that the administration of high-cost case management departs from these patterns, this largely positive assessment may not hold. For instance, if the case manager offers the patient and family a choice between loss of coverage and implementation of an alternative treatment plan, then the program may be perceived negatively. Likewise, if the family must take on substantial extra burdens of care but the assistance of special home services is denied, then high-cost case management may add rather than relieve stress. And poor administration of a program—by virtue of poorly selected and trained staff, inadequate documentation of conditions and decisions, and weak assessment and monitoring of alternative providers—can easily undermine the potential positive features of high-cost case management. The committee notes these possibilities but does not have evidence that they now constitute real problems.

Effects on Health Care Providers

Although the pattern of effects on health care providers may be somewhat more mixed than they are for patients and families, the committee believes that high-cost case management has probably had a preponderance of positive effects. For the attending physician and hospital discharge planner, the case manager can often bring to bear a more specialized knowledge of certain alternative treatments and providers and a more intensive assessment of patient circumstances and options. For example, the case manager may know more about innovative rehabilitation services or specialized home care options and have established relationships with these providers so that it is easier to tailor services for particular patients. The committee has no information about the administrative costs that high-cost case management creates for physicians and hospitals, but the interactions described by those involved suggest that it imposes few additional costs and may, in some cases, substitute its resources for those of the physician or hospital.

Physicians and hospital discharge planners faced with high-cost case management for the first time may feel somewhat threatened, but familiarity seems to mitigate initial sensitivities. Most firms say that they try very hard to select and train case managers to work constructively with physicians and hospital staffs. One potential source of conflict with providers is the contractual or other preferential arrangements with particular health care institutions that some case management organizations have established. Selective arrangements, per se, may create hard feelings, but the charge that high-cost case management companies may have a conflict of interest and may be channeling patients to lower-quality institutions is a more serious charge. The committee was unable to find specific evidence on this point and heard only a few references to this possibility during its deliberations.

Effects on Purchasers

Although the benefits of case management can be identified in the abstract, it seems that purchasers have sometimes been surprised at how positive the reactions from employees have been. The personalized nature of most high-cost case management may make the benefits more tangible to both employers and employees. And it promises more support for access and quality care than it poses threats. However, the lack of concrete, reliable information on whether high-cost case management is saving money is an irritant to purchasers. There is some suspicion that savings are overestimated and that more time is being charged than is strictly necessary. The committee heard few complaints about the lack of empirical data on health outcomes, patient satisfaction, or the impact of alternative program designs. On balance, high-cost case management seems to be regarded by purchasers as more of a "win/win" program than other utilization management and cost-containment programs are.

QUESTIONS ABOUT AVAILABLE EVIDENCE

As the study committee discovered for other utilization management programs, much of the evidence cited in support of high-cost case management is of questionable value—for many of the same methodological and organizational reasons. (Table 5-2 summarizes measures of impact commonly reported for high-cost case management programs and notes some of their limitations.) On the other hand, certain characteristics of case management programs can make their evaluation easier.

One characteristic of high-cost case management that facilitates evaluation of utilization and savings is the explicit focus on the cost-effectiveness of proposed alternative care. For each case, an estimate is made of the cost of alternative care versus that of care that is likely to be provided without case management. These cost estimates are sounder when they rely on information about the specific hospitals, home health agencies, and other providers that are involved or likely to be involved with the patient. Some programs track billing data during the period of active case management to determine the actual cost of care. Since alternative treatment plans may be changed, complications may arise, and other divergences from the projected course of care may occur, this sort of follow-up is important in assessing cost and other impacts.[4] Such tracking and follow-up may be easier when the high-cost case management and claims administration functions are managed by the same organization.

Certainly, the case-by-case projections of use and costs incurred and avoided by high-cost case management may be flawed in various respects.

---

[4]Predetermination programs, in contrast, rarely if ever attempt any case-by-case assessment of whether outpatient surgery will likely be less expensive than inpatient care in a specific case. That is, the probable expenditure for inpatient care at a particular hospital is not compared with the probable outlay for a particular alternative site of care. The assumption has been that, on average, the alternative care will be cheaper—an assumption that is no longer taken for granted.

The program may take credit for treatment strategies that would have been adopted anyway. For example, home care is often arranged for terminally ill patients through family, physician, and hospital initiatives without the involvement of a third-party case manager. In these situations, net savings may still occur from case management if the program produces earlier and

TABLE 5-2 Measures of High-Cost Case Management Impact

ACTIVITY DATA
    Number of cases referred for assessment
    Number of cases initiated
    Number of cases closed
    Number of cases ongoing
    Average length of case management
    Source
        Review organization
    Comments
    •   Are not impact measures.
    •   Cannot be used to evaluate efficiency absent additional information on characteristics of cases, client preferences, cases missed or identified late, etc.

UTILIZATION
    Inpatient days of care projected without case management
    Alternative services (projected or actual)
        Home health
        Skilled nursing facility
        Durable medical equipment
        Other
    Source
        Claims data
        Review organization
    Comments
    •   Projected utilization of hospital care is easy to overstate, particularly during periods of changing practice patterns.
    •   Projected use of alternative services is less satisfactory than are reports based on actual claims data.
    •   Generally focused on short-term costs and savings.

BENEFIT COSTS
    Projected costs of care without case management
    Projected or actual cost of substituted services
    Cost of services for which contract limitations are waived
    Source
        Claims data
        Bills submitted for special services
        Review organization
    Comments
    •   See comments on utilization projections.
    •   Cost estimates may not differentiate between more expensive early days of stay and less expensive (typically) later days and, thereby, may overestimate savings from reduced length of stay.

TABLE 5-2 (continued)

ADMINISTRATIVE COSTS
  Billed services during specified period
  Per contract charge for all contracts
  Source
    Review organization
  Comments
  •   Charges to client may not reflect the real administrative cost of the program,
      particularly in a multiservice organization that has not done cost studies for the
      service.
  •   Do not reflect any costs to patient or providers.
  •   May not always be billed separately from other utilization or benefits
      management services.

SAVINGS
  Projected cost of care without intervention minus high-cost case management benefit and
  administrative costs
  Ratio of benefit savings to benefit and administrative costs
  Source
    Claims data
    Review organization
  Comments
  •   See comments on use and cost measures.
  •   Needed to assess net impact of high-cost case management on purchaser costs.
  •   Do not include any costs or savings for patient or provider.

---

more successful transfers (consistent with physician and patient preferences) and if administrative fees do not exceed savings.

Some projections of averted costs are more plausible than others. To cite one case, during the process of planning a case management program, staff for one insurer examined computer printouts to locate patients who had generated very high costs in recent years. In the process, they discovered a child with muscular dystrophy who was ventilator dependent and had been hospitalized continuously for 8 years. The parents' benefit plan had covered the care and would have covered continued hospitalization. With the family's and physician's cooperation, the insurer arranged appropriate home care and waived contract provisions restricting payment for some of these services. The insurer's intervention clearly precipitated the move to home care for this child and reduced expenditures for the insurance plan (Thomas, personal communication, 1988).

Nevertheless, trying to assess more generally the savings produced through case management is difficult without some assessment of comparable groups not subject to the program. Clearly, practice patterns are changing for many reasons—new technologies, more sophisticated resources for out-of-hospital care, expanded health plan coverage of such care, and new methods for paying institutions and physicians. In the absence of comparative data, it is hard to know what savings attributed to high-cost case management may really be due to other factors.

The committee was unable to discover any studies that included comparison of a group subject to case management with one having no such program. Researchers at Brandeis University attempted such comparisons in their work with one insurer, but limitations in the claims data precluded it (Henderson, personal communication, 1988).

The relatively small number of cases subject to case management compared with the large numbers processed through predetermination programs and the relatively intense nature of the case management process do ease some burdens of projecting and comparing use and costs. However, the time horizon for assessment still tends to be constrained, partly for practical reasons, such as lack of historical data and a short program life span, and occasionally for policy reasons, in particular, a preference for being conservative in projecting savings.

One example of this conservatism can be found in the Brandeis University research just mentioned. The researchers concentrated in their initial reports on short-term savings that "would be realized within six months of implementation of the case management plan" and that "were clearly documented and supported by medical record data and physician input" (Henderson, 1987, p. 44). Longer-term savings were not studied in the initial assessment because they were both harder to track *and* more speculative.[5]

Although the relatively small number of patients in most high-cost case management programs has some advantages for evaluation purposes, it also means that the mix of cases—and program effects—can fluctuate for reasons unrelated to the program or to other systematic influences. Case mix and program results can also be affected by program design.

For instance, how cases are targeted and screened for acceptance into case management programs can systematically affect the composition of a group subject to case management. A program that does not accept a case unless there is potential for short-term savings could be expected to show higher per-case savings than one that accepted cases with potential for long-term savings only. Programs that accept cases with little potential for cost savings but considerable potential for improving patient and family quality of life would also show lower per-case savings. Ignoring such program

---

[5] The potential for longer-term savings seems reasonable in some cases, such as chronically ill patients who, with careful management, can avoid repeated hospitalizations. The possibility that long-term effects could include *higher* costs because of inappropriate short-term treatment under the case management plan does not seem to be expected. This may be because the intensive nature of the management process and the communication with the attending physician and the voluntary aspect of high-cost case management is thought to make this prospect unlikely.

features could lead to incomplete judgments about the effectiveness of particular programs. However, these details may not be identified explicitly in the program description or assessment.

In addition, the potential impact of other cost-containment initiatives may be not be considered. For example, if a purchaser or insurer moved to a per-case payment method with limited provision for outlier payments at the same time that it implemented high-cost case management, it might find case management of little or no marginal value. The results under these circumstances should not be generalized to programs associated with more traditional provider payment methods. (Note that Medicare does not have a high-cost case management feature, although demonstration projects are being planned.)

LEARNING CURVE IN HIGH-COST CASE MANAGEMENT

One reason that relatively little objective evidence is available on the impact of high-cost case management is that the programs are relatively new. Most are still evolving. Savings may grow, administrative costs may drop, and documentation of results may become more specific and realistic. Such improvements seem likely because of several types of changes in case management programs. These include

- better targeting and earlier identification of cases,
- elimination of overlapping cost-containment efforts,
- increases in administrative efficiency and computer support,
- development of standardized clinical protocols to guide the management of more cases, and
- establishment of more economical and effective arrangements with health care providers.

As organizations gain familiarity with high-cost case management, they generally look for ways to improve case identification and screening. In some cases, this means adding new conditions to their lists of target diagnoses or problems, for example, AIDS cases, spinal cord injuries, and psychiatric cases. Or certain target diagnoses may be eliminated, and some diagnoses may be subject to more up-front screening for associated diagnoses, past hospitalizations, or other indicators of high-cost potential.

Yet another targeting strategy is to examine whether certain services can be more effectively managed as part of the basic benefit plan rather than through an exceptions process. A manager for Caterpillar tractor said that adding a regular home care benefit in April 1988 "almost put their case management program out of business" (William Beale, Caterpillar, Inc., personal communication, November 30, 1985). Patients recuperating from relatively straightforward acute problems are now rarely seen by case managers whose smaller caseload consists mostly of chronically and terminally ill individuals.

Another way organizations try to improve their results is through earlier identification of potential cases when more options for lower-cost care may be considered.[6] Links to precertification and continued-stay review, informational mailings and seminars for health care providers, and involvement of employer personnel offices are common strategies. These steps involve closer integration of high-cost case management, claims administration, provider relations, and human resources functions, which can be difficult even when the first three functions are handled by a single organization.

As links to other aspects of utilization management are developed, it is sometimes possible to gain administrative efficiencies. For example, continued-stay review is unnecessary for cases already accepted for case management. Other administrative efficiencies are possible through refinement of information collection procedures and routinization of some communications with health care providers. Better computer support can increase efficiency at all stages in the case management process, from case identification and screening through outcome documentation and reporting.

Standardized protocols for managing certain kinds of cases (for example, substance abuse or AIDS) may minimize the need for intensive involvement of a case manager in the clinical assessment of the patient and the development of a treatment plan (Henderson and Wallack, 1987). If methods for identifying when monitoring or intervention is no longer cost-effective can be improved, cases may be closed more promptly, resulting in lower administrative and benefit costs.

Experience can also help case managers develop greater sensitivity and efficiency in handling certain kinds of difficult cases, for example, AIDS patients with dementia or nonaccepting families. In addition, as relationships with providers are established and reinforced over time, the identification of good alternative sources of care requires less effort. The prospects for negotiating reduced prices for care or other special arrangements increase.

---

[6] For example, AIDS cases are thought to be good targets for case management to reduce costs and improve patient quality of life (DiBlase, 1987; Health Insurance Association of America, 1988; Taravella, 1987). However, the immediate cause of hospitalization is generally a problem such as pneumonia, and there are understandable reasons an explicit AIDS diagnosis may not be mentioned in information provided to an insurer, employer, or utilization management firm. A diagnosis-based method for identifying probable high-cost cases will not, absent other information, pick up such cases. Therefore, some case management programs are trying to develop better early identification strategies such as having predetermination software screen each pneumonia case for age and sex of patient and any previous admissions. Sensitivity to confidentiality is a particular concern for this kind of approach, but confidentiality issues are significant for many high-cost care management cases.

POTENTIAL LEGAL ISSUES

There is virtually no case law, legislation, or regulation that specifically delineates the responsibilities and liabilities of organizations involved in high-cost case management. However, three areas of potential concern can be identified.

First, there are several questions about liability for harm to a patient. Because high-cost case management can shape the course of treatment for a patient, the possibility exists that a patient or family who has suffered a bad outcome will claim that case management contributed, and a jury may agree. The case of *Wickline* v. *the State of California*, discussed in the paper by William A. Helvestine in Appendix A of this report, makes it clear that organizations engaged in utilization management may be held liable for their failure to exercise due care in designing and administering a program. Although not mentioned in the *Wickline* case, a number of cases involving claims payment administration suggest that an organization would also have to act in "good faith" in administering a case management program. Some employers, citing sensitivity about perceived conflicts of interest, are reluctant to have their own physicians or other employees involved in high-cost case management and prefer to hire outside firms instead.

Actions that might put an organization at risk are the use of poorly selected and trained personnel, negligent referrals to particular providers, and poor protocols for collecting information about patients' conditions. A capricious refusal to make an exception to a benefit contract might also give rise to a legal challenge. Good documentation of decisions and rationales, as well as reliance on written protocols for developing treatment plans and referrals, help demonstrate the exercise of due care and good faith (Saue, 1988). The degree to which the attending physician and the patient are involved in developing and consenting to the treatment plan may also be relevant in assessing liability.

A somewhat different risk may arise if a case manager becomes aware of improper treatment by a patient's physician. One commentator believes that the case manager may be responsible for discussing such problems with attending physicians and, if that does not work, notifying the quality assurance committee of the hospital or medical society (Blum, 1989).[7]

A second legal concern about high-cost case management is whether exceptions that are made to limits in benefit contracts will set a precedent

---

[7] One question not raised in the site visits or hearings is whether a nurse case manager might be practicing beyond the scope of his or her nursing license. Blum (1989) raises this question but suggests that problems are unlikely so long as a nurse manager does not attempt to control treatment decisions. Blum does, however, raise doubts about whether the use of licensed practical nurses rather than registered nurses as case managers is appropriate.

that undermines the contract. For instance, if a patient for whom exceptions have been made, say, to cover special home care services, reaches the maximum dollar coverage of the benefit plan, that patient might argue that since some limits had already been waived, the limit on maximum benefits should not be enforced.[8] Such situations do not appear to be very common, but case management organizations do report a few sensitive cases. Written agreements among parties describing the nature and limits of any benefit exceptions are a recommended protection (Saue, 1988). Another way organizations can minimize problems when coverage maximums are being approached is to work with patients and their families, state Medicaid agencies, and charitable organizations to arrange a smooth transition to other sources of financing and avoid disruption in the plan of treatment.

A third concern is that an individual whose request for an exception to contract restrictions was denied could try to argue unfair treatment because exceptions had been made for others covered under the same plan. A related worry is that a claim of discriminatory treatment might be prompted under Section 89 of the Internal Revenue Service Code, which forbids discrimination between more and less highly paid employees. In order to protect against a successful charge of discrimination, some organizations involved in high-cost case management are improving their case documentation, clarifying contract provisions, securing written agreements to contract exceptions, and tracking the characteristics of employees assisted by case management (Cologero, personal communication, 1988).

In general, reasonable administrative procedures should be in place to guide any prospective or retrospective case-by-case decisions about benefits. And these procedures should be implemented responsibly and documented systematically for both routine and exceptional cases. Evidence of careless, biased, and uninformed decision making is hazardous whether a complaint involves a routine payment denial, a bad health outcome, or a charge of discriminatory treatment.

CONCLUSION

Case management has become a popular utilization management strategy in a very short period of time. Although it has been the subject of even less systematic research than prior review techniques, claims of positive impact for case management appear to be generally accepted. The committee believes that several characteristics of high-cost case management

---

[8]Some plans set no limit on the maximum total amount that may be paid under the contract. Where limits exist, they vary from less than $250,000 in some groups to more than $1,000,000 in others. Many plans set lower limits—often $50,000—on psychiatric benefits.

account for this acceptance: the relatively personalized and intensive assessment of patient situations; the explicit attention to the cost-effectiveness of alternative care; the potential for patients to receive extra benefits; and the emphasis on consensus in arranging alternative treatment. During the committee's deliberations, few concerns were raised about high-cost case management specifically. In the concluding chapter, the committee's concerns focus less on case management and more on issues involving the less individualized methods of prior review.

REFERENCES

Alexandre, Leslie M., "Who Are the High Cost Cases in a Health Benefits Plan?," *Medical Benefits*, September 15, 1988, p. 7.

Berk, Marc L., Monheit, Alan C., and Hagen, Michael H., "How the U.S. Spent its Health Care Dollar, 1929-80," *Health Affairs*, Fall 1988, pp. 46-60.

Blum, John D., "An Analysis of Legal Liability in Healthcare: Utilization Review and Case Management," *Houston Law Review*, January 1989, pp. 191-228.

Corporate Health Strategies, *The Health Poll*, Fall 1988, p. 1.

DiBlase, Donna, "AIDS Claims Hard to Track for Insurers," *Business Insurance*, September 7, 1987, p. 22.

Equitable Life Assurance Society of the United States, *The Equitable Health Care Survey: Options for Controlling Costs*, conducted by Lou Harris and Associates, Inc., New York, August 1983.

Health Insurance Association of America, *AIDS Case Management: What Health Insurance Companies Are Doing*, Washington, DC, 1988.

Henderson, Mary, and Collard, Anne, "Measuring Quality in Medical Case Management Programs," *Quality Review Bulletin*, February 1988, pp. 33-39.

Henderson, Mary, and Wallack, Stanley, "Evaluating Case Management for Catastrophic Illness," *Business and Health*, January 1987, pp. 7-11.

Henderson, Mary G., Souder, Barbara A., and Bergman, Andrew, "Measuring Efficiencies of Managed Care," *Business and Health*, October 1987, pp. 43-46.

Independence Blue Cross and Pennsylvania Blue Shield, *Independence and Leadership in Health Care: Community Health Care Report 1988*, Philadelphia, June 1988.

Mazoway, Jackie M., "Early Intervention in High Cost Care," *Business and Health*, January 1987, pp. 12-16.

Merrill, Jeffrey C., "Defining Case Management," *Business and Health*, July/August 1985, pp. 5-9.

Monroe County Long Term Care Program, Inc., "Direct Assessment vs. Brokerage: A Comparison of Case Management Models," Final Report for Robert Wood Johnson Foundation, East Rochester, NY, October 1986.

Ricklefs, Roger, "Firms Turn to 'Case Management' To Bring Down Health-Care Costs," *Wall Street Journal*, February 7, 1988, p. D1.

Rosenbloom, David, and Gertman, Paul M., "An Intervention Strategy for Controlling Costly Care," *Business and Health*, July/August 1984, pp. 17-21.

Saue, Jacqueline M., "Legal Issues Related to Case Management," *Quality Review Bulletin*, August 1988, pp. 239-244.

Service Employees International Union, "Utilization Review and Case Management in Employee Benefit Plans," Washington, DC, July 1988.

Taravella, Steve, "Coping with AIDS," *Business Insurance*, September 7, 1987, pp. 1, 20-22.

Tonsfeldt, Lynne, "Using Medical Case Management to Reduce Catastrophic Injury and Chronic Illness Coverage Costs," *FORUM*, 1986.

6
Conclusions and Recommendations

Utilization management is part of a complex balancing act created by society's struggles with two important questions. First, how do we ensure that people get needed medical care without spending so much that other social objectives are compromised? Second, how do we discourage unnecessary and inappropriate medical services without jeopardizing necessary, high-quality care?

Experience indicates that these questions have no fixed answers. Rather, as suggested by the first two chapters of this report, we find a series of working hypotheses and partial solutions that are continually revised, discarded, and even reinvented as medical technology, social values, economic conditions, and other circumstances change. In this preliminary report, the committee has examined one current working hypothesis—that externally applied assessments (those occurring outside the relationship between the patient and physician) of the appropriateness of proposed medical services can improve how care is provided and, as a consequence, help constrain health benefit costs. The validity of this hypothesis is of interest to everyone involved with health care—patients and potential patients, providers, employers, unions, insurers, and public policymakers.

Although attempts to manage the use of health services on a prospective case-by-case basis are not inventions of the 1980s, the application of utilization management techniques in private health benefit plans has become widespread only during the last half-dozen years. Its growth reflects purchasers' dismay over continuing rapid rises in health care costs and their perception that much care is unnecessary.

The Institute of Medicine is studying utilization management not only because the field is expanding but also because it has important implications for the delivery of medical care that have not been systematically investigated. On the one hand, utilization management has features that make it an attractive strategy for managing health benefits. When successfully implemented, utilization management takes the clinical circumstances of individual patients into account and gives patients and providers its assessments about whether services are appropriate before rather than after care is provided. It does not involve across-the-board limitations on health plan coverage. On the other hand, utilization management has certain unattractive aspects. It adds to the administrative demands on both patients and providers and employs criteria for decision making that are sometimes vague or even secret.

In this first phase of its work, the committee has examined two major methods of utilization management: (1) prior review of the appropriateness of proposed medical services and (2) high-cost case management. The first category includes several techniques—preadmission review, admission review, continued-stay or concurrent review, discharge planning, and second surgical opinion.

One of the committee's basic findings is that there is limited empirical evidence on which to make authoritative conclusions about the impact of utilization management at this time. Most private sector programs are relatively new, and the field has been changing rapidly. Therefore, the committee has tried initially to frame the important questions, offer reasoned judgments about the state of utilization management, and suggest directions for the future. As stated in the Preface, the committee has based its judgments and projections on reviews of published and unpublished reports on the workings and effects of utilization management, site visits by the committee to several utilization management organizations, and hearings and discussions involving consumers, providers, purchasers, and others. Judgments also reflect the committee members' extensive and diverse experience in health care delivery and financing.

This chapter summarizes the committee's findings about the current status of utilization management and its evolution. It identifies some issues raised by that assessment and recommends what prudent decision makers can do to promote the positive potential of utilization management.

CURRENT STATUS OF UTILIZATION MANAGEMENT

Several features of utilization management are important to keep in mind: (1) its great diversity, (2) its limited scope, and (3) its relative lack of regulatory oversight. First, utilization management, as it currently operates in the private sector, is highly variable, which makes generalization about it difficult. Some variations may reflect the industry's youth, for example, the growing but uneven extent of computerization. Other variations, such as those involving links with providers and claims payment arrangements, may depend on whether the utilization management function is freestanding or integrated into an insurance or prepaid health plan.

Second, utilization management has, until recently, emphasized the site, duration, and timing of medical care. The unnecessary and inappropriate use of the hospital, and not the actual need for a particular procedure, has been the main focus. Review organizations vary in their willingness to tackle new issues of appropriate care, but they generally appear to follow the lead of researchers and medical groups in adopting criteria or selecting targets for review. Also, as a general rule, prior review programs have not made case-by-case assessments of the comparative costs of alternative treatments or sites of care. In contrast, high-cost case management programs have built such assessments into their evaluations of proposed courses of treatment. The main strategy has been to discuss and negotiate appropriate care rather than to refuse prior authorization of benefits explicitly. Denials rates appear to run about 1 to 2 percent of cases with some later changed upon appeal.

Third, utilization management in the private sector operates under few explicit regulatory restrictions. There is, however, considerable awareness among review organizations and major purchasers of the legal risks inherent in efforts to influence patient care decisions and operationalize the terms of health benefit plans. And there appears to be growing recognition of the conventional—but not infallible—protections offered against liability by good management, good judgment, good faith, and good documentation.

As discussed in Chapters 4 and 5, empirical evidence on the effects of utilization management is limited and suffers from a number of methodological weaknesses. Although the number of comparative multivariate analyses is increasing, there still is little or no evidence about the consequences of specific differences in the way utilization management is conducted by different organizations.

Despite these limitations, the committee believes that the available reports and studies, taken together, suggest that purchasers who have adopted utilization management have experienced some changes in health care use and costs. Specifically:

- Utilization management has helped to reduce inpatient hospital use and limit inpatient costs for some purchasers beyond what could be expected from other factors such as growth in outpatient resources, changes in benefit plan design, and shifts in methods for paying hospitals. Groups with higher initial levels of hospital use tend to show more change than groups with lower initial hospital utilization.

- The impact of utilization management on net benefit costs is less clear. Savings on inpatient care have been partially offset by increased spending for outpatient care and program administration. Some of this offset is an expected and acceptable result of utilization management (and other factors), and some is an unwanted consequence of moving care to outpatient settings where there are fewer controls on use and price.
- Although utilization management probably has reduced the level of expenditures for some purchasers, it—like other cost-control strategies—does not appear to have altered the long-term rate of increase in health care costs. Employers who saw some short-term moderation in benefit expenditures are seeing a return to previous trends.

Systematic evidence about the impact of utilization management methods on the quality of care and on patient and provider costs (both economic and noneconomic) is virtually nonexistent. Purchasers have not demanded such evidence, and researchers have found the measurement of these effects more costly, time-consuming, and uncertain than measuring effects on purchaser's costs. During the course of this study, the committee did not locate documented cases to suggest that prior review programs in the private sector are jeopardizing patient safety, although some physicians believe they are. They may also cause anxiety and inconvenience to some patients. Utilization management does add to the administrative burdens on practitioners and institutional providers and contributes to resentments about reduced professional autonomy and satisfaction.[1] More positively, the committee has some confidence that high-cost case management, as currently practiced on a voluntary basis, is easing some financial and emotional burdens on catastrophically ill patients and those who care for them.

The lack of good research on the effectiveness and impact of utilization management is a frequent theme in this report. The gaps and deficiencies in clinical research on the effectiveness of many medical procedures also must be emphasized. As utilization management moves toward more review of the actual need for specific procedures, the clinical bases for these kinds of assessments become more important. (This is not, however, to assert that utilization management programs are making sufficient use of clinical information that is already available.) Later in this chapter, the committee recommends greater public and private involvement in both program evaluation and clinical outcomes research.

---

[1] However, the committee found it difficult to be certain (1) when complaints about utilization management programs stemmed specifically from private programs rather than Medicare, Medicaid, or internal hospital programs or (2) when they really involved prior review or case management rather than basic exclusions in benefit plans, retrospective claims denials, or provider payment methodologies.

HOW UTILIZATION MANAGEMENT IS EVOLVING

The continuing evolution of utilization management is most evident in two areas: its scope and its operational efficiency. There are several reasons for this evolution. First, the initial savings from shifting the site and timing of care have largely been realized in may places, and the survival of utilization management programs may depend on their ability to continue to have an impact on use and costs. Second, review organizations are being influenced by researchers' belief that a significant amount of care is still inappropriate and unnecessary. Third, the administrative costs of review programs and the provider and patient relations problems they create make simplification and efficiency important objectives.

Scope of Review

The emphasis of utilization management is beginning to expand from the site and duration of care to include more evaluation of the actual need for specific types of inpatient and outpatient services. The question is not only whether the hospital is the appropriate site for a proposed procedure but whether the procedure is clinically indicated. The procedures targeted for this kind of assessment are a mix of very expensive and relatively high-risk services, such as coronary artery bypass surgery, and less expensive and less risky procedures, such as bunionectomy. The assessments themselves tend to involve more questions about patient history and previously tried treatments than do site-of-care reviews.

As the focus of utilization management expands, the development of sound clinical criteria for assessments of medical necessity is becoming increasingly important. When the question is not where someone will get care but whether or not a particular treatment is necessary at all, the stakes for the patient, the practitioner, and the purchaser tend to be higher and the soundness of the criteria and their application more critical. The generation of useful criteria requires at least three steps: (1) the development of clinical and other evidence of treatment effects for particular procedures and services; (2) the formulation of guidelines for treating specific conditions or using specific procedures; and (3) the delineation of review criteria based on clinical evidence and practice guidelines. The research on feedback and education strategies to influence physician decisions on patient care suggests that the criteria used to make medical necessity assessments will be more likely to win acceptance and change behavior if they are based on good clinical evidence from respected academic and professional sources and if the medical community is involved in the process of criteria development.

Operational Efficiency

With respect to administrative costs, utilization management organizations have a strong self-interest in measures that can reduce their own costs—particularly since the short-term impact of their programs seems to be diminishing and the ratio of savings to administrative costs appears to be dropping. Frequently mentioned priorities include greater computerization, expanded use of treatment protocols in high-cost case management, and greater targeting of reviews to high-payoff categories of problems and services. To some extent, gains in operational efficiency for review organizations could also reduce administrative burdens on patients and providers.

In addition, some moves are being made that may standardize certain aspects of utilization management and reduce the variability and ambiguity now complained of by both purchasers and providers of care. One example, described in Chapter 4, is the effort initiated by the American Medical Association, the Health Insurance Association of America, and the Blue Cross and Blue Shield Association to develop guidelines for the conduct of prior review programs. The American Hospital Association also has been working with insurers to establish guidelines for on-site review of medical records by insurers, utilization management organizations, and others.

It seems likely that much of the clinical and administrative technology of utilization management will be increasingly integrated into health benefit programs, although the details will continue to vary across HMOs, PPOs, and fee-for-service plans. However, to the extent that clinical standards for medical decision-making are expanded and then internalized by practitioners, third parties at risk for the costs of medical care may be able to focus their utilization management programs more narrowly and reduce the burdens on patients and providers.

In addition, redesign and more careful specification of health benefits may, in certain situations, eliminate the need for some case-by-case prospective review of services and for some forms of case management.

Rationing

At this time, the committee does not see utilization management moving toward intentional rationing of clinically necessary medical services. A decision not to approve payment for a medically unnecessary service is not rationing, per se. Nurse and physician reviewers do not make explicit case-by-case assessments of whether the expected clinical benefits of a hospital admission or other proposed service for a specific patient are, in some way, worth not only the clinical risks but also the economic costs. Reviewers also do not make decisions, like those sometimes involved in emergency care or transplant services, to allocate limited medical resources to those most in need or most likely to benefit. The committee recognizes, however, that there may be some instances when a review nurse or physician may apply implicit cost-effectiveness judgments to discourage proposed care that may have only marginal clinical value in a specific case.

The committee notes that high-cost case management may assess whether making an exception to routine coverage restrictions will be less expensive for a specific patient than enforcing the contract provision. This might be considered a form of rationing. If so, it is a peculiar form in that it adds resources where they normally would be restricted rather than restricting resources that would otherwise be available.

It is useful to draw a distinction between *micro* and *macro-level* resource allocation decisions. Micro-level decision-making operates at the individual level, for example, to determine who gets a heart transplant when organs are in short supply. Macro-level decision-making operates at an aggregate level, as when health plans decide to cover only 30 days of inpatient psychiatric care. It is possible that prior review could become a micro-level rationing tool, but the committee found no evidence of such a development at this time. In contrast, employers and others already make a wide range of macro-level allocation judgments in benefit plan design.

ISSUES FOR THE FUTURE

In Chapters 3, 4, and 5, the committee identified some shortcomings in utilization management or gaps in our knowledge that raise concerns about patient protection, particularly given the course now being charted by purchasers and utilization management organizations. If the positive potential of utilization management is to be encouraged, then the committee believes that several issues need attention.

- Methods and resources for evaluating the impact of utilization management on health care costs, use, and quality are limited and must be strengthened. All those involved in health care delivery and financing need to feel more confident about what works and what does not under what circumstances.
- The criteria used by those engaged in utilization management (including hospitals and HMOs) should be available for outside scrutiny. Physicians, purchasers, and others should know the basis for judgments about the site, timing, and need for care.
- Systematic investigation of the effects of utilization management not only on purchaser costs but also on patient and provider costs and attitudes should be a higher priority. A more complete picture of costs and benefits is needed.
- The opportunities for patients and providers to appeal utilization

management judgments should be clearly described and free from unreasonable complexity or other barriers. This is an essential protection for patients.

• The explicit links between utilization management and quality assurance mechanisms need to be clarified and strengthened. Utilization management organizations should have standard operating procedures for responding to the quality problems they uncover.

RECOMMENDATIONS FOR THE NEAR TERM

The committee believes that utilization management has sufficient promise that a number of short- and long-term efforts should be made to promote its positive potential and guard against its shortcomings. A prudent course for the near future is for the parties involved in utilization management—purchasers, review organizations, health care providers, and patients—to accept greater responsibility for the reasonable and fair conduct of utilization management and the appropriate use of medical care.

The concepts of prudence, fairness, and responsibility described below are supported by a framework of general rights, duties, and obligations created by state and federal legislation, regulation, and judicial decisions. The most important examples include tort and contract law. Depending on the model of utilization management used and whether it involves a self-insured employer, an HMO, or other arrangement, different legal rules may apply. Little case law and not much legislation or regulation apply explicitly to utilization management. However, it is reasonable to expect that utilization management will be subject to standards of prudent conduct similar to those affecting other areas of health plan administration.

Responsibilities of Employers and Purchasers

As financers of both utilization management and health services, employers are in the best position to exert influence on the conduct of prior review and high-cost case management programs. They have a direct interest in programs that work fairly and effectively to ensure the value of their investment in employee health benefits. The committee, however, recognizes that there are practical limits to what individual employers can do, particularly small employers with limited administrative resources, expertise, and leverage.

In general, purchasers should investigate the operating procedures and capabilities of the organization or organizations from which they purchase utilization management services. This investigation should include organizations such as HMOs that provide prior review and high-cost case management as part of a broader package of services. Benefits managers can visit review organizations, request detailed information and references from current and former clients, and seek advice from business coalitions, consultants, and similar resources.

Table 6-1 lists the types of information a purchaser may want to request. This kind of information can help purchasers assess in broad terms a review organization's experience, its investment in staff and information technology, and its sensitivity to purchaser, patient, and provider concerns. The exercise can also help purchasers to think through their own preferences for different styles of utilization management. Unfortunately, this preliminary report cannot offer purchasers the equivalent for utilization management of the crashworthiness tests for automobiles or the nutritional quality evaluations for foods that commonly appear in consumer magazines. Again, the absence of research on the impact of variations in program structure and operations is a limiting factor.

As prudent managers of a total program of health benefits, employers should also examine other aspects of their benefit plans for impediments to the appropriate use of medical services or the rational payment for these services. For example, if reviewers are judging hospitalization to be unnecessary for intravenous (IV) therapy, is outpatient IV therapy a covered benefit? Are fees paid for necessary IV therapy in an outpatient setting subject to fewer controls than for those paid for inpatient therapy? What is provided to help employees understand what their benefit plan will pay for or how much they may pay out-of-pocket for selecting one provider or service rather than another? A benefit plan's scope of coverage, levels of cost-sharing, provisions for retrospective claims review and profiling, and methods of paying providers can all affect the impact of utilization management programs on health care costs and quality.

Although employers have the right and duty to take vigorous actions to manage the costs of employee health benefits, they should respect both the confidentiality of medical information about employees and the primary obligations of physicians to serve their patients. In their own business interest and to protect employees, employers should see that workers are informed of their responsibilities and rights. Key means of reaching employees include orientation for new employees, clearly written and eye-catching brochures explaining responsibilities, and health plan identification cards with clear notice of utilization management requirements. Human resources staff should be trained to respond to employee questions, assist with problems, and handle grievances.

Responsibilities of Utilization Management Organizations

Any supplier of services has responsibilities to purchasers that are intrinsic to the concept of a buyer-seller relationship. It is in the business

TABLE 6-1 Types of Information That May Be Requested by Purchasers of Utilization Management Services

1. Organization experience and range of services
    a. Years in operation
    b. Origins/affiliations (insurance company, PRO, etc.)
    c. Services offered, for example:
        (1) Utilization management
        (2) Claims administration
        (3) Insurance
        (4) Data analysis and consulting
    d. Number of clients for utilization management services by category of service (preadmission review, high-cost case management, etc.)
    e. Contract turnover rate--new, renewed, lost
    f. Number of individuals covered
    g. Other (Medicare contracts, etc.)
    h. References from current and past clients
    i. Record of lawsuits or judgments
    k. Extent of liability insurance
2. Facilities and operations
    a. Geographic locations
    b. Telephone and other communications capabilities (monitoring and tracking options, frequency of calls lost, flexibility)
    c. Computer hardware and software
        (1) On-line access to eligibility, coverage data
        (2) Link to claims payment system for monitoring compliance and reporting data
3. Personnel
    a. Primary reviewers or case managers
        (1) Number (full-time and part-time employees or contractors) and location
        (2) Education and experience requirements
        (3) Responsibilities and resources
        (4) Training program and supervision
        (5) Ratio of reviewers to covered individuals
    b. Physician reviewers (if not primary reviewers)
        (1) Number (full-time and part-time employees or contractors) and location
        (2) Clinical qualifications and experience
        (3) Responsibilities and resources
        (4) Training program and oversight
        (5) Ratio to covered individuals
4. Clinical criteria for assessing medical services
    a. Primary external sources of criteria
    b. Internally developed criteria (request information about development process, qualifications of clinicians and others involved, updating mechanisms)
    c. Availability for review by purchaser, attending physician, other
5. Patient or employee role
    a. Responsibilities for initiating review
    b. Recommended policy for noncompliance with process
    c. Involvement of patient or family in case management
    d. Access to utilization management organization for consumer information
    e. Information and education provided by organization
    f. Survey or other follow-up of employees or patients
    g. Complaint handling (volume, process, resolution)

TABLE 6.1 (continued)

6. Physician or hospital role
   a. Responsibilities for initiating review
   b. Recommended policy for noncompliance with process
   c. Involvement of practitioner in case management
   d. Information and education provided by organization
   e. Survey or other follow-up of practitioner
7. Preferred employer role
   a. Identification of potential high-cost cases
   b. Agreement to exceptions to benefit contracts
   c. Involvement in appeals of prior review decisions
8. Policies on confidentiality of medical and other data
9. Pattern of prior review decisions: volume or rate of
   a. Denials
   b. Appeals
   c. Appeals approved or denied
10. Pattern of high-cost case management decisions
   a. Percentage and types of cases accepted
   b. Average cost of cases and benefits exceptions
11. Appeals process
   a. Procedure for patient and provider appeals
   b. Decision maker and relation to organization and original reviewers
12. Reporting
   a. Activity reports (content, frequency, source)
   b. Utilization reports (content, frequency, source)
   c. Savings reports (content, frequency, source)
13. Basis and level of charges for services

interest of utilization management organizations to anticipate and respond to purchaser demands for information about the organization, its services, and its results. Further, it is in the legal interest of these organizations to manage their activities rationally, to act in good faith, and to maintain careful records.

Although good business and legal judgment should dictate prudent behavior, those who provide utilization management services also have a moral obligation not to harm the patients whose medical care they review and influence. Harm includes discouraging appropriate care and mishandling confidential information. When organizations perform prior review and high-cost case management for individually purchased insurance plans (with no employer sponsorship), they have a particular responsibility to provide good educational materials and appeals processes for beneficiaries who have no employer or other sponsor to act as their agent and aid.

With respect to physicians and other providers of care, good business sense should dictate that review organizations encourage provider acceptance and cooperation, although their incentives to do so are less strong than the incentives to respond to client wishes. Chapters 3, 4, and 5 suggest that utilization management organizations can increase physician acceptance by

- involving the medical community in the development and evaluation of review criteria;
- making the bases for review decisions open for examination by purchasers, physicians, and others;
- clarifying and improving the process for discussing cases and appealing negative decisions; and
- minimizing the administrative burdens placed on hospitals and physicians.

Given the diversity and competition now evident in utilization management programs, significant progress in these two directions will probably require ongoing cooperation between elements of the utilization management industry and provider groups to identify problem areas and propose operating procedures that avoid unreasonable demands on providers. Currently, there is no natural focal point to coordinate and promote these efforts or monitor progress. However, the cooperative efforts of organizations like the American Medical Association, American Hospital Association, Blue Cross and Blue Shield Association, and Health Insurance Association of America to develop guidelines for review are encouraging.

The committee is aware that further steps, particularly making clinical criteria available, raise difficulties given the competitive environment of benefit plan administration. Organizations that have invested their own resources in developing criteria will be reluctant, on the one hand, to make them available to competitors with less initiative and, on the other hand, to reveal some details to practitioners and institutions for fear of their "gaming the criteria." Although these are reasonable concerns, on balance, they are outweighed by the need to move toward open criteria and standards.

It is inevitable that utilization management organizations will occasionally identify cases of apparent malpractice or other quality-of-care problems. These cases may involve a proposed treatment for a single patient or a pattern of behavior. The experience that the Health Care Financing Administration has had in developing regulations and procedures for PROs that have uncovered quality problems indicates that balancing patient protection against due process for providers is a difficult political and legal issue. Nonetheless, review organizations should prepare guidelines for dealing with clear quality-of-care problems, at a minimum, having their medical director discuss the situation with the provider in question and, perhaps, raise the matter with the local PRO.

Responsibilities of Health Care Practitioners and Institutions

The committee found the responsibilities of health care practitioners and institutions most troublesome to analyze and define. In this respect, utilization management mirrors the situation with many other questions of provider responsibility and ethics, whether the questions involve the limits of heroic efforts to maintain life, the provision of care to those who are unable to pay, or the recognition of patient preferences about treatment alternatives.

The narrowest area of controversy involves physician self-interest versus the patient's well-being, where law and ethics have long agreed that the latter should prevail. Broader controversy and lack of agreement surround the questions of whether and how physicians should consider societal interests in making patient care decisions. Intermediate in scope are issues involving the physician's responsibilities when third parties are paying for patient care. For example, is it acceptable to shade the truth in order to obtain prior certification or retrospective payment for services? Is it legitimate to refuse to disclose information needed by review organizations or claims administrators? When should a physician challenge a negative payment decision? Is the physician obligated to provide a service he or she believes is necessary when a review organization, HMO, or hospital disagrees? What role should patient preferences play?

With respect to third-party payment, the committee agreed that health care practitioners and institutions are responsible for

- cooperating with payers' reasonable efforts, including utilization management, to assure that they are paying for appropriate care within the terms of their benefit plans, but
- constructively challenging unreasonable review programs and specific decisions that threaten patient safety or damage patient privacy.

Although some difficult situations with insurers and review organizations may be more conveniently and quickly dealt with in the short term by misrepresenting patient symptoms, diagnoses, or treatments, the committee believes it is in the patient's, physician's, and society's interest over the long term for physicians to deal honestly with reviewers and claims administrators and to challenge questionable criteria, procedures, and decisions directly. Manipulation and evasion can have serious risks. Specifically, incorrect information may enter the patient's medical records or insurance history with later negative consequences for the patient. Moreover, perceptions by purchasers that physicians are gaming the system undermine professional credibility and stimulate the sorts of auditing, second-guessing, and external oversight to which practitioners object.

With respect to patients, the committee sees additional responsibilities for practitioners. These include informing patients about treatment options, risks, and benefits and then considering their preferences. Insofar as is feasible and desired by the patient, the physician should also try to ensure that the patient gets care when a review organization denies precertification for services that the physician believes are medically necessary. This may mean locating an alternative source of care if the patient cannot pay and the physician cannot provide free care.

In the context of this committee's consideration of appropriate medical practice, an obvious responsibility for health care practitioners is to stay current with scientific literature on the necessity and effectiveness of medical services in their area of practice. (Many researchers would add that practicing physicians should, if at all possible, participate in the clinical trials and other research on which this literature rests.) As research results accumulate on the effectiveness and appropriateness of specific diagnostic and treatment methods, the committee sees an enormous implementation challenge to make knowledge more readily usable by busy practitioners. Meeting this challenge will require continued initiatives in such areas as the development and dissemination of practice guidelines, continuing medical education, and office-accessible computer resources for physicians. Utilization management can play a role in supporting these initiatives.

Responsibilities of Patients

In many respects, patients and potential patients are the weakest strand in the web of responsibilities for the prudent use of medical services. One person's view of appropriate patient responsibility can seem like "victim-blaming" to others. Although it is now a cliché among sophisticated consumers that more medical care is not necessarily better medical care, people may not be able to act in an informed and prudent way when they are ill. Furthermore, individuals may find both their benefit plans and their medical care difficult to understand and evaluate even when they are not stressed by illness. Education levels, family support systems, employer communication efforts, and other factors may all affect how much information people can understand and use. Nonetheless, health plan members should try to understand their responsibilities under their plan and their responsibilities for protecting their own health.

The challenge for those involved in health care delivery and financing is to help all kinds of patients make informed decisions about getting or not getting care. Concepts of probability, differential diagnosis, and risk-benefit trade-offs are not part of most people's everyday vocabulary. Fortunately, new tools, such as the video disk recently developed to explain prostatectomy risks, benefits, and alternatives, have promise in making complex issues more understandable for patients. It is not inconceivable that protocols used by review organizations to assess a proposed treatment might one day ask not only whether certain clinical steps (for example, a trial of antibiotic therapy) have been taken but whether and how the patient has been informed of risks, benefits, and alternatives for the proposed treatment.

RECOMMENDATIONS AND QUESTIONS FOR THE LONGER TERM

Early in this chapter, the committee observed that utilization management, per se, is essentially a working hypothesis, one of several partial and overlapping strategies for balancing health care expenditures, access, and quality. As knowledge advances, economic conditions change, and social values shift, these partial strategies are revised, integrated, and sometimes discarded. However, even if some of the techniques now employed by utilization management organizations are abandoned or the organizations themselves change, improvements in the criteria for judging appropriate care and for monitoring the provision of care will continue to be relevant. The longer-term recommendations of the committee focus on the foundations for such judgments: knowledge development, knowledge application, and value clarification.

The following discussion examines three issues:

- research on the effectiveness of medical services *and* the effectiveness of utilization management and related techniques,
- formulation and dissemination of guidelines for medical practice and criteria for utilization review, and
- oversight of utilization management.

Research on Effectiveness

Utilization management can be no better than the clinical evidence and expertise on which it is based. Although review organizations may not be effectively using all available research now, they are still constrained by the large areas of undocumented impact and clinical uncertainty involving many major medical procedures and services.

Policymakers are increasingly recognizing that the free-market system is unlikely to invest sufficiently in effectiveness research and data collection because those making the investment cannot capture all the benefit but must share much of it with those who have not invested. Since the public gains from investments in such research, a major public role in financing and priority setting is appropriate. It should add to, not replace, initiatives being undertaken by private researchers, health care organizations, and others.

The creation of an agenda to strengthen knowledge of what is effective in medical care is well under way, and the committee joins the many other public and private groups that support these efforts. Nonetheless, compared with the resources invested in biological research and health care delivery, the promised investment in effectiveness research is still relatively small.

However, while more investment in research is desirable, it is important to have realistic expectations. First, there are practical and ethical limits on clinical research—too few researchers, long time horizons, and numerous instances in which clinicians would balk at research protocols that require withholding treatments generally thought to be useful or providing treatments generally thought to be inappropriate.

Second, much research does not really focus on the effectiveness of care in an average setting or population, nor does it evaluate the impact of care on quality of life and many other outcomes that are now considered important. What is needed are longitudinal observations of natural variations in the use and outcomes of economically and clinically important medical technologies in different practice situations. Clinical, claims, and other data bases need to be designed, and parallel attention needs to be given to the methodological issues in interpreting and disseminating research findings.

Third, effectiveness research that relies on existing claims and other records, while less expensive and time-consuming than most clinical trials, is not necessarily quick nor suitable for providing answers to many questions. Effectiveness research needs to be complemented by judgmental strategies, such as consensus panels, that use but go beyond scientific literature and empirical data. Many times the practical results of these processes will be imperfect. However, in the past 10 years, we have learned that the best randomized clinical trials have weaknesses and that these weaknesses are accepted, sometimes too readily. Intelligent compromise with perfection is necessary.

Fourth, research cannot resolve some questions. For example, researchers may be able to assess the clinical benefits and risks in using cataract surgery to correct a 20/40 vision defect. They cannot tell us whether such use of resources is wise given other uses to which those resources might (but not necessarily would) be put.

Fifth, sound clinical research does not automatically affect behavior. The research on what works in medical care should be complemented by research on how best to ensure that such knowledge is used effectively and efficiently. Such programmatic research is, for the most part, a low priority today. It is expensive, methodologically troublesome, and slow to pay off. As part of the overall strategy for containing total health care costs and improving the appropriateness of health care for all citizens, the committee urges federal and private consideration of carefully targeted research projects to test utilization management strategies and build methodologies for documenting the effects of existing programs.

Practice Guidelines and Review Criteria

To a very considerable extent in the past, medical practice guidelines have been implicit and have been linked to the amorphous concept of community standards of practice. The medical profession has historically resisted setting standards that are both explicit and national in scope. This resistance has been challenged by the research on practice variations and inappropriate use discussed in Chapter 2. The increasing emphasis on effectiveness research is also adding to the momentum for developing better and more extensive guidelines for patient care.

Translating clinical and other research into valid, reliable, and usable guidelines for medical practice and utilization management is a complicated enterprise that can take many forms. One approach is the development of clinical protocols that specify the tests, procedures, and other medical services that should be provided to patients with a specific clinical problem. Another approach is more proscriptive than prescriptive. It essentially sets boundaries outside which specific services for specific medical conditions are defined as inappropriate. Within the boundaries, guidelines may allow considerable room for an individual practitioner's judgment about the value of alternative courses of treatment. The two latter approaches have provided the bases for explicit and implicit review criteria used in utilization management organizations, but review organizations appear to have made little use of explicit clinical protocols.

The committee has cited analyses that show that some practice guidelines do not match relevant empirical research very well, and the fit between practice guidelines and criteria for utilization management may likewise be poor. The committee has identified a number of questions about the process of developing, disseminating, and updating practice guidelines and review criteria that need attention. They include the following:

- Should there be some kind of oversight of guidelines developed by different sources—a sort of quality review mechanism that assesses both the method and the substance of specific guidelines? What should happen when different sources develop conflicting guidelines?
- To what extent should patient preferences or cost-effectiveness analyses be considered in the development of practice guidelines? How should these issues of value be dealt with in the application of guidelines or in other strategies?
- Should adherence to guidelines provide physicians with protection against malpractice charges?

- Over the long term, should a role for community or local standards continue?
- What considerations should apply in translating guidelines into criteria for prospective or retrospective review programs?
- Should private review organizations be encouraged to invest in criteria development if the results are open to outside examination?

These questions are relevant to much of the Institute of Medicine's agenda. Further investigation of these issues is now underway. It will draw not only on the Committee on Utilization Management by Third Parties, but also on the Committee to Design a Quality Assurance Strategy for Medicare and the Council on Health Care Technology, as well as outside groups such as the Health Care Financing Administration and the Physician Payment Review Commission.

Oversight of Utilization Management

Whether additional mechanisms for oversight of utilization management are needed to weed out incompetent organizations and programs was a question the committee discussed at considerable length. The protections offered by caveat emptor, self-regulation, and tort liability, although important, do not respond to all concerns about the impact of utilization management on patients, providers, and overall health care costs. Moreover, the current lack of oversight poses some risks to utilization management as a promising strategy for managing benefit costs. Misbehavior by a few organizations could harm patients, infuriate practitioners, and seriously damage acceptance and cooperation from patients and providers. On the other hand, premature or misguided regulation could stifle worthwhile innovations in technique and lock in inefficient or ineffective methods. Purchasers might then abandon utilization management for more onerous techniques of cost containment. As this report has emphasized, utilization management is still relatively new, is evolving quite rapidly, and works quite differently depending on the delivery and financing mechanism it serves.

At this time, the committee is not prepared to make recommendations about where oversight may be appropriate or what oversight strategies may offer a workable balancing of the conflicting values, interests, and needs of different parties. Rather, the committee has posed several questions about the oversight of utilization management that it will be considering further.

- How do we decide whether oversight is necessary and feasible?
- If an oversight mechanism is necessary and feasible, should it be public or private? If public, should all 50 states make their own policies or should the federal government impose uniform standards?[2]

---

[2] As noted in the discussion of PROs in Chapter 2, federal regulation does not guarantee uniform

- What should be the focus of oversight? Should the clinical criteria for assessing care and the mechanisms for appealing decisions be the main concerns? What about staffing, training, outcome reporting, and so on?
- Should utilization management conducted by different kinds of organizations, for example, PPOs versus staff model HMOs, be subject to different kinds of oversight? Should utilization management of some services—for example, mental health care—be subject to different kinds or levels of oversight?
- Can anything be learned from government oversight of PROs or the accreditation process managed by the Joint Commission on the Accreditation of Health Care Organizations?

These are not simple questions. Answering them demands more information and more thoughtful debate over how to judge the strengths and weaknesses of utilization management versus other strategies to control costs and influence patient care decisions and how to weigh the legitimate but sometimes conflicting needs, interests, and values of the parties involved in utilization management. At this time, the committee advises caution to public policymakers currently considering proposals to regulate and limit utilization management.

CONCLUSION

Utilization management needs to better demonstrate that it reduces the wasteful use of resources, improves the appropriateness of patient care, and imposes only reasonable burdens on patients and providers. It is important that it be given a chance to prove itself because if it works, it offers a means of accommodating individual patient circumstances that is more sensitive than many other cost-containment strategies, for example, those that rely on across-the-board restrictions in benefits.

However, the limits of utilization management and any other single strategy, even any combination of strategies, also need to be recognized. The issue is not whether utilization management does everything that needs to be done but whether it produces desirable results in reasonable ways at an acceptable cost. Is it, on balance, better to use it than discard it? And if utilization management is helpful, how can provider payment methods, retrospective utilization review and feedback techniques, resource planning mechanisms, and other tools be used to reinforce utilization management and deal with problems—such as distorted payment rates or excessive use of low-cost, high-volume services—not effectively addressed by utilization

---

practice. And as noted in Chapter 3, proposed state regulations vary enormously and, in some cases, could make prior review and high-cost case management infeasible.

management? This report has provided initial views on some of these questions.

The Institute of Medicine will continue its efforts to better define what role utilization management might play in helping society find an acceptable balance of efficiency, access, and appropriateness in health care. This clearly must be a shared venture. Fortunately, the quest to know what is useful and how to apply it universally are now central issues in medical research and public policy.

Acknowledgments

The participants in an initial meeting to plan this project provided valuable direction and stimulating ideas for committee investigation. The meeting was chaired by Stanley B. Jones and included Rhoda Abrahms, U.S. Department of Health and Human Services; Robert A. Berenson; John M. Burns, Honeywell, Inc.; E. Langdon Burwell, Falmouth Medical Associates; John W. Bussman, Oregon Health Sciences University; Priscilla Dasse, Beth Israel Hospital; John T. Dunlop, Harvard University; Paul Gertman, Health Data Institute; Nathan Hershey, University of Pittsburgh; William Hoffman, United Auto Workers; John K. Iglehart, *Health Affairs*; Karen Ignani, American Federation of Labor and Congress of Industrial Organizations (AFL-CIO); Arnold Milstein, National Medical Audit; David Ottensmeyer, Equicor; Robert Patricelli, ValuCare, Inc.; Mindy Pellissier, Scripps Clinic and Research Foundation; Gail J. Povar, George Washington University School of Medicine; David Rosenbloom, Health Data Institute; Richard S. Sharpe, John A. Hartford Foundation; David N. Sundwall, U.S. Department of Health and Human Services, and Jeffrey Weiner, U.S. HealthCare.

In June 1988 the committee heard much helpful testimony from a range of medical, consumer, purchaser, insurer, and other organizations. A brief summary of that meeting and a list of the participants are included in Appendix D of the report.

The committee cannot identify the 12 organizations that it visited; it agreed to keep that information confidential. Many individuals from those organizations spent considerable time answering questions, showing their facilities, reviewing summaries of the visits, and generally responding to follow-up inquiries. Several committee members were involved in the site visits: Alice G. Gosfield, Robert A. Berenson, John M. Burns, John M. Eisenberg, Nathan Hershey, Carol Ann Lockhart, Cynthia L. Polich, and Bruce S. Wolff.

The authors of three commissioned papers also contributed to the committee's understanding of issues. Two papers are published in Appendixes A and B of the report. One other paper, which is not included but is available from the committee upon request, also provided useful background information in an area that was not dealt with explicitly by the committee. This paper on Medicaid cost-containment strategies was prepared by Robert E. Hurley, Pennsylvania State University, and Deborah Anne Freund, a member of the committee. During regular meetings, the committee heard presentations on utilization management from several individuals: Ed Zalta, CaPP Care; Paul Gertman, ClinMan, Inc.; and Marcia Gold, Group Health Association of America.

Several committee members drafted materials to assist in developing the report. Neil Hollander reviewed problems with evaluating the savings claimed for utilization management programs. Nathan Hershey developed an analysis of the contents of contracts between utilization management organizations and their clients. Alice G. Gosfield prepared a background paper on utilization management in peer review organizations, and Michael Herbert provided background discussion on utilization management in health maintenance organizations. Suggestions about what purchasers should look for in utilization management organizations were contributed by Robert Patricelli, Karen Ignani, Michael E. Herbert, Alice G. Gosfield, John M. Burns, and Howard L. Bailit. Alan R. Nelson discussed physician concerns and responsibilities.

For the first year of the project, Richard H. Egdahl chaired the committee. Dr. Egdahl has since continued to serve as a member of the committee and kindly extended invitations to committee staff to attend meetings organized for Pew Foundation Corporate Fellows at Boston University. During the second year, Jerome H. Grossman chaired the committee as it developed its conclusions, outlined the report, and planned next steps.

The initial idea for this project came from Bradford H. Gray, who secured much of its funding, organized the planning session, and served as study director through December 1988. The project would not have existed without his initiative. When Dr. Gray left for Yale University, Marilyn J. Field joined the project as the committee defined its views, and she took major responsibility for drafting the report. Dr. Field will continue as study director for further work by the committee. Margaret Walkover was research associate for the early months of the project. Susan E. Sherman, who served as research associate during the summer of 1987, went on all the site visits, and assisted in preparing the site visit summaries. Eileen Connor of Boston University contributed much to the project as a consultant, and Sharon Rosen of the New England Medical Center assisted Dr. Grossman and the committee during its final months.

As project secretary, Don Tiller provided much needed continuity as well as exemplary support for the committee. The ongoing guidance of Karl D. Yordy, director of the Division of Health Care Services, was important for the project, particularly given the changes in committee and staff leadership.

A great many people helped the committee with information and insights about utilization management. Particularly useful was a meeting in January 1989, arranged by Marion Ein Lewin of the IOM, with executives from clients of review organizations: H. Dean Belk, ALCOA; Jo Anne Brown, Service Employees International Union; Jerry Clark, UMWA Health and Retirement Fund; Richard Ekstrom, Westinghouse; Jeanne Kardos, Southern New England Telephone; Walter B. Maher, Chrysler; William J. Schneider, J.P. Morgan; Elizabeth Solem, 3-M Company; Julia Smith, Bank of America; and Loring Wood, NYNEX. Others include Harris Allen, Richard Bondi, and Constance Winslow (Aetna Life and Casualty); Mark Chassin, Jacqueline Kosecoff, and Leslie Michaelson (Value Health Sciences, Inc.); Michael Cologero, Robert Snyder, and Eileen Thomas (Blue Cross and Blue Shield Association); Jon Gable, Al Minor, and Thomas Muscow (Health Insurance Association of America); David Bergohlz and Mary Ann Sevick (Pittsburgh Program for Affordable Health Care); Mary Henderson (Brandeis University); Gail Beiber (American Medical Association); Howard Birnbaum, Deborah Kottler, and Len Vernick (Health Data Institute); John Blum (Loyola University, Chicago); Joan Trauner (Coopers & Lybrand); Robert Beale and Richard Wright (Caterpillar, Inc.); Jill Bernstein (Physician Payment Review Commission); Shan Haley (American Hospital Association); JoAnne Brown (Service Employees International Union); Ronald Hurst (Association of Preferred Provider Organizations); Joseph Restuccia (Boston University), Shelley Greenfield (New England Medical Center); Steven Sieverts (Blue Cross and Blue Shield of the National Capital Area); Deborah Chollet (Employee Benefits Research Institute); and Spencer Vibbert (McGraw-Hill). The library staff of several organizations provided information or sources on a number of issues: American Hospital Association, American Medical Association, Blue Cross and Blue Shield Association, Health Insurance Association of America, and Group Health Association of America.

Appendixes

Appendix A
Legal Implications of Utilization Review

William A. Helvestine*

The recent decade has seen a dramatic increase in the use of utilization review (UR) programs in an effort to stem the tide of rising health care costs. UR serves to verify the medical necessity of hospital admissions and specific medical procedures. However, by intruding into the traditional physician-patient relationship, UR programs raise a host of liability issues.[1]

INTRODUCTION

This paper reviews the rights and responsibilities of the parties involved in UR decisions in an effort to determine what legal guidelines exist and which areas remain unsettled.

The Types of Utilization Review

UR is used in one form or another by government payers such as Medicare, private insurers, health maintenance organizations (HMOs), and self-insured employers. Some payers perform the review in-house; others contract with independent entities to perform all or part of the review. If the physician's treatment plan is approved, the patient is fully covered

*William A. Helvestine is a Partner at Epstein Becker Stromberg & Green in San Francisco. The author gratefully acknowledges the assistance of Dena R. Belinkoff, an attorney with Epstein Becker Stromberg & Green, in the preparation of this paper.

to the limits of the plan; if not, the patient's financial coverage may be reduced or denied altogether. Many physicians criticize the intrusion of UR programs, while most payers claim they reduce health care costs.

Under traditional indemnity plans, UR occurs retrospectively. That is, claims for payment are reviewed after the treatment is rendered. Recently, prospective and concurrent review programs have become more prevalent. A prospective review program requires the physician to obtain prior certification from the payer before providing treatment. In concurrent review, the payer monitors a patient's treatment (usually the length of a hospital stay) and specifies the last day for which payment is authorized.

Because these programs can directly affect the medical care of the patient, they increase the potential for harm and, consequently, the potential for liability arising out of the UR program. Prospective and concurrent UR decisions also pose dilemmas for the treating physicians and hospitals. If a treatment plan is disapproved, is the physician free to abandon the plan? To what extent is the physician or hospital obligated to provide the treatment despite the risk of nonpayment? How vigorously must the physician pursue any appeal rights to contest the UR decision?

The patient is also left in a quandary. The patient faces conflicting judgments by two medical professionals: the treating physician and the UR consultant. Should the patient rely on the treating physician's opinion, go forward with treatment and accept the resultant benefit penalties, or should he limit treatment to that which the payer will cover? Who is ultimately responsible for such decisions, and where should liability fall if the decision results in injury to the patient?

There are two leading court decisions regarding liability for UR decisions, *Sarchett* v. *Blue Shield of California* 43 Cal. 3d 1, 233 Cal. Rptr. 76, 729 P. 2d 267, (1987), and *Wickline* v. *California* 192 Cal. App. 3d 1630, 239 Cal. Rptr. 810 (1986). *Sarchett*, a retrospective review case, upheld the fundamental right of an insurer to challenge the treating physician's determination of medical necessity. *Wickline*, a case involving concurrent review, addressed the reviewer's potential liability to the patient for harm resulting from prospective or concurrent review decisions.

The *Sarchett* Decision

The most important aspect of the California Supreme Court's decision in *Sarchett* v. *Blue Shield of California, supra,* was that it affirmed an insurer's right to disagree with the treating physician's determination of medical necessity. The decision also made it clear that if coverage is denied, the insurer must inform the insured of any contractual rights to reconsideration or independent review, such as by arbitration.

The plaintiff, John Sarchett, was hospitalized for 3 days by his family physician. Blue Shield reviewed the hospital records and determined that the hospitalization appeared to be for diagnostic purposes only. It denied coverage based on two policy exclusions: first, an exclusion for hospitalization that is primarily diagnostic, and second, an exclusion for nonmedically necessary services.

The California Supreme Court upheld Blue Shield's right to challenge the medical necessity of hospitalization, even though the patient had relied on the recommendation of the treating physician. The court squarely rejected the plaintiff's argument that the treating physician is the final arbiter of medical necessity. It found retrospective review to be an implied right of the insurance relationship, even though the policy does not expressly state that the insurer may conduct retrospective review.[2]

In the *Sarchett* case, the court also commented favorably on the increasing practice of health care payers to require preauthorization for elective procedures. However, lest payers become too aggressive in coverage decisions, the decision included a reminder that any doubts and uncertainties in an insurance policy will be construed in favor of coverage for the insured. As a result, the decision of a treating physician will rarely be reversed as being unreasonable or contrary to good medical practice, the court predicted.[3]

The *Wickline* Decision

Although the decision in *Wickline* v. *California, supra*, was only an intermediate appellate ruling in California, it promises to be a seminal decision in the area of UR liability. Mrs. Wickline was being treated for problems associated with her back and legs, and her physicians recommended surgery. While her hospitalization and treatment were covered by Medi-Cal (California's Medicaid program), Medi-Cal required precertification for hospital admission and assigned an approved length of stay for the admission. Any extension of the approved length of stay had to be authorized. Medi-Cal approved Wickline's surgery and authorized a 10-day length of stay, with payment approved until January 17, 1977.

Mrs. Wickline suffered complications after the original surgery, and two additional surgeries were performed. Her treating physician determined that she should remain in the hospital 8 days beyond her scheduled discharge date and filled out a Medi-Cal form requesting an extension. The Medi-Cal on-site nurse reviewer, after consulting with a Medi-Cal physician adviser, approved only a 4-day extension. While there were appropriate spaces on the form for the on-site nurse's recommendation and the reason for disapproval by the physician adviser, both were left blank.

The attending surgeon discharged Wickline to her home when the 4-day extension period expired. All three of her treating physicians were aware that there was a process whereby the Medi-Cal decision could be appealed, but none of them appealed. A week after discharge one of the physicians examined her and found nothing remarkable. Then, nine days after discharge, Wickline was readmitted to the hospital with severe pain and discoloration of her right leg, which eventually had to be amputated at the hip. Wickline brought an action alleging that her injuries were caused by Medi-Cal's negligence in failing to authorize the full 8-day extension. A jury awarded her $500,000.

The Court of Appeal reversed the jury verdict, reasoning that although the state's preauthorization program played a role in the decision to discharge Wickline, this role was not determinative. Rather, the decision to discharge Wickline was made by the attending physicians. The court held that Medi-Cal was not a party to that medical decision and could not be held liable if that decision were negligently made. In refusing to find liability for the review decision, the court placed responsibility for the hospital discharge on the attending physicians and implicitly criticized them for not appealing the Medi-Cal denial decision if they disagreed with it.

The fact that the *Wickline* court based its holding on the lack of causation by the UR decision, rather than on any other available alternative basis, suggests that the court was particularly sensitive to the danger of holding the UR organization liable. Viewed in this light, the *Wickline* decision is not merely an ordinary application of the law of causation, but represents a precedent against UR liability. The *Wickline* case provides judicial recognition of the need for and the importance of UR as a check and balance in a system in which health care costs typically are paid by third parties rather than by the patient.[4]

At the same time, the court clearly stated that third-party payers could be held liable for "defects in the design or implementation of cost containment mechanisms" that result in the denial of medically necessary services. The decision recognizes that negligent UR decisions may result in denial of needed treatment, thereby causing injury to the patient. It thus sets the stage for further development of the allocation of responsibilities in this area.

The Elusive Concept of Medical Necessity

A UR decision invariably turns on whether a treatment or service is "medically necessary." This term is not only difficult to define but it also is frequently confused with other terms or limitations of the insurance policy. Failure to isolate the "medical necessity" aspects of a decision can easily result in wrong decisions, and hence potential liability for the reviewer.

Examples of such confusion are cases in which coverage is denied because the procedure is "cosmetic" or "experimental."[5] Often, a procedure will be "cosmetic" only because it is not "medically necessary" under the circumstances. Plastic surgery that otherwise would be cosmetic becomes medically necessary following a disfiguring accident. And, yet, a reviewer may attempt to deny the surgery as cosmetic, without determining whether it is medically necessary under the circumstances. When the issue is whether something is "experimental," it is generally presumed that some medical treatment is necessary. However, since the concept of "experimental" depends in part on whether the treatment is customary, the considerations are often similar to those used in determining medical necessity.

Definitions of "medical necessity" vary greatly.[6] Some policies define medical necessity simply, such as "such services . . . as are reasonably intended, in the exercise of good medical practice, for the treatment of illness or injury."[7]

Other policies provide more lengthy criteria.[8] Regardless of the definition, a determination of medical necessity is always a judgment call, and the reviewer must be careful not to apply an overly restrictive standard.[9]

An independent review organization is generally able to limit its decisions to whether something is "medically necessary." Where the review is conducted in-house by an insurance company or HMO, there may be more of a tendency to confuse a medical necessity determination with other coverage decisions. Care should be taken to delineate clearly the different reasons for a denial, even though the considerations may overlap.

In some cases, the UR entity's contract may require it to apply certain benefit restrictions, for example, in cases which the health plan covers certain procedures only if they are provided on an outpatient basis. In that situation, the UR entity is not making a decision as to medical necessity, but is simply applying nondiscretionary criteria. Presumably, the benefits restrictions satisfy any applicable regulatory requirements for minimum plan benefits. In such a case, the UR entity should not be held responsible for applying nondiscretionary criteria, since it is not making a medical necessity determination.

In some arrangements, the UR entity may be required to apply criteria, but has the latitude to deviate from the criteria in cases in which an exception is medically necessary, for example, when an outpatient procedure would be particularly risky for an elderly patient. Under this arrangement, the UR entity is exposed to liability because it must balance individual medical necessity against the standard criteria in each case. Of course, if such standard criteria appear in a variety of health plans, the very existence of the criteria may be evidence of the community standard of care.

LIABILITY OF THE REVIEW ORGANIZATION

Potential liability for the review organization exists under various legal theories, which are discussed in this section. One of the more unsettled areas is the extent to which Employee Retirement Income Security Act (ERISA) preemption applies. In a case in which ERISA applies, none of the common law claims discussed in this section would be available, and the plaintiff would be limited to ERISA remedies (see the section ERISA Preemption below).

Regardless of the legal theory, two factors weigh heavily in any case. The first factor is whether financial considerations influence the decision on medical necessity. A payer who conducts a review in-house may be more susceptible to improper fiscal considerations. For example, in one unreported case there was evidence that the medical director began systematically denying coverage for a particular treatment after attending a finance committee meeting where the costs for this treatment were singled out as being over budget. Independent review organizations may be less likely to be influenced by financial considerations, because the relationship between an independent reviewer's UR decision and the reviewer's compensation is indirect. However, the review organization's method of compensation may alter this conclusion. Most independent review organizations are compensated on a per-person or per-review basis. But if the review organization's compensation is based on the savings it realizes for its clients, then financial considerations might influence its decisions.

The second important factor in any UR liability case is causation. *Wickline* is a prime example of a case in which the plaintiff failed on the issue of causation. Regardless of the legal theory, causation typically is the biggest obstacle in the plaintiff's case.

Aside from these factors, the outcome of any liability case against a UR organization is likely to be influenced by the inherent sympathies of the jury, as illustrated by the *Wickline* case. That is, an injured individual generally will evoke more sympathy than the corporate review organization or insurance company.

The evidence in *Wickline* was overwhelming that Mrs. Wickline did not require continued hospitalization beyond the date of her discharge. Her bodily functions were all normal. She had commenced rehabilitation treatment. There was no open infection or open wound. No new symptoms had appeared, and she did not appear to be in any danger. Her initial length of stay had been extended for 4 days for general observation. Her treating physician testified that at the time of discharge, her condition was neither critical nor deteriorating. If it had been, he testified, he would have kept her in the hospital regardless of the Medi-Cal decision. Moreover, she was examined a full week after her discharge by one of her physicians, who noted nothing remarkable in her condition.

How, then, did the jury assess liability against the utilization reviewer for half a million dollars? The answer is easy—the jury system protects the individual against faceless bureaucracies. The jurors were presented with a tragic situation in which, through no fault of her own, Mrs. Wickline lost her leg, suffered greatly, and would continue to suffer greatly for the rest of her life. Yet, the Medi-Cal reviewer could not even remember why he had denied the hospital stay extension. It should come as no surprise that the jurors who have the legless and tearful Mrs. Wickline and her family sitting before them day after day will be inclined to ignore fine distinctions in the evidence and compensate Mrs. Wickline for her suffering. From this perspective, the $500,000 verdict does not seem so large.

The *Wickline* case illustrates the basic difficulty in defending cases of this nature. Utilization review, when viewed most favorably, solves the broad societal goal of containing health care costs. But the plaintiff's attorneys are likely to cast UR as simply a tool of insurance companies to make more money. The review organization's paper forms, the inability to remember specific cases, and the inevitable failure to gather every detail and other indicia of bureaucracy, coupled with the inescapable fact that reducing the amount of medical care saves money for the insurer, will always embellish the plaintiff's case. Moreover, unlike a malpractice case in which evidence of a physician's coverage is carefully shielded from the jury, in a UR case, the insurance company itself is usually the named defendant. For these reasons, the role of the jury cannot be ignored in any assessment of utilization review liability.

Negligence

Negligence is likely to be the principal cause of action against both a payer and an independent review organization for a UR decision. If the case involves a payer's in-house review, the plaintiff will probably proceed also on theories of breach of contract and breach of the implied covenant of good faith and fair dealing. In *Wickline*, a case involving in-house review, the only cause of action was negligence, and the court did not discuss any other potential theories. To establish negligence, the plaintiff must show that the defendant owed the plaintiff a duty of reasonable care, that the defendant breached the duty, and that the breach proximately caused the plaintiff's injury.

Existence of a Duty of Care

Whether a duty of care extends from an independent review organization to the patient depends on a variety of factors, but the courts are likely to find that a duty exists.[10] A primary factor in determining whether a duty of care exists is foreseeability of harm. When a review organization denies authorization for a treatment program, it is certainly foreseeable that the patient may forego treatment. The review organization may argue that its determination is for payment purposes only and is not to be relied upon as medical advice.[11] Nevertheless, the UR decision inevitably will have some affect on the decision whether to proceed with treatment. At the least, the UR decision may be a factor for the patient to consider and in many cases, it will be the decisive factor. The argument that the UR decision affects payment only is more persuasive on the issue of causation than on the issue of duty, as discussed in the section Causation below.

Wickline clearly recognizes that a duty of care exists for UR decisions made in-house by a payer.[12] However, there is also good reason for finding that the duty is owed by an independent review organization, given that the potential harm to the patient is just as foreseeable. The technical distinction that the independent review organization may not be in direct privity of contract with the patient should not prevent the imposition of a duty of care for tort law purposes.

The Standard of Care

The next issue in a negligence action is to define the standard of care.[13] There are two subissues involved here. First, the review organization may be liable if a defect in its procedures resulted in harm to the patient. Second, even if the organization's procedures were adequate, the duty of care may be breached if the decision on medical necessity did not meet proper standards.

The standard of care for the procedural aspects of a UR decision is likely to be based on the standards followed by review organizations generally, that is, the standard of care in the community of consultants in the same business. Overall, UR procedures must be sufficient to obtain enough information to make an informed decision and to enable a timely dialogue and/or appeal if the treating physician or patient disagrees.

In *Wickline* the physician consultant reviewed only the Medi-Cal form completed by the treating physician. He did not review the patient's chart or consult with the treating physician or a specialist consultant before rejecting the requested hospital extension.[14] The plaintiff attempted to show that these procedures were insufficient. The *Wickline* decision did not criticize the review procedure, thereby implicitly accepting the argument that the reviewer was entitled to rely on the information on the Medi-Cal form and that the burden was on the attending physician to justify the request by including all pertinent information on the form.[15] Nonetheless, there is no doubt that the defendant's sloppy recordkeeping, including the failure to document any reasons whatsoever for the denial, played a persuasive role in the trial court.

The procedural safeguards for review organizations are increasingly the subject of articles and seminars. As a result, the industry appears to have developed minimum standards that are consistently suggested for review organizations and would be put forth by plaintiff's attorneys in a UR case.[16] These standards include the following:

1. review decisions should be made by qualified medical professionals, and any denial decisions should be made only by licensed physicians;

2. reviewers should consult with specialist physicians as appropriate;

3. efforts should be made to obtain all necessary information, for example, by reviewing the patient's charts and consulting with treating physicians as appropriate;

4. the reasons for decisions should be clearly documented;

5. there should be a well-publicized and readily available appeal mechanism; and

6. decisions and appeals should be made in a timely manner as required by the exigencies of the situation.

Finally, the review organization should be careful to follow its own procedures. The failure to follow one's own procedures exposes the entity to potential liability, regardless of whether the particular review decision was correct.[17]

The other standard of care in a UR liability case is the standard for the substantive decision on medical necessity. The duty of care for this medical judgment is likely to be the same as that for physicians generally. By using the expertise of physicians, UR organizations hold themselves out as having a special skill in the evaluation of medical treatment. The UR organization, through its individual physician and nurse review consultants, will likely be held to a professional standard of care.[18] In other words, a UR consultant should authorize treatment if a physician applying the community standard of care would recommend this procedure as medically necessary.[19]

Many review organizations use standardized criteria to determine the appropriate treatment and length of hospitalization. A statistical methodology may be used to measure inappropriate treatment, admission, or length of stay.[20] Of course, the criteria need to be based on an appropriate standard of care and should be reviewed periodically to ensure that they do not become outdated.

Some believe that the fear of liability may deter UR organizations from adopting well-reasoned criteria that deviate from the existing community standard of care, even if it can be demonstrated that the community standard may lead to unnecessary care. There is no doubt that because of liability concerns, close cases tend to be resolved in favor of allowing care based on the existing community standard. At the same time, it seems clear that UR reduces the volume of certain types of care, for example, inpatient hospital days for HMO enrollees. To some extent, the adoption of criteria is self-validating; that is, as the use of the criteria becomes more widespread, the criteria themselves become evidence of the community standard of care.

The development and refinement of utilization criteria is a fluid process. Even though a UR organization is held to the community standard of care, the community standard is rarely a bright line, but is more often a consensus of judgment. In a close case, the UR organization is well advised to research the literature or data on particular criteria before making a final decision, in order to assess how strong the expert testimony will be if the decision is challenged. If the literature or data are strong, there is a good likelihood of being able to defend successfully if the case is taken to trial. On the other hand, if the criteria are based on weak data, an obscure article, or an article that recognizes that the procedure is new and unverified, then the UR organization should give the benefit of the doubt to the patient and await further evidence before adopting a more restrictive standard.

Standardized criteria have the beneficial effect of providing a uniform basis for screening all cases initially. Some UR organizations, particularly payers performing UR in-house, develop criteria from their own enrollment population and physicians. Such statistical models may provide valid screening tools for initial decisions, but their use may lead to inappropriate decisions in individual cases posing variations from the statistical norm. If criteria are used, there should be procedures available to allow the reviewer to deviate from them in individual cases of medical necessity.[21]

Another danger in the use of utilization criteria is the possibility that overzealous and mechanical application of the criteria may contradict explicit coverage provisions in the policy. As long as the criteria are limited to quantitative considerations, such as statistical determinations of lengths of stay or lists of procedures ordinarily done on an outpatient basis, the criteria serve a useful purpose. However, a too sweeping exclusion may result in the denial of services that are medically necessary and, therefore, that are covered under the basic policy.[22]

Causation

The third issue in a negligence action against a review organization is whether the denial of coverage proximately caused the patient's injury. Causation was the decisive issue in *Wickline* and promises to be the single largest hurdle in most UR liability cases.

In *Wickline*, the treating physician failed to take any steps to contest the initial denial. In fact, he signed the hospital discharge order and testified at trial that Mrs. Wickline's condition at the time of discharge was neither critical nor deteriorating. The fact that the physician may have been intimidated by the Medi-Cal program did not mean that he was incapable of contesting the decision if he disagreed with it. Thus, the court concluded that Medi-Cal did not participate in the medical decision to discharge Mrs. Wickline from the hospital and could not be held responsible for that decision.[23]

An alternative basis for the *Wickline* decision might have been that, wholly aside from the hospital discharge, the Medi-Cal decision was too remote from the infection and gangrene that eventually set in. In other words, the same harm would have befallen Mrs. Wickline even if she had remained in the hospital for the additional 4 days. One of her doctors testified that he examined her in his office a full week after the discharge (that is, 3 days beyond the extension that Medi-Cal denied) and that he did not note any material or substantial change in her condition.[24]

While *Wickline* provides an excellent description of the facts, its legal analysis is not as crisp. The holding could have been reached on any number of points, but the court's case law analysis is limited to a general recitation of overall negligence principles.[25] The court does not specifically discuss proximate cause, superseding intervening cause, or how the principles of comparative fault may apply. The court simply concludes as a factual matter that the Medi-Cal decision had nothing to do with the hospital discharge.

There remains an infinite variety of fact situations in which the causation issue has yet to be explored. What if Mrs. Wickline's infection had set in only 1 or 2 days after discharge instead of 10 days? At that time, she still would have been in the hospital if Medi-Cal had not denied the extension. Based on the court's analysis, Medi-Cal still would have been absolved of liability because, according to the court's analysis, Medi-Cal did not participate in the discharge decision.

Breach of Contract

A UR organization may be liable under contract theories as well as under tort theories. A contract typically exists between the patient and the third-party payer to pay for medically necessary services. When the payer performs UR in-house, an improper review decision that results in nonpayment is a direct breach of contract.

When the payer delegates UR to an independent review organization and improperly denies benefits based on the UR decision, a contract remedy against the payer would still be available to the patient, even though the utilization review was undertaken by the independent review organization.[26] The absence of a contractual relationship between the patient and the UR organization does not insulate the payer from contract liability for the UR organization's actions.[27] In addition, the patient may assert a contract claim directly against the independent entity if the patient is a third-party beneficiary of the contract between the UR entity and the payer. This contract often sets forth the scope of services to be rendered and the standards for review. A third-party beneficiary relationship exists if the contract between the payer and the UR entity was intended to benefit the patient.[28] The review organization will argue that its contract with the payer was not intended to benefit the patient, but was simply to provide services to the payer and to benefit the payer exclusively.[29]

The measure of damages for breach of contract is all damages reasonably foreseeable from the breach.[30] In prior or concurrent review, since it is foreseeable that denying authorization will result in the patient foregoing medical services, the defendant potentially is liable for injury or death caused to the patient.

The critical issue in a contract action, just as in a negligence claim, is causation. The plaintiff still must show that the review decision proximately caused the harm. Thus, in the final analysis, the pivotal issue in a contract claim is likely to be the same as in a negligence claim.

Insurance Bad Faith

Many states recognize tort liability against an insurance company for breach of the implied covenant of good faith and fair dealing. This cause of action exposes the defendant to punitive damages that ordinarily would not be available in a simple negligence or breach of contract case.[31] Insurance bad faith theories are also useful to the plaintiff because they inquire directly into the process used to reach a coverage decision, and not merely the correctness of the decision itself.[32] Similarly, the failure to provide adequate appeal rights may itself be the basis for bad faith liability.[33]

Insurers performing UR in-house have direct exposure to this liability. When the payer delegates the UR function to an independent entity, both the payor and the reviewer, as its agent, are potentially exposed to bad faith liability. When the payer ratifies the reviewer's decision, or leaves the decision primarily in the reviewer's hands, the courts are likely to hold the payer responsible to the plaintiff for the reviewer's mistakes.[34]

Whether the independent review organization is directly liable for insurance bad faith is a more complicated question. The legal basis for bad faith liability is unique because it contemplates a tort—the breach of a duty of care—arising from a special contractual relationship. In contrast, the tort of negligence is not based in contract, but arises out of the finding that a duty of care is owed directly by one party to another. The difficulty in applying the bad faith tort theory in the UR context is the absence of the direct contractual relationship on which the tort is based between the plaintiff (the insured) and the independent UR organization. Furthermore, an independent review entity, unlike an insurance company, does not stand in an established "special" or fiduciary relationship to the insured. The nature of the relationship between the insurer and the insured is one reason the courts have sanctioned the development of the bad faith doctrine. Also, as long as a reviewer's compensation is not incentive-based, the reviewer is not subject to the insurance company's inherent conflict of interest, namely, making more money by denying more care.

Despite these differences between the status of the insurance company and the independent reviewer vis à vis the insured, there are arguments that the reviewer should be subject to the same risk of bad faith liability as the insurer. First, the review organization makes decisions that directly affect the level of insurance benefits, and thus cause the same kind of harm as insurance company decisions do. Moreover, the harm is foreseeable, and the potential magnitude of the harm is great. Like the relationship between the insurance company and the insured, the relationship between the review organization and the insured is reflected in a nonnegotiable "adhesion" contract. As a practical matter, the insured cannot bargain with the reviewer over the nature of their relationship and, therefore, is forced to accept the reviewer's terms. Finally, the reviewer is acting in the role of an insurance company. For these reasons, an independent reviewer may be exposed to bad faith liability, even though the direct contractual link is absent.

While the courts generally have not imposed bad faith liability on the agents and contractors of insurance companies,[35] at least one case found liability despite the lack of contractual privity. In *Delos* v. *Farmers Insurance Group*,[36] the management company for a reciprocal insurer was liable under the implied covenant of good faith and fair dealing for bad faith handling of a claim. The court found that the management company was acting in the capacity of an insurer by processing claims. The case may be distinguishable from other cases because the management company was, in fact, an arm of the insurer and was the attorney-in-fact and, therefore, a fiduciary with respect to each insured. Nevertheless, the case is significant because the court wanted to prevent the insurer from insulating itself from liability by forming a management company, and consequently, the absence of contractual privity did not prevent the bad faith tort remedy. In addition, there is a possibility that an independent reviewer could be sued for conspiracy with the insurer to breach the implied covenant of good faith and fair dealing.[37]

As a practical matter, a plaintiff is likely to seek the punitive damages available for bad faith liability from the "deep pocket," which is the insurer, rather than the independent reviewer. However, there is a definite risk that an independent reviewer would be exposed to such liability or forced to defend against such claims.

Infliction of Emotional Distress

A review organization is potentially exposed to claims for infliction of emotional distress. In states where the intentional tort is recognized, proof is required of (1) extreme and outrageous conduct, (2) intent to cause severe emotional distress to the insured or reckless disregard of the probability that such distress would result, and (3) severe emotional distress suffered by the plaintiff as a proximate result of the defendant's conduct.[38] The intentional tort has been interpreted to require proof that the defendant's acts were "so extreme as to exceed all bounds of that usually tolerated in civilized community."[39] Since such extreme misconduct is not likely to arise in the UR context, the more likely cause of action against a UR entity would be negligent infliction of emotional distress. The negligence tort requires a showing of (1) negligent conduct by the review organization, (2) severe emotional distress suffered by the patient, and (3) proximate causation.

Warranty Theories

Consumer materials from the payer or the review organization frequently will tout the beneficial services performed by UR or emphasize the quality aspects of the UR procedure. Such materials may support a claim for breach of warranty. The question generally will be whether the consumer materials were intended to warrant a specific result as opposed to being generalized sales puffing.[40]

An independent UR organization is well advised to specify in its payer contracts that the payer must include in its consumer documents certain provisions relating to UR. This is particularly important for UR organizations contracting with self-insured employers who may not be as sophisticated as large insurers in preparing consumer documents. At a minimum, the UR organization will want to make sure that the consumer materials reference the insured's consent to UR, clarify that the UR system is the payer's enterprise, and spell out the rights and obligations of the UR process. Another provision would state that the UR entity does not make medical decisions but only advises on payment questions, and that the patient and physician are solely responsible for deciding what medical treatment is provided. Although such statements may not be strictly enforceable, they can be helpful to a UR organization in defending against various liability theories.

Products Liability

The increasing use of computer software programs by UR organizations to determine the appropriateness of admissions may give rise to claims focusing on the design of the software. A plaintiff could attempt to fashion an argument that he or she suffered damages resulting from an erroneous denial that was made by using a defectively designed software program. By arguing under a products liability theory that the software is a defectively designed product, the plaintiff need not prove that any party acted negligently. Products liability cases require proof only that the product was defective and that the defect caused the injury.[41] In addition, the fact that the UR organization did not develop the software, but merely acquired it from a software vendor, may not insulate the UR entity from liability. The products liability doctrine casts a wide net over prospective defendants, permitting plaintiffs to sue virtually every party in the chain of the manufacture and distribution of a product.[42]

A key issue in a products liability case would be whether the use of the software program constitutes a product or a service. Products liability theories do not apply to services, but the distinction between a product and a service is not clearly defined in the law.[43] Moreover, it appears that there is little precedent for finding that products liability applies to claims arising out of the use of computer software programs. However, there are cases finding that, for example, instrument approach charts used by pilots for landing are considered products for purposes of product liability claims brought in wrongful death actions against the manufacturers of the charts.[44] Plaintiffs may try to extend these cases by analogy to software programs.

Defamation and Interference with Contractual Advantage

The UR entity's liability is not limited to potential claims by the patient. Physicians or other providers who are harmed by UR decisions may also bring suit. Typically, these actions would be for defamation or, potentially, for interference with the physician's contractual relationship with the patient.[45]

In *Slaughter* v. *Friedman*,[46] plaintiff Slaughter was an oral surgeon who brought an action against a dental insurance company and its dental director for defamation and intentional interference with prospective advantage. In denying claims for Slaughter's services, the insurer enclosed a letter to the patients that described Slaughter's work as "unnecessary," claimed that Slaughter had been "overcharging," and stated that the insurance company would report him to a dental association for disciplinary proceedings. The letters also advised the patients to make no further payments to Slaughter. The California Supreme Court upheld Slaughter's right to sue for defamation (the interference claim was not before the court).

Whenever a UR program informs a patient that the treating physician rendered, or proposes to render, treatment which is not medically necessary, a potential defamation claim exists. The UR decision carries a stamp of authenticity and may cause a patient to question the doctor's medical judgment and capability. In addition, a finding that services were not medically necessary may justify the patient's decision not to pay for the services.

The UR entity would have available in a defamation action the defense of qualified privilege that applies to communications between persons with a mutual interest in the subject matter.[47] The privilege is not absolute, however, and may be defeated by showing that the communication was made with malice. In the *Slaughter* case, the court found that the pleadings sufficiently raised the issue of malice to allow the complaint to stand.[48] For these reasons, a UR organization should be careful to limit its communications simply to the basis for its denial decisions and should avoid unnecessary embellishments or inflammatory language.

Antitrust

A full discussion of potential antitrust liabilities is beyond the scope of this paper. However, a few points are worth noting.

For the review organization that does medical necessity determinations, antitrust is a relatively lesser threat than the other potential liabilities reviewed above are. Antitrust is a more immediate concern for entities that set uniform fee schedules or that limit or exclude providers, such as HMOs or preferred provider organizations (PPOs). When a closed-panel system such as an HMO excludes a physician because of high utilization, there is some potential for antitrust liability. As a general rule, the conduct will not be illegal per se but will be tested under the rule of reason. Under the rule of reason test, the challenged activity will be upheld when the legitimate, procompetitive interests outweigh the potential anticompetitive effects.[49] As long as the defendant succeeds in having the court apply the rule of reason test, the beneficial effects of limiting the provider panel to cost-effective physicians are likely to prevail over the interest of a single physician in remaining on the panel, at least in cases in which the defendant's market share is within reasonable bounds.[50]

The difficulties in defending a provider exclusion case tend to be the inevitable problems of proving that a physician is a high utilizer. The excluded physician often attempts to show that he or she was singled out because of some personal animus by his or her competitors on the review committee. Often, the defendant's records are not as precise as the attorney would hope and the statistics are not consistent or are incomplete. Other physicians who have not been excluded may have equally bad or worse utilization records, thereby raising the question of unequal treatment. The excluded physician may have an outstanding reputation for quality, or may claim that his or her patients tend to be sicker than the average population. All of these problems make the defense of the antitrust case more difficult, but there is nothing inherently illegal in excluding a provider based on utilization data.

For UR entities doing medical necessity determinations, the principal source of antitrust claims lies in restricting the availability of new or controversial treatments. Because UR applies a community standard of care, there is a built-in bias against new treatments that do not have widespread acceptance in the medical community. For example, various antitrust cases have been brought by purveyors of dimethyl sulfoxide and laetrile claiming that third-party payers and their reviewers were unlawfully refusing coverage for these new "miracle" cures. For a less controversial example, consider heart transplants. It is likely that utilization review entities continued to deny transplants as "experimental" or not medically necessary for some period of time beyond the point when transplants became relatively safe and even commonplace in sophisticated areas of practice.

In this kind of antitrust case, one of the biggest hurdles is to show that a combination or conspiracy exists to deny coverage. Unilateral action is insufficient to establish a violation under Section 1 of the Sherman Act; there must be a "contract combination or conspiracy in restraint of trade."[51] The fact that several employees or even a committee of reviewers participated in a denial of coverage generally is not enough to establish antitrust liability because they all work under a single corporate entity.[52] The plaintiff will want to show that a number of payers are conspiring to deny coverage of a new treatment. While the plaintiff often can show that a number of payers actually do deny coverage, it is a rare case when the plaintiff can establish an agreement among the payers to deny coverage.[53]

Liability of Consultants and Employees

The consultants and employees of the review organization may be found liable for torts in which they participated, just as is the case for any other individuals who work for a corporation. Their protection lies in proper insurance and in their right to indemnity from the corporation.

Many states have statutes that provide immunity from liability for certain peer review activities. However, these statutes generally do not protect the physician consultants of independent review organizations. The statutes generally are limited to certain types of peer review, such as hospital review committees, medical society committees, and certain committees of HMOs; and they generally focus on peer review of quality of care rather than medical necessity determinations for private payers.[54] The immunity is usually a qualified rather than absolute immunity, meaning that the participant who acts with malice is not shielded from liability.

When a physician provides independent consultant services to a UR entity, the physician's malpractice insurance may or may not cover those services.[55] The UR entity's policy probably does not cover independent contractors and may also exclude claims arising from the provision or failure to provide medical services. Liability insurance needs to be clarified by both the physician consultant and the UR entity.

An employee of a corporation who is personally named in a lawsuit and is successful in the defense of the suit may have the right to indemnity from his or her employer under the applicable Corporations Code, unless it is shown that he or she did not act in good faith or acted against the best interests of the corporation.[56] A corporation will generally have the option of indemnifying an agent for actions taken in good faith and with the reasonable belief that the actions were in the corporation's best interests.[57] As a practical matter, employees generally expect the corporation to assume any liability in a situation such as that in the case of *Wickline*. However, cases will arise in which the corporation will not indemnify, the corporate insurance is exhausted, or the corporation is otherwise without assets. A physician consultant, therefore, is well advised to examine carefully the corporation's liability policy and to review his or her own consultant contract in light of the corporation's liability policy and the applicable law on indemnity.

State Regulation

The design of UR procedures is increasingly the subject of state regulation. The state of Maryland enacted legislation in early 1988 requiring a UR organization to obtain a certificate from a state agency before conducting UR.[58] The application process requires, among other things, submission of a UR plan, including a description of review standards and procedures, the circumstances in which UR may be delegated to a hospital UR program; and the appeal mechanism for patients, providers, and hospitals. The legislation does not specify any detailed requirements for standards and procedures, and no regulations have been promulgated as of this writing.

Minnesota also enacted in 1988 a provision requiring prospective utilization review decisions to be made within ten business days. The time period does not run until all information reasonably necessary to the decision has been made available.[59]

Maine requires insurers with prospective review requirements to file annual reports setting forth the number and type of such review decisions.

The reports also must include a summary of denials and any appeals or lawsuits related to the prospective review.[60]

Louisiana presently has the most comprehensive legislation regarding prospective utilization review requirements.[61] The Louisiana statute expressly permits a damages action for "unreasonable delay, reduction or denial" of services, and sets certain standards for prospective utilization review decisions. Decisions made within two working days are deemed to be timely; however, longer time periods may be justified under some circumstances. The statute further provides that decisions on medical necessity must be based on "nationally accepted current medical criteria," but the statute fails to give any further guidance as to what medical necessity means.

While the Louisiana statute expressly authorizes damages actions, it also limits the potential recovery. Damages for prospective review decisions are limited solely to physical injuries, which excludes punitive damages and also may be interpreted to exclude emotional distress damages. However, the prevailing plaintiff may recover reasonable attorneys' fees. The statute also imposes on the plaintiff a strict causation requirement, and limits damages solely to injuries that are the "direct and proximate cause" of the unreasonable delay, reduction, or denial. Thus, although some may view the Louisiana statute as unwanted regulation, the statute actually provides certain safeguards to the insurance industry and limits the amount of recoverable damages.

ERISA Preemption

In *Pilot Life Insurance Co. v. Dedeaux*,[62] the U.S. Supreme Court held that when insurance is provided through an ERISA plan, common law actions by an insured for bad faith denial of insurance coverage and related state law tort claims are preempted by ERISA.[63] Most private employers' benefits plans are covered by ERISA.[64] Thus, many of the liability theories discussed above are subject to an ERISA preemption defense. However, the courts are still grappling with the scope of preemption, and there remain areas of uncertainty.[65]

When a utilization review case is brought directly against an ERISA payer based on a denial of benefits or mishandling of a claim, the action should be preempted. The alleged wrong at issue is the denial of benefits provided by the ERISA plan, which is the same as the wrong involved in the *Pilot Life* case. The fact that consequential damages flowed from the denial of benefits (for example, Mrs. Wickline's loss of a leg) should not distinguish the case from that of *Pilot Life*.

When the defendant is an independent review entity, the ERISA preemption issue will turn on whether the review entity is deemed to be a "fiduciary" under ERISA. A person or entity performs fiduciary functions, and is therefore deemed to be a fiduciary under ERISA, if it exercises discretionary authority or control over the plan.[66] When the review entity makes the initial determination on coverage, for example, by refusing to authorize surgery or refusing to extend a hospital length of stay, a court is likely to hold that the review entity is exercising a fiduciary function. If the review entity is held to be a fiduciary, then ERISA preemption would apply.

However, if the court finds that the review entity is not a fiduciary, it is not clear whether ERISA preemption would apply.[67] This area is one of continuing development following the *Pilot Life* decision.

ERISA preemption does not leave the plaintiff entirely without a remedy. However, the remedies available under ERISA may be severely restricted and may preclude the plaintiff from recovering consequential damages such as pain and suffering or, in a situation like that of *Wickline*, the cost of living a life as an amputee. The monetary remedy available to a plan participant in an ERISA action is limited generally to recovery of plan benefits, and consequential damages are not permitted.[68] The court does have discretion under ERISA to fashion broad equitable relief,[69] and given the right set of facts, a creative court may well attempt to fashion an equitable remedy to provide adequate compensation for the plaintiff.

Two other features of an ERISA action are worth noting. First, to the plaintiff's advantage, attorneys' fees may be awarded under ERISA. Second, to the plaintiff's general disadvantage, there is no right to a jury trial under ERISA.[71]

The recognition of ERISA preemption as a defense to state common law torts may lead plaintiffs to resort to other innovative theories to avoid preemption. One such theory would rely on a federal racketeer influenced and corrupt organization (RICO) action,[72] which permits a prevailing plaintiff to recover treble damages and attorneys' fees. Since RICO is a federal action, it is not preempted by ERISA. Some courts have permitted a RICO cause of action against an insurance company for denying coverage.[73] The plaintiff's theory is that the insurer misrepresented the coverage at the time the policy was issued. Since the insurer used the mails in selling the policies, the alleged misrepresentation constituted mail fraud, which is one of the predicate acts for RICO liability. Although these cases did not involve health insurance, similar allegations could arise in the health insurance context.

LIABILITY OF THE EMPLOYER OR PAYER

If utilization review is performed in-house, then the employer or payer is directly liable for the consequences of review decisions.[74] This section addresses the liability of the payer or employer that contracts with an independent review entity. In that situation, the payer has the potential for direct liability or vicarious liability.

The principal practical distinction between direct and vicarious liability is whether the payer will be fully indemnified by the review entity. A principal who is found to be vicariously liable for the torts of its agent is entitled to full indemnity from the agent.[75] However, if the payer is found to be directly liable for the harm, the damages will be allocated proportionately between the payer and the review entity based on their respective faults. Thus, the payer will want to avoid direct liability, if possible, and shift as much responsibility as possible to the review entity.

Direct Liability

The employer or payer may be directly liable under several theories. First, if the payer acts on the reviewer's decision and denies coverage, there is potential liability for breach of contract. If a bad faith insurance claim is available, then the payer may also become liable for tort damages in cases which it adopts or ratifies the reviewer's decision. An insurance company may not escape liability by delegating its responsibilities to an outside entity.[76] When the payer is not an insurance company but is, for example, a self-insured employer, the employer may still be liable for breach of its contract to pay benefits (or under ERISA for denial of benefits).

In a contract action, the payer could not avoid liability by showing that the review entity was an independent contractor. A party to a contract does not avoid contractual liability by delegating contractual obligations to another unless the delegate assumes liability and the obligee consents to the assumption.[77] Few, if any, review contracts would qualify as an assignment.

A payer also may be liable directly in tort if it participates in the design of a faulty UR system or if the payer fails to exercise due care in selecting the independent review entity. The latter theory, negligent selection, is being increasingly recognized in a variety of fields.[78] For this reason, a payer should inquire into the reputation of the independent review organization, inquire directly about any lawsuits or judgments, and document the results of its inquiry as evidence of the exercise of due care.

Vicarious Liability

A payer also may be found vicariously liable for the torts of the review entity under traditional principles of agency. It is frequently suggested that a payer may avoid vicarious liability in cases in which the review organization serves as an independent contractor, rather than as an agent, as UR contracts almost universally contain independent contractor provisions.

While this distinction is theoretically possible, the independent contractor defense is difficult to sustain in practice. Not only is the independent contractor doctrine viewed with disfavor today,[79] but it also may be difficult to prove independent contractor status.[80]

Even if the review entity is an independent contractor, the plaintiff may still be able to prevail under the doctrine of ostensible agency. Ostensible agency exists when one either intentionally or negligently allows another to believe that an agency relationship exists.[81] In cases in which the review entity tells a hospitalized patient that the payer's benefits are terminating or tells the patient who wants an operation that the procedure is not medically necessary, the patient is likely to assume that the reviewer is the "agent" of the payer. A payer might be able to avoid ostensible agency by clearly emphasizing in its consumer documents that the review entity is entirely separate and independent. Even so, a court may be reluctant to allow the payer to escape liability entirely.

Indemnity

The most important protection for a payer is to insist that the reviewer carry adequate liability insurance. Ideally, the payer will be named as an additional insured on the review entity's policy, and the insurance company will be required to notify the payer directly of any change in coverage or cancellation. The payer should also review the terms of the reviewer's policy to see that it covers the various types of liability that can arise in the utilization review context.

Many payers also insist on indemnity and hold harmless provisions in the contract with the review entity. Such clauses are likely to be much less helpful without an adequate liability policy. Without insurance, the review entity may not be able financially to satisfy its indemnity obligation. Also, when one defendant is insured or is otherwise financially viable and the other defendant is uninsured, the plaintiff will try to tailor the case toward the financially viable defendant. Thus, the payer who otherwise may be a secondary defendant may find itself the primary target if the review entity is uninsured.

LIABILITY OF THE TREATING PHYSICIAN

The impact of UR has fallen most heavily on practicing physicians. While a physician is accustomed to having some services questioned by retrospective claims review, the more intrusive forms of prior or concurrent review meddle directly in the physician's course of treatment of the patient. A review consultant, who usually and has never seen the patient, is questioning the physician's judgment as to what is medically necessary. Then, as in the *Wickline* decision, the judicial system blamed the treating physician for failing to protest strongly enough against the reviewer's decision.

On a philosophical level, many physicians have cried foul. UR usurps the considered, professional judgment of the physician. It interferes with the essential relationship of trust between the physician and patient. It is Big Brother watching. Nevertheless, UR appears to be firmly entrenched in the U.S. medical system, and the courts will be forced to continue to grapple with the respective obligations of the parties.

Defining the obligations of treating physicians presents the largest area of unanswered questions.[82] A UR denial places the physician at risk of nonpayment if he or she proceeds with the proposed treatment. Assuming that the physician appeals the UR decision, is he or she safe to defer to the reviewer and withhold treatment if the appeal is denied? Can the physician simply withdraw from treating the patient if the review decision is adverse and the patient cannot pay for the treatment? If the physician withholds treatment and harm results to the patient, does the UR decision provide the physician with a defense to a malpractice action?

Wickline suggests that a physician may not avoid a malpractice claim simply by acquiescing in a UR decision. *Wickline* held that the responsibility for the hospital discharge was solely that of the physicians. In that case, of course, the physicians did not protest Medi-Cal's denial, and by their testimony they agreed that the discharge was appropriate at the time. But *Wickline* did not say how far a physician must go in appealing a denial decision. Would the court have upheld Medi-Cal liability if the treating physicians had simply requested reconsideration and Medi-Cal had denied the request? Were the treating physicians required to pursue all available avenues of appeal, including an administrative review hearing and even a court challenge to the decision? Was it even possible for these avenues of appeal to be resolved in the limited time before the patient was to be discharged? If, after contesting the decision, the physician still believed it was unsafe to discharge Mrs. Wickline from the hospital, were they required to keep her in the hospital and risk nonpayment?

Hard cases will arise when the physician vigorously appeals the denial, to no avail. In this situation, the risk of nonpayment is even clearer than it is at the time of the initial decision. At the same time, by protesting the initial decision, the physician may have created substantial evidence that the treatment is medically necessary—evidence that will be used against the physician if he or she then withholds treatment and harm occurs. At some point, if the physician's appeal is strong enough, a court is likely to hold the review entity responsible for causing at least part of the harm.[83] But the possibility of sharing liability with another defendant is little solace to the treating physician, who still remains a clear potential defendant if he or she withholds treatment.

Most of these questions focus on the physician's obligation to provide treatment to a patient who cannot pay. When the physician has not commenced treatment, he or she is relatively free to turn away the case.[84] Most UR cases, however, involve an established physician-patient relationship. Terminating this relationship may constitute the tort of medical abandonment.

The essence of abandonment is unilateral nonconsensual termination by the medical practitioner.[85] The two elements required to avoid a claim of abandonment are (1) notice and (2) opportunity to secure alternative medical services. When a UR denial applies to a truly elective procedure, there is generally ample opportunity for the physician to satisfy these two elements before foregoing the course of treatment. However, when the patient is hospitalized and a certified length of stay expires, as in the *Wickline* case, there is little or no practical opportunity to give notice and to seek alternative treatment. The responsibility remains on the physician to provide care, or to keep the patient in the hospital, if the physician believes that the community standard would require such action.[86]

The physician also has increased exposure to claims of lack of informed consent.[87] When a proposed treatment is denied, the physician must be careful to explain to the patient the options and the risks. The patient then must decide whether to go ahead with the treatment and pay for it out of his or her own pocket. Even if the risks inherent in the treatment are minimal, the financial pressure on the patient to forego treatment makes it particularly important for the physician to explain carefully the medical risks of foregoing the treatment.

Many physicians complain that they often are unable to learn the basis for a UR organization's denial decision. However, the appeals process should provide a means for obtaining the basis for the decision. In view of the responsibility placed by *Wickline* on the physician to appeal adverse decisions, the physician should demand the basis for the UR decision on the grounds that he or she needs it to respond adequately in the grievance or appeals process.[88] Also, in this writer's opinion, it is generally good practice for the UR appeals committee to prepare a written statement of its decision. A written statement demonstrates a good faith, reasoned approach to the problem. Even if the patient or the physician disagrees with the conclusion, a well-reasoned written decision serves to dampen the sense of frustration and anger generated by a terse rejection of the appeal.

In any case in which a reviewer denies care, the physician, of course, is free to explain the denial and obtain the patient's consent to treatment and to pay for the care, notwithstanding the denial. However, a physician should take precautions to ensure that the patient understands fully the financial implications of such consent.

LEGAL ISSUES FOR THE PATIENT

The patient, of course, lies at the heart of the controversy. Aside from the various liability issues discussed above, the most pressing issue for the patient is how to obtain timely review of a UR denial. The other issue for the patient is whether he or she must pay for physician services that the reviewer determines were not medically necessary.

The Need for Expedited Review

Consider Mrs. Wickline's situation when she was lying in the hospital recovering from multiple surgeries and was told that Medi-Cal would not cover further hospitalization. She could have either gone home, which would have been against the initial advice of her physician, or she could have remained in the hospital and risked the devastating possibility of having to pay for it herself.

This situation highlights a major weakness in most UR systems—the ability to resolve appeals in a timely manner. Most UR appeals systems are designed for retrospective review. They include multiple levels of in-house review, followed by an independent decision by an arbitrator, a court, or an administrative law judge. It may be weeks, months, or even years before a UR decision is reviewed by an independent third party.

While such a system may suffice for retrospective review, in a prior or concurrent review situation the patient's medical care is directly at stake. To be effective, the appeal process must occur within a time frame consistent with the patient's medical condition. For example, in cases in which the challenged decision is the discharge of a sick infant from the hospital to the home, it should be possible to complete the appeal before the infant is sent home and complications can set in. Another example is when an HMO patient needs urgent treatment of a specialized nature. If a question arises whether the patient needs to go out of the HMO plan to secure specialized services, there should be a means to resolve the question in the short time span dictated by the patient's medical needs.

One answer may be to seek expedited judicial relief. While immediate independent review has certain advantages, it also creates a cumbersome burden on the courts and results in the substitution of judicial judgment for medical judgment. Although physicians would say that the courts have not shied away from substituting their own judgment in the past, the prospect of reviewing a number of UR decisions on an expedited basis is not something the judicial system will welcome.

An analogous burden was thrust upon the courts in cases involving decisions to disconnect life support systems. Many courts resisted having to make these decisions.[89] However, there is a difference between court review of decisions to forego treatment of terminally ill patients and court review of UR decisions. Whereas the former decisions frequently border on the philosophical, decisions in UR cases often simply resolve disputes between two professionals' judgment of medical necessity. The latter dispute is similar to what the courts are asked to do in many routine cases. Nevertheless, the courts can be expected to resist the added burden on the judicial system of having to review UR denials, particularly if the review is expedited while the patient's treatment hangs in the balance.

Another means of resolving the problem of expedited review of UR decisions is to allocate the burden of payment prospectively to the payer. If care were deemed medically necessary until the conclusion of the review process, UR organizations would have a significant financial incentive to make careful, reasoned decisions and to expedite the review process. If a denial were subsequently upheld, the patient would incur the debt for the treatment rendered.

Payment for Unnecessary Medical Services

Another issue for the patient is whether the physician can collect payment from the patient for services that are determined to be medically unnecessary. Or, phrased differently, the issue is who should bear the risk of payment for claims that the payer denies because they are not medically necessary under the payer's rubric? One solution would be to allocate this risk by recognizing a new implied covenant in the physician-patient relationship obligating the physician to advise the patient on whether the physician's assessment of the medical necessity of services conforms with, or is defensible under, the insurance company's definition of medical necessity.[90] As the interpreter of "medical necessity," the physician is placed at financial risk for the cost of unnecessary services.

The rationale for adopting an implied covenant of medical necessity is to create a disincentive for physicians to overutilize medical services. It would also motivate physicians to appeal questionable UR denials out of self-interest, thereby enhancing the protection of the patient. The concept is supported by the disparity in knowledge between the physician and patient regarding medical necessity.[91]

Theoretically, both the review organization and the treating physician should operate under the same standard of medical necessity, which, by definition, should be determined by the community standard of care. There is a danger, of course, that a review organization would apply a standard in the middle to low range of the community standard of care. However, the judicial inclination to construe insurance policies against the insurer, and the general deference given to the judgment of the treating physician, tend to minimize this problem. In addition, the effect of the implied covenant on the behavior of physicians could alter the community standard of care, as physicians become more cautious in recommending treatments for fear that they will be liable for payment to other providers and will not receive their physician fees.

As a practical matter, and without an implied covenant of medical necessity, if the physician, patient, and insurer are all joined in a single action in a case in which medical necessity is the issue, the patient is virtually certain to escape any payment obligation. The trier of fact can be expected to place the burden either on the physician or the payer, but not on the patient.[92]

When the patient is an HMO member, the question of payment for unnecessary services does not arise, at least for services from a participating physician, because the physician is prohibited from direct billing for covered benefits. The HMO system thus protects the patient by excluding him or her from payment disputes.

It is conceivable that legislation could mandate the same result in the indemnity insurance context. Such legislation would prohibit physicians from collecting for services determined to be medically unnecessary, in effect, codifying the implied covenant in the physician-patient relationship suggested above. There would be two problems with such legislation. First, it would be necessary to clarify the point at which there is a final determination that services were not medically necessary. This issue in itself could increase the volume of litigation as physicians scramble to obtain final determinations of medical necessity in order to support their bills. Second, such legislation could work to the detriment of patients by effectively prohibiting physicians from rendering care that may ultimately be beneficial, even though it cannot be shown to be medically necessary under standards of insurance coverage. A patient who can afford to pay for treatment should not be precluded from using his or her own funds to purchase the services he or she wants, even if the insurer will not pay for them.

CONCLUSION

If the current trends continue, the placement of liability for UR ultimately will be sorted out by the courts. However, many of the issues raised in this paper may not be developed thoroughly for judicial review because of the broad sweep of ERISA preemption of common law actions. Moreover, in cases in which the allocation of UR liability arises in an HMO context, the issues are likely to be resolved by arbitration and never reach the courts because of the binding arbitration clauses that are frequently found in HMO consumer documents and physician contracts.

When a UR case does reach the courts, the plaintiff has a range of legal theories to test and several potential defendants, including the provider, the payer, and the utilization review organization, to bring into the lawsuit. Given the increased use of UR by cost-conscious payers, it is likely that opportunities for testing the various legal theories will be plentiful. In anticipation of this uncharted development of the law, the health care industry would do well to begin addressing the liability issues internally.

At the heart of one UR liability debate is the fundamental question of who should bear the risk of UR decisions and whether and how that risk can be allocated without resorting to the judicial system. A secondary, but perhaps more immediate, question is how to provide for expedited review of UR decisions, so that bad decisions are reversed before they have an immediate impact on the patient's medical care.

REFERENCES

1. See generally Byrnes, "Corporation's Institution of Healthcare Utilization Review," *Medical Trial Technique Quarterly* (Spring 1987), at 478; Carabillo, "The Manageable Risks of Managed Care," *Health Cost Management*, Vol. 3, No. 6 (Nov./Dec. 1986), at 1; Eisenberg and Rosoff, "Physician Responsibility for the Cost of Unnecessary Medical Services," *New England Journal of Medicine*, Vol. 299 (July 13, 1978), at 776; Hershey, "Fourth-Party Audit Organizations: Practical and Legal Considerations," *Law Medicine & Health Care*, Vol. 14, No. 2, at 54; Lanzafame, *Provider Liability Under Public Law 98-21: The Medicare Prospective Payment System in Light of Wickline v. State*, 34 Buffalo L. Rev. 1011 (1985); Jespersen and Kendall, "Utilization Review: Avoiding Liability While Controlling Health Costs," *HEALTHSPAN*, Vol. 4, No. 7, at 3 (July 1987).

2. For a contrary decision, see *Van Vactor* v. *Blue Cross Association*, 50 Ill. App. 3d 709, 8 Ill. Dec. 400, 365 N.E. 2d 638 (1977), which found no justification for the denial of benefits solely on the ground that the insurer disagrees with the honest judgment of the treating physician. The court concluded that decisions of medical necessity are "vested solely and exclusively in the judgment and discretion of the treating physician." *Id.* 365 N.E. 2d, at 647.

3. The court also concluded that Blue Shield acted in bad faith when it failed to inform the insured of his right to impartial review and arbitration as provided in the policy. Although this aspect of the case turned on the particular conduct of Blue Shield, which went beyond a simple failure to inform of appeal rights, the decision emphasized the duty of the insurer to protect the rights of the insured at least equally with its own. 233 Cal. Rptr., at 84-86. Thus, even if the insurance policy contains clear and conspicuous language regarding remedial rights, the insurer should take affirmative steps to inform the insured of his or her rights if a denial of coverage is disputed.

4. The decision proceeds to review the beneficial aspects of the Medi-Cal program and the Medi-Cal regulations providing for prior authorization for hospitalization. *Id.*, 228 Cal. Rptr., at 671. Although the court may have been citing this material in connection with the alternative defense of immunity raised by the state, the court states that it declines to address the immunity defense. See 228 Cal. Rptr. 669, at

672. The purpose of discussing the Medi-Cal regulations appears to be simply to show that prior review is an integral part of the payer's system.

5. Several courts have held an exclusion for "experimental" procedures to be inherently ambiguous, and hence unenforceable. See *Johnson* v. *District 2 Marine Engineers Beneficial Assoc.*, 857F. 2d 514 (9th Cir., July 11, 1988); *DiDomenico* v. *Employers Cooperative Industry Trust*, 676 F. Supp. 903 (N.D. Ind. 1987).

6. Some policies simply use the term but do not define it. These policies run the risk that a denial based on medical necessity will not be upheld because the term is not adequately defined. See, e.g., *Dallis* v. *Aetna Life Insurance Co.*, 100 F.R.D. 765 (N.D. Ga. 1984); *Zuckerberg* v. *Blue Cross Blue Shield of Greater New York*, 119 Misc. 2d 834, 464 N.Y.S. 2d 678 (1983), rev'd on other grounds. 487 N.Y.S. 2d 595, 108 A.D. 2d 56 (1985).

7. *Sarchett, supra*, 233 Cal. Rptr., at 78.

8. One plan defines "medically necessary services" as those which are:

"(1) Appropriate for the symptoms and diagnosis or treatment of a condition, illness or injury.

(2) Provided for the diagnosis, or the direct care and treatment of the condition, illness or injury.

(3) In accordance with the standards of good medical practice.

(4) Not primarily for the convenience of the Member, or the Member's physician and surgeon, or the provider.

(5) The most appropriate supply or level of service which can safely be provided to the Member.

When applied to hospitalization, this further means that the member requires acute care as a bed patient due to the nature of the services rendered or the member's condition, and the Member cannot receive safe and adequate care as an outpatient."

9. *Hughes* v. *Blue Cross*, 199 Cal. App. 3d 318, 245 Cal. Rptr. 273 (1988), upheld liability against an insurer which applied a standard of medical necessity which was more restrictive than that of the medical community. Citing *Sarchett*, the court emphasized that the term *medically necessary* must be construed liberally so that uncertainties are resolved in favor of coverage. The court noted that by employing a standard of medical necessity significantly at variance with the medical standards of the community, the insurer places the insured at risk of incurring unforeseen liability, which is contrary to the insured's reasonable expectations. "[G]ood faith demands a construction of medical necessity consistent with community medical standards that will minimize the patient's uncertainty of coverage in accepting his physician's recommended treatment." *Id.* 245 Cal. Rptr., at 279.

10. See *Wickline, supra*, 228 Cal. Rptr., at 669; *Rowland* v. *Christian*, 69 Cal. 2d 108, 70 Cal. Rptr. 97, 443 P. 2d 561 (1968). Rowland lists the following factors as the major considerations in determining whether a duty exists: "The foreseeability for harm to the plaintiff, the degree of certainty that the plaintiff suffered injury, the closeness of the connection between the defendant's conduct and the injury suffered, the moral blame attached to the defendant's conduct, the policy of preventing future harm, the extent of the burden to the defendant and consequences to the community of imposing a duty to exercise care with resulting liability for breach, and the availability, cost and prevalence of insurance for the risk involved." *Id.* 69 Cal. 2d, at 112. Although the *Wickline* decision states that these factors lead it not to find liability, it appears that *Wickline's* holding is based on lack of causation rather than on the nonexistence of a duty. This is evident from a statement later in *Wickline* to the effect that third-party payers may be held liable for medically inappropriate decisions resulting from their cost-containment program. 228 Cal. Rptr., at 670.

11. UR contracts usually expressly distinguish between the role of the UR organization in determining the availability of coverage, the roles of the payer in making payment decisions, and the roles of the provider and patient in deciding whether to proceed with treatment. One UR contract states that the UR provider "shall not determine a participant's eligibility for benefits under the Group Contract. Group shall have final and sole authority for all benefit determinations." Another contract states that "the decision or determination to obtain or deliver any health care service is always made only by the [patient] and/or his or her physician, and any decisions made by the [UR organization] . . . or the health benefit insurer . . . shall relate only to the obligation for payment for any such service under the terms of the group insurance policy. . . ."

12. The patient who requires treatment and is harmed when care that should have been provided is not provided should recover for the injuries suffered from all those responsible for the deprivation of such care, including, when appropriate, health care payers. Third-party payers or health care services can be held legally accountable when medically inappropriate decisions result from defects in the design or implementation of cost-containment mechanisms, as, for example, when appeals made on a patient's behalf for medical or hospital care are arbitrarily ignored or unreasonably disregarded or overridden. *Wickline, supra,* 228 Cal. Rptr., at 670-671.

13. Every person or entity is expected to exercise the care that the ordinary, reasonable person of common skill and prudence would use under the circumstances of the case. The standard of care is heightened if the person causing the injury enjoys some specialized skill or knowledge. Professionals such as doctors and lawyers are expected to use the skill and care common to their professions, not merely that of the "ordinary person." Prosser and Keeton, *The Law of Torts,* Section 32, at 185-186 (1984).

14. *Wickline, supra,* 228 Cal. Rptr., at 666.

15. *Wickline's* suggestion that the burden is on the treating physician to provide the reviewer with sufficient information is not a panacea for every utilization review liability case. In *Hughes* v. *Blue Cross of Northern California,* 199 Cal. App. 3d 318, 245 Cal. Rptr. 273 (1988), the reviewing physician consultant testified, in explaining why his file lacked complete medical information, that he felt it was the responsibility of the treating doctor or the hospital to submit any information they felt was important. The court nevertheless upheld liability for bad faith claims denial, noting that the letters sent to the treating physician did not explain the medical basis for denial and failed to advise what information the reviewer already had and what additional information would be useful. *Id.* 245 Cal. Rptr., at 280.

16. See generally Jesperson and Kendall, *supra* note 1, at 7.

17. For a discussion of state regulation, see the section State Regulation.

18. See the sections Liablity of Consultants and Employees and Liability of the Treating Physician *infra* regarding the vicarious liability of the UR organization for the torts of its agents.

19. See *Hughes* v. *Blue Cross,* 199 Cal. App. 3d 318, 245 Cal. Rptr. 273 (1988) (bad faith verdict upheld in a case in which the insurer applied a standard of medical necessity that was more restrictive than the community standard).

20. See generally J. Restuccia, "The Appropriateness of Hospital Use," *Health Affairs,* at 130 (Summer 1984).

21. See the section The Elusive Concept of Medical Necessity for a discussion of situations in which criteria are expressly included as part of the plan benefits.

22. For example, a criteria that disallows all fertility services under an HMO plan that covers all medically necessary physician services may be too sweeping an exclusion.

23. *Wickline, supra,* 228 Cal. Rptr., at 671.

24. *Id.* 228 Cal. Rptr., at 668.
25. *Id.* 228 Cal. Rptr., at 669.
26. The payer's liability for tort damages resulting from the negligent act of an independent review organization may be more complicated, depending on whether the UR entity is viewed as an independent contractor or an agent or employee of the payor (see Liability of the Treating Physician).
27. When a contractual duty is delegated, the obligor remains liable to the obligee, unless the delegate assumes the obligations and the assumption is accepted by the obligee in substitution for the original obligor. See Calamari and Perillo, *The Law of Contracts*, Sections 277-280 (1970) and *Restatement (2d) of Contracts*, Section 150(3). There also would be a significant question of whether the duty to perform UR functions is a delegable duty under the law. See Calamari and Perillo, *supra*, Section 278; *Hughes* v. *Blue Cross*, 199 Cal. App. 3d 318, 245 Cal. Rptr. 273, (1988) (an insurance company generally cannot delegate its responsibilities to the insured).
28. See Calamari and Perillo, *Restatement (2d) of Contracts*, Section 302. The court will look to the surrounding circumstances to determine whether the patient is an appropriate third-party beneficiary. In cases in which the benefit literature describes the UR program as a beneficial service for the insureds, for example, in helping to avoid unnecessary hospitalization, the employee has a better chance of establishing a third-party beneficiary relationship.
29. This issue is likely not to be of much practical importance, since the patient can probably assert a negligence claim directly against the review organization. Whatever benefits the patient can obtain from a contract action, such as an action for breach of the implied covenant of good faith and fair dealing, ordinarily can be obtained in an action directly against the payor.
30. *Restatement (2d) of Contracts*, Section 351.
31. See generally *Pilot Life Insurance Co.* v. *Dedeaux*, 107 S. Ct. 1549 (1987); *Fletcher* v. *Western National Life Ins. Co.*, 10 Cal. 3d 376, 401, 89 Cal. Rptr. 78, 93 (1970).
32. See, e.g., *Egan* v. *Mutual of Omaha*, 24 Cal. 3d 809, 157 Cal. Rptr. 482, 598 P. 2d 452 (1979) (bad faith failure to properly investigate claim); *Taylor* v. *Prudential Ins. Co. of America*, 775 F. 2d 1457 (11th Cir. 1985) (reversing summary judgment for the insurer on the issue of bad faith where the insurer relied on a Medicare determination of no medical necessity without making its own investigation); *Hughes* v. *Blue Cross*, 199 Cal. App. 3d 318, 245 Cal. Rptr. 273 (1988) (bad faith verdict upheld where insurer denied claims without reviewing all relevant medical records, applied a standard of medical necessity that was more restrictive than a community standard, failed to explain medical grounds for denial of coverage, and failed to advise treating physician of what additional information would be useful for decision); *Mordecai* v. *Blue Cross/Blue Shield of Alabama*, 474 So. 2d 95 (Ala. 1985) (bad faith allegations arising from failure to consider portions of nurses' notes and to consult with treating nurses and physicians); *AEtna Life Insurance* v. *LaVov*, 470 So. 2d 1060 (Ala. 1984) (bad faith claim upheld where insurer misrepresented the extent of its medical review in denying the claim).
33. See generally *Sarchett* v. *Blue Shield, supra*; *Davis* v. *Blue Cross of Northern California*, 25 Cal. 3d 418, 158 Cal. Rptr. 828 (1979) (bad faith upheld in a case in which the insurer failed to inform the insured of rights to appeal an arbitration).
34. In such a case, the payer could seek indemnity from the reviewer, unless prohibited by some provision of the contract between the payer and reviewer. See *Hughes* v. *Blue Cross*, 199 Cal. App. 3d 318, 245 Cal. Rptr. 273 (1988).
35. *Gruenberg* v. *AEtna*, 9 Cal. 3d 566 (1973) (demurrer sustained as to bad faith liability of insurer's independent contractor adjusters and attorneys who were not party to the

insurance contract); *Iversen* v. *Sup. Ct.*, 57 Cal. App. 3d 168, 127 Cal. Rptr. 49 (1976) (reversal of judgment against claims supervisor and claims examiner, both found to be independent contractors, because they were not party to insurance contract); *Hale* v. *Farmers Insurance*, 42 Cal. App. 3d 681, 117 Cal. Rptr. 146 (1974) (insurer not liable for employee's bad faith handling of claim where insurer has not ratified employee's acts). See also *Reiderscheid* v. *Comorecare. Inc.*, 667 P. 2d 766 (Colo. Ct. App. 1983) ("The test of bad faith failure to exercise due care in discharge of a contractual duty and the granting of damages for mental anguish caused by a willful and wanton breach of contract are grounded in basic common law, and not solely in the area of insurance law."); *Taylor* v. *Prudential Ins. Co. of America*, 775 F. 2d 1457 (11th Cir. 1985) (upholding cause of action against insurer for bad faith and emphasizing the weight to be given to treating physician's opinion); *Linthicum* v. *Nationwide Ins. Co.*, 723 P. 2d 675 (Sup. Ct. Ariz. 1986) (punitive damages may be recoverable against insurer for failure to disclose medical basis for denial or failure to seek direct input from treating physician).

36.   93 Cal. App. 3d 642, 155 Cal. Rptr. 843 (1979).

37.   See *Sprague* v. *Equifax Inc.*, 166 Cal. App. 3d 1012, 213 Cal. Rptr. 69 (1985); *Younan* v. *Equifax Inc.*, 111 Cal. App. 3d 498, 169 Cal. Rptr. 478 (1980).

38.   *Fletcher* v. *Western National Life Ins. Co.*, 10 Cal. App. 3d 376, 89 Cal. Rptr. 78 (1970).

39.   See *Schlauch* v. *Hartford Acc. & Indem. Co.*, 146 Cal. App. 3d 926, 936, 194 Cal. Rptr. 658, 665 (1983), quoting *Ricard* v. *Pacific Indem. Co.*, 132 Cal. App. 3d 886, 895, 183 Cal. Rptr. 502, 507 (1982).

40.   See *Pulvers* v. *Kaiser Foundation Health Plan*, 99 Cal. App. 3d 560, 160 Cal. Rptr. 392 (1979) (advertisement of "high standards" of medical service held not to warrant a specific result, but was generalized "puffing," to the effect that physicians would exercise good judgment in care).

41.   The *Restatement (2d) of Torts*, Section 402A, states as follows: ". . . One who sells any product in a defective condition unreasonably dangerous to the user or consumer or to his property is subject to liability for physical harm thereby caused to the ultimate user or consumer, or to his property, if (a) the seller is engaged in the business of selling such a product, and (b) it is expected to and does reach the user or consumer without substantial change in the condition in which it is sold." In California, the plaintiff need not show that the product was "unreasonably dangerous," but only that the product was "defective." See *Cronin* v. *J.B.E. Olson*, 8 Cal. 3d 121, 104 Cal. Rptr. 433 (1972).

42.   See *Restatement (2d) of Torts*, Section 402A, Comment f.

43.   See generally *CCH Products Liability Reporter*, Section 4235.

44.   See *AEtna Casualty and Surety Co.* v. *Jeppesen & Co.*, 642 F. 2d 339 (9th Cir. 1981); *Brocklesby* v. *United States*, 767 F. 2d 1288 (9th Cir. 1985), *cert. denied sub nom*, 106 S. Ct. 882 (1986).

45.   See *Slaughter* v. *Friedman*, 32 Cal. 3d 148, 185 Cal. Rptr. 244, 649 P. 2d 996 (1982) (defamation; interference with prospective economic advantage); *Teale* v. *American Manufacturers Mutual Ins. Co.*, 687 S.W. 2d 218 (Mo. Ct. App. 1985) (tortious interference); *Moore & Assoc.* v. *Metropolitan Life Ins. Co.*, 604 S.W. 2d 487 (Tex. Civ. App. 1980) (claim stated for tortious interference with doctor-patient relationship by association of anesthesiologists against group medical insurer for insurer's letters to former patients advising that claims would not be paid in full because associaton's charges were excessive).

46.   *Supra.*

47.   See, e.g., California Civil Code, Section 47(3).

48. Slaughter, *supra*, 185 Cal. Rptr., at 248-249. The court pointed out that defendants were only required "to inform dental patients of the basis for rejection of their claims; they were not required additionally to defame plaintiff with accusations regarding his dental practices."

49. See *Chicago Board of Trade* v. *U.S.*, 246 U.S. 231 (1981); *Dos Santos* v. *Columbus-Cuneo-Cabrini Medical Center*, 684 F. 2d 1346 (7th Cir. 1982) (under rule of reason analysis, the hospital was permitted to grant exclusive privileges where policy is grounded in ensuring quality patient care and necessary hospital services).

50. See generally *Northwest Wholesale Stationers. Inc.* v. *Pacific Stationery Printing*, 105 S. Ct. 2613 (1985) (unless an organization possesses market power or controls access to an element essential for competition, expulsion for failure to follow reasonable rules is not per se illegal); see generally remarks of Charles F. Rule, Assistant Attorney General, U.S. Department of Justice, March 11, 1988.

51. 15 U.S.C., Section 1.

52. Cf. *Copperweld Corp.* v. *Independent Tube Corp.*, 467 U.S. 752, 104 S. Ct. 2731, 81 L. Ed. 2d 628 (1984).

53. Plaintiffs often attempt to rely on the doctrine of "conscious parallelism." Conscious parallelism is easy to allege but exceedingly difficult to prove. It requires proof that the parallel conduct was against the defendant's self-interest and was not based on good faith business judgment. See *Supermarket of Homes* v. *San Fernando Valley Board of Realtors*, 786 F. 2d 1400 (9th Cir. 1986); *Proctor* v. *State Farm Mutual Ins. Co.*. 675 F. 2d 308 (D.C. Cir.), cert. denied, 459 U.S. 839 (1982).

54. See, e.g., California Civil Code, Sections 43.7, 43.8; California Health & Safety Code, Section 1370.

55. For example, Norcal Mutual Insurance Company's malpractice policy only covers claims alleging negligence in "direct patient treatment" or involving professional committee activities (which are limited to hospital staff committees or American Medical Association or medical society committees). Coverage is specifically excluded for "the performance of administrative duties, which are not direct patient treatment, as a medical director." If liability is found against an independent physician reviewer in a *Wickline*-type case, it is not clear whether the coverage for "direct patient treatment" applies. The physician providing consultant services should seek clarification from the carrier.

56. See, e.g., California Corp. Code, Section 317(d).57.

57. See, e.g., California Corp. Code, Section 317(b).

58. Md. Health Code Ann., Sections 19-1301 *et seq.*

59. Minn. Stat. 1988, Section 72A.20(4a).

60. Maine Ins. Code Title 24-A, Section 2679. Maine also has legislation pending that, if enacted, would impose certain criteria on independent review organizations, such as requiring prospective UR decisions to be made within a set time.

61. La. Revised Stat. 22:657(D).

62. 107 Sup. Ct. 1549 (1987).

63. See 29 U.S.C., Section 1144. See generally Helvestine, "ERISA Preempts Insurance Bad Faith Actions," *HEALTHSPAN*, Vol. 4, No. 10, at 8 (Dec. 1987).

64. Significant exceptions to ERISA coverage are government employee plans (including local government plans, such as school districts), certain church plans, and certain statutorily required workers' compensation, unemployment, and disability laws. UR cases will not be preempted when they arise under these kind of plans. See 29 U.S.C., Section 1003(b).

65. One major area of uncertainty has been whether ERISA preempts causes of action based on state statutes governing unfair insurance practices, such as California

Insurance Code, Section 790.03(h). In *Kanne* v. *Connecticut General Life Ins. Co.*, 857 F. 2d 96, No. 85-5641, 5642 (9th Cir., Oct. 4, 1988), the Ninth Circuit held that ERISA preempts such claims. This issue is of considerably less importance following the California Supreme Court's decision in *Moradi-Shalal* v. *Fireman's Fund Ins. Co.*, 46 Cal. 3d 287, 250 Cal. Rptr. 116 (1988), which overturned 10 years of precedent and held that no private right of action exists under Section 790.03(h). At this time, only Montana and West Virginia continue to recognize private actions under unfair insurance practices statutes. See *Moradi-Shalal, supra,* 250 Cal. Rptr., at 121 and note 6.

66. 29 U.S.C., Section 1002(21)(A); see *Stanton* v. *Shearson Lehman/American Express, Inc.*, 631 F. Supp. 100, 102 (N.D. Ga. 1986).

67. See *Nieto* v. *Ecker*, 945 F. 2d 868 (9th Cir. 1988) (rejecting a theory of liability under ERISA for aiding and abetting a fiduciary); *So. Cal. Meat Cutters Unions* v. *Investors Research*, 687 F. Supp. 506 (C.D. Cal. 1988) (ERISA only applies to those defendants against whom ERISA provides a statutory right of action); *Munoz* v. *Prudential Ins. Co. of America*, 633 F. Supp. 564 (D. Colo. 1986) (same findings as previous case).

68. See 29 U.S.C., Section 1132(a)(1)(B); *Massachusetts Mut. Life Ins. Co.* v. *Russell*, 473 U.S. 134, 105 S. Ct. 3085 (1985) (emotional distress damages prohibited); *Sokol* v. *Bernstein*, 803 F. 2d 532 (9th Cir. 1986) (same findings as previous case).

69. See 29 U.S.C., Section 1132 (a)(3).

70. *Id.* Section 1132 (a)(3).

71. See, e.g., *Blau* v. *Del Monte Corp.*, 748 F. 2d 1348 (9th Cir. 1984).

72. 18 U.S.C., Section 1961 *et seq.*

73. See *Marcial* v. *Coronet Ins. Co.*, No. 87C 3072 (N.D. Ill., 1987 WL 19532); *Unocal Corp.* v. *Superior Court (Harbor Ins. Corp.)*, 198 Cal. App. 3d 1245, 244 Cal. Rptr. 540 (2d Dist. 1988), decertified (June 2, 1988).

74. Under the theory of *respondeat superior*, an employer may be held liable for the torts of its agents or employees acting within the scope of their employment. See Witkin, *Agency and Employment*, Sections 113 *et seq.*; California Civil Code, Section 2338.

75. See Witkin, *supra, Agency and Employment*, Section 61, at 67.

76. See *Hughes* v. *Blue Cross*, 199 Cal. App. 3d 318, 245 Cal. Rptr. 273 (1988).

77. See note 24, *supra.*

78. See, e.g., *Restatement (2d) of Torts*, Section 411; *Elam* v. *College Park Hospital*, 132 Cal. App. 3d 332, 183 Cal. Rptr. 156 (1982) (hospital negligently allowed podiatrist to remain on staff despite malpractice complaints). See Burch 122 Mich. App. 798, 333 N.W. 2d 140 (Mich. 1983); *Kendall* v. *Gore Properties*, 236 F. 2d 673 (D.C. Cir. 1956); *Giles* v. *Shell Oil Corp.*, 487 A. 2d 610 (D.C. 1985) (employer responsible for harm caused by employee in a case in which the employer negligently failed to screen the employee's background).

79. The general rule that parties are not liable for the torts of their independent contractors is riddled with exceptions. When the plaintiff can show that one party retains control over the enterprise, benefits from it, selects the independent contractor, and is free to require indemnity and insurance from the contractor, that party may be found vicariously liable for the torts of its independent contractor. Also, when the plaintiff can demonstrate a "special relationship" giving rise to an affirmative duty of care owed by the defendant, vicarious liability may result. See Witkin, *supra, Torts*, Section 997. An insurance company is likely to be found to have a special relationship with its insureds, thus increasing the likelihood of liability for the acts of independent contractor UR organizations.

80. The fact that the contract between the payer and reviewer specifies independent contractor status is not dispositive. The reviewer may be considered an independent

contractor for purposes of its relationship with the payor, and yet be considered an agent of the payor in matters involving the patient. Cf. *Arthur* v. *St. Peter's Hospital*, 169 N.J. Super. 575, 405 A. 2d 443 (1979) (physician may be considered an independent contractor in his relations with the hospital, but be deemed an employee of the hospital in his relations with the patient). The principal factor in distinguishing an independent contractor from an employee is the freedom from control by the employer over the details of the work. See Witkin, *supra, Agency and Employment*, Sections 12, 14, at 28-31; Prosser and Keaton, *The Law of Torts* (5th ed., 1984) for a discussion of the doctrine generally and a suggestion that it is disfavored.

81. See *Restatement (2d) of Agency*, Sections 8, 159 (apparent authority of agent); California Civil Code, Section 2300; *Quintal* v. *Laurel Grove Hospital*, 62 Cal. 2d 154, 41 Cal. Rptr. 577, 397 P. 2d 161 (1964) (whether the physician was ostensible agent of the hospital is a jury question); *Mduba* v. *Benedictine Hospital*, 384 N.Y.S. 2d 527, 52 App. Div. 2d 450 (1976) (emergency room physicians may be named agents of the hospital despite independent contractor language in their contracts).

82. Many of the same dilemmas discussed in this section apply to hospitals as well. Indeed, in a concurrent review situation like *Wickline*, the hospital has the largest financial stake in the patient's discharge because it is the hospital bills that would remain unpaid. The rights and responsibilities of a hospital are similar to those of a physician and are not treated separately for the purposes of this paper.

83. If the physician is named in a lawsuit, he or she may cross-complain against the review entity for indemnity or contribution. Likewise, a review entity named in a *Wickline* type of case will consider cross-complaining against the treating physician.

84. See, e.g., *Goldman* v. *Ambro*, 512 N.Y.S. 2d 636 (1987); *Harper* v. *Baptist Medical Center-Princeton*, 341 So. 2d 133 (Ala. 1976). In *Harper*, the Alabama Supreme Court held that a doctor and hospital who rendered emergency treatment to the plaintiff, but refused to accept him as a patient because he did not have insurance, were not liable for subsequent injuries because the plaintiff had not been accepted as a patient. Until a professional doctor-patient relationship is established, the physician's only duty is to provide emergency care; there is no duty to accept a patient under other circumstances.

85. See generally, Mains, "Medical Abandonment," *Medical Trial Technique Quarterly*, at 306 (1985).

86. See, e.g., *Meiselman* v. *Crown Heights Hospital*, 285 N.Y. 389, 34 N.E. 2d 367, 217 N.Y.S. 2d 12 (1941) (liability against hospital where the patient was discharged prematurely because he was unable to pay for further care). See generally Lanzafame, *supra*, note 1, at 1023-1030.

87. Informed consent requires disclosure of all information that the patient would consider material in deciding whether to undergo the treatment. See *Canterbury* v. *Spence*, 464 F. 2d 772 (D.C. Cir. 1972). Presumably, economic consequences would be a material consideration for the patient.

88. Physicians should be mindful, however, of the UR organization's legitimate concerns regarding the disclosure of its review criteria and systems, which are usually considered protectable trade secrets.

89. See *In Re Quinlan*, 70 N.J. 10, 355 A. 2d 647, 649, cert. denied, 429 U.S. 922 (1976) (review would be "inappropriate," not only because that would be a gratuitous encroachment upon the medical profession's field of competence, but because it would be impossibly cumbersome").

90. For a thoughtful treatment of this issue, see Eisenberg and Rosoff, *supra*, note 1.

91. The implied covenant of medical necessity should not, however, supplant the patient as the final decision maker in matters of medical care. Rather, it obligates the

physician to add a new economic dimension to the physician's determination of medical necessity, which must be communicated to the patient.

92. In one case, the court apparently refused to relieve the patient of payment responsibility, even though the insurer denied coverage because the treatment was not medically necessary. *Albert Einstein Medical Center* v. *Lipoff*, No. 3872X (Ct. of Common Pleas, Phila., Apr. 23, 1973), described in Eisenberg and Rosoff, *supra*, note 1. In that case, the patient sought to hold her physician contractually liable for the hospital bill. The court denied her claim, reasoning that her claim sounded in tort and that she could recover only by proving that the doctor's treatment was medically unsound. That it was economically unsound was irrelevant to a tort claim.

Appendix B
Utilization Management and Quality Assurance in Health Maintenance Organizations: An Operational Assessment

Joan B. Trauner and Sibyl Tilson*

In the 1980s, health care payers in the public and private sectors have relied increasingly on utilization management to help control health care costs. As a result, the autonomy of health care providers—hospitals and professionals—has been curtailed as payers have applied predetermined criteria to judge the appropriateness of care. The medical community, in turn, has expressed concerns about the design of the clinical standards or algorithms governing utilization review decisions by health insurers, Blue Cross and Blue Shield plans, third-party administrators, and health maintenance organizations (HMOs). In particular, as payers seek to control costs more aggressively, physician organizations are seeking to review the criteria used for denial of services under second-opinion and prior authorization programs.[1]

At the same time, federal and state legislators, health policy analysts, and consumer groups are concerned about the impact of physician incentive plans on quality of care and accessibility to services in prepaid delivery systems. This concern was prompted, in part, by concerns about the quality of care delivered to Medicare beneficiaries enrolled in International Medical Centers Inc. (IMC), a for-profit HMO located in south Florida.[2] The well-publicized IMC scandals raised a number of public policy issues, including enrollee understanding of benefit restrictions in HMOs,[3] ineffective

---

*The authors are members of the accounting firm Coopers & Lybrand, San Francisco, Calif., and Washington, D.C.

quality assurance monitoring in HMOs (both internally by HMO staff and externally by regulatory agencies), and the impact of financial incentives on ordering of services and specialty referrals by HMO physicians.[4] The intent of this paper is to describe the range of utilization management and quality assurance strategies that are used by HMOs and then to evaluate their actual implementation. The paper begins with a brief discussion of the methodology used in preparing this paper. The second section describes the organizational structure of existing HMOs, and the third discusses market, structural, and operational factors affecting HMO performance. The fourth section discusses the approaches to utilization management and quality assurance, and the fifth section evaluates the performance of utilization management and quality assurance programs in HMOs. In the sixth section, there is a review of existing research on physician risk incentives in HMOs, while the seventh section addresses some additional policy and research issues. The final section of this paper contains five condensed case histories.

Except for the discussions on the organizational structure of licensed HMOs, the term HMO is generically in this paper to cover all closed systems in which physicians are partly or fully capitated for delivery of care and where enrollees may receive services only from contracting providers.[5] All state-licensed prepaid medical plans are included in this definition, regardless of whether they are federally qualified and offer a full range of benefits.

METHODOLOGY

This paper reflects the authors' experience as health care consultants for an international accounting firm. During the past 3 years, we have had the opportunity to analyze the health benefits offered by numerous employers in both the public and private sectors and to help design their managed care programs. (By managed care, we refer to any program that channels patients to a specific set of health care providers.) During the same time, we and our associates have conducted operational reviews of over 20 HMOs, ranging from local to regional and multistate plans. In general, the HMO reviews have involved an analysis of financial, actuarial, enrollment, and utilization trends in the context of benefit design, premium pricing, marketing practices, claims processing procedures, contractual arrangements with providers, utilization review, and management reporting procedures.

This managed care and HMO consulting experience provides the background for this paper. To supplement our experience, we reviewed the health services research literature for HMO-related studies. In describing our personal experience, we do not purport to review a statistically representative sample of HMOs. In fact, because many of the plans that we studied are in transition, the paper may magnify some of the problems facing the HMO industry.[6] The crucial advantage of an experiential analysis, however, is that it offers an internal view of HMO operations at all organizational levels that is not available through standard survey instruments or through a review of documents filed with regulatory agencies.[7]

In our HMO discussions, we do not refer to any plans by name, nor do we provide any information on exact plan size, geographic location, plan age, or precise sponsorship in order to preserve client confidentiality. The brief case histories for five plans that appear at the end of this paper do not include any plan identifiers, but do contain actual descriptions of the utilization management programs in place at the time that the operational reviews were conducted. We present these studies to show the range of operational problems that can undermine the structural design of utilization management and quality assurance programs.

HMO ORGANIZATIONAL STRUCTURE

According to the current InterStudy classification of HMOs, there are four types: staff, group, network, and individual practice association (IPA) model plans.[8] Staff model HMOs deliver health services through physicians who are under salary to the plan. Group model HMOs contract with one independent multispecialty group practice, whereas network model HMOs contract with two or more multispecialty groups. IPAs contract with physicians in private practice, either as individuals, through their group practices, or through separate physician associations.

Under the mandating process established by the HMO Act of 1973, an employer is required to offer only one group or staff model HMO and one IPA in a given service area. (The network classification did not exist under the original HMO Act.) In some geographic areas, HMOs have used a model designation that allows them to take advantage of the mandating process, rather than one that strictly corresponds to their underlying structure. For example, plans that contract almost exclusively with multispecialty groups have sought IPA designations to compete against long-established group or staff model plans. Therefore, any analysis of HMOs requires an assessment of the underlying contractual arrangement with physicians, rather than the plans own self-designation.[9]

More recently, ICF, Inc. has categorized HMOs as having two-tier or three-tier organizational structures.[10] In the two-tier structure (Figure B-1), the HMO contracts directly with individual physicians; in the three-tier structure (Figure B-2), the HMO makes capitation or fee-for-service payments to the IPA or group, which, in turn, contracts with individual

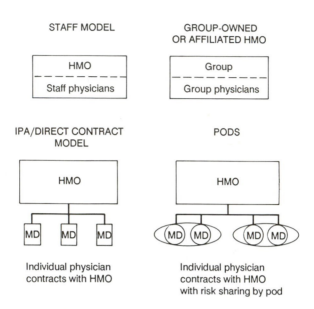

FIGURE B-1 Organizational structures within HMOs: two-tier structures.

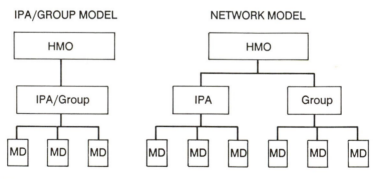

FIGURE B-2 Organizational structures within HMOs: three-tier structures.

physicians. ICF originally included only staff model plans and direct contract IPAs in the two-tier classification. In Figure B-1, we have added two additional categories: HMOs owned by group practices and HMOs in which physicians contract directly with the HMO but are arbitrarily grouped into risk-sharing pools or "pods."

As described in the literature, a two-tier structure may facilitate contracting in areas where physicians are geographically dispersed (that is, suburban or rural areas) or where physicians have not developed their own

IPAs. According to the literature, some HMOs elect to use a two-tier structure purposely to forestall physicians from creating IPAs, which, in turn, can function as bargaining units to provide physicians with higher fees.[11]

Lately, we have come across a new two-tier contractual arrangement involving those HMOs that contract directly with individual physicians and then create arbitrary physician risk pools, or pods. In these arrangements, the financial risk is shared with other providers with whom the physician may or may not have direct contact in daily practice.[12] Depending upon the local market, pods may sometimes be organized by group practice or hospital affiliation; in other areas, physicians may be assigned to a pod solely on the basis of practice location.

In this paper, we use the two- and three-tier structure as the basis for much of our analysis. This approach allows us to focus on where responsibility for utilization management decisions actually rests. For example, in two-tier IPA arrangements, most decision-making resides at the HMO level, whereas in three-tier arrangements those entities that contract with the HMO (for example, IPAs and multispecialty groups) may take over many of these responsibilities. In determining how plans are classified, we ignore the self-designated HMO plan type and instead examine the underlying contractual relationship that exists with participating physicians. In this way, we can describe more precisely utilization management activities in those plans that have contractual arrangements with varying types of provider entities (for example, plans that have group-, staff-, and hospital-based IPA arrangements).

MARKET, STRUCTURAL, AND OPERATIONAL FACTORS AFFECTING HMO PERFORMANCE

We believe that any review of HMO performance that focuses exclusively on structural measures will have serious limitations. The HMO market is in a state of flux. Not only are many plans reporting financial losses, but they are having to contend with employer demands regarding the provision of data and experience rating and with provider concerns about reimbursement rates and design of utilization review programs. In this section, we briefly describe the relationship of the health care marketplace to HMO structure and operations. The intent of the analysis is to show that plan performance, as measured by financial, utilization, and quality indicators, is a function of multiple variables, many of which are beyond the control of HMO management.

The Health Care Marketplace

An HMO both reacts to and helps shape the health care market in which it operates. For example, the regulatory environment establishes parameters for benefit design, premium pricing, and marketing practices. The employment market determines eligibility for health benefits, level of employer contributions, and design and pricing of indemnity benefits. Demographic and geographic factors, such as the size of Medicare and Medicaid populations, the location of local industry, and commuting patterns, affect product development and the boundaries of HMO service areas.

The use of a two- or three-tier contracting structure by an HMO is dependent upon existing alternatives to individual physician contracting, such as the presence of multispecialty group practices or hospital-sponsored IPAs, and the prior experience of local providers in working with other HMOs or managed care programs. Negotiation of reimbursement rates, capitation payments, and risk-sharing arrangements are dependent upon (1) hospital and physician supply, (2) the presence of competing HMOs and the design of their payment and risk arrangements, and (3) utilization and cost trends within the local market. In return, as an HMO becomes established, it will have an impact on the design and pricing of health benefits and health services in the local market, as well as on the structure of hospital and physician relationships (including the emergence of new IPAs, group practices, and joint ventures).

HMO Structure

HMO structure, in part, reflects plan sponsorship, consumer orientation date of entry into the market, and short- and long-term financial goals. The adoption of nonprofit or for-profit status may reflect the history of the sponsoring entity, the availability of capital, and the marketability of the program to investors or joint venture partners. Management's perspective on provider behavior, plus the existence of other HMOs in the local market, help to determine the operating model (staff, group, network, IPA, or hybrid), the approach to contracting (direct contract versus three-tier arrangement), and the extent of any risk-sharing arrangements.

Except in markets with a large oversupply of physicians and hospitals, there generally is some give and take in contract negotiations between an HMO and the provider community. While quality of care is always a concern in these negotiations, actual discussions usually end up focusing on economic considerations. As noted by Gnessin,[13] there is an inherent conflict between the goals of any HMO's management and those of its participating physicians. Gnessin defines six goals for HMOs: (1) profit maximization; (2) capital appreciation; (3) enrollment growth; (4) shift of financial risk to third parties; (5) maximum utilization control with minimum malpractice exposure; and (6) control over all components of HMO operations, including the actual health care delivery system. For physicians, Gnessin defines five goals: (1) maximum autonomy in the practice of medicine; (2) minimal loss of existing patient base or patient volume; (3) expansion of patient base and volume; (4) minimal financial risk; and (5) increased income from new revenue sources (other than the direct provision of health services).

It is the tension between these two perspectives that establishes the setting for the negotiation and implementation of financial incentives. According to Gnessin's "fairness doctrine," at any given time either HMO management or HMO providers may be in a superior bargaining position. However, when the dominant party imposes its will unilaterally on the other, this strategy usually proves successful only in the short term; in the long term the imbalance in power will result in acrimony and disintegration of the relationship. In other words, a plan that transfers risk to providers without reimbursing them adequately or providing them with data to manage their practices runs the risk of losing physician participation in the long run. Conversely, a plan that accedes completely to physician demands and pays them market rates without changing practice patterns may price itself out of the marketplace or require the plan sponsors to absorb large operating losses.

HMO Operations

An HMO cannot transfer risk fairly to providers and deliver quality care in a cost-effective manner without (1) effective management information systems for tracking enrollment, premiums, and utilization and for providing usable and timely reports to management and participating providers; (2) efficient claims processing procedures to ensure prompt payment to providers and the accurate capture of procedural and diagnostic data; (3) accurate actuarial and underwriting procedures for reliable projection of utilization and delivery costs by provider class (hospital, primary care provider, specialist, and other ancillary providers); (4) representation of professional staff and/or a medical director at the HMO's upper management level; and (5) adequate professional staffing to support a utilization management and quality assurance program.

In Figures B-1 and B-2, we described two- and three-tier physician contracting arrangements, as first defined by ICF. There is considerable variation within these two- and three-tier arrangements, however, depending upon how much control any HMO wishes to retain for itself or to delegate to contracting providers. Broadly speaking, there are three issues that influence the HMO's decision-making process: (1) how physician groups and IPAs are organized in the local market in terms of the cost-effectiveness of their delivery networks, the design of their data systems, and their management capabilities; (2) how institutional and professional providers are reimbursed and whether the HMO wishes to retain control over the claims payment process; and (3) whether the HMOs believe that the physicians can discipline themselves effectively through the utilization review and peer review process.

As shown in Table B-1, which describes operational responsibilities, there are two control models for two-tier organizations and three control models for three-tier organizations. Responsibilities for utilization management and financial operations may rest almost entirely with the HMOs (Model 1), may be shared between the HMOs and providers (Model 2), or may be assumed largely by providers (Model 3). In two-tier arrangements, in which the physicians either are not independent contractors (for example, staff model, group-owned, or affiliated HMOs) or are fee-for-service providers contracting directly with the HMO, an arrangement like that in Model 3 is not feasible. Moreover, any sharing of services with providers is more limited in two-tier plans than it is in three-tier plans. Typically, sharing of services involves those utilization management and claims payment activities that revolve around the gatekeeper role of contracting primary care physicians (for example, preadmission authorizations and specialty referrals). In pod-type situations in which primary care physicians are capitated, the physicians may review claims from specialty providers before authorizing them for payment. In rare cases, when providers are individually capitated and have direct control over their own specialty funds, they may actually pay for specialty claims.

In three-tier organizations, HMOs are usually not responsible for physician selection and peer review, as these responsibilities rest with contracting IPAs or groups. In Model 1, the IPA or group may share limited utilization review functions with the HMO. For example, an IPA may receive utilization and financial reports from the HMO's claims system; the IPA, in turn, uses these reports as the basis for remedial action against errant providers. In Model 1, all physician payments and all risk incentives are calculated by the HMO.

In Model 2, the HMO creates a medical (physician) fund, which is then handled by the IPA or groups; this fund may represent a capitated payment or a budget allocation based upon anticipated fee-for-service charges. The IPA or group then processes and pays claims for services rendered by its member physicians, while the HMO continues to pay for hospital services and emergency and out-of-area claims. The IPA or group provides feedback on utilization patterns to contracting providers and provides encounter data

TABLE B-1 Operational Responsibilities in Two- and Three-Tier Organizational Structures by Control Model

| | Two-Tier Organizations (with Pods) | | | |
| | MODEL 1 | | MODEL 2 | |
	HMO	MD	HMO	MD
Marketing	X		X	
Enrollment/underwriting	X		X	
Utilization review	X		X	X
Claims payment	X		X	X
Encounter data				X
Data analysis	X		X	
Provider feedback	X		X	
Peer review	X		X	
Quality assurance	X		X	

| | Three-Tier Organizations | | | | | |
| | MODEL 1 | | MODEL 2 | | MODEL 3 | |
	HMO	IPA/Grp	HMO	IPA/Grp	HMO	IPA/Grp
Marketing	X		X		X	
Enrollment/underwriting	X		X		X	
Utilization review	X	X	X	X		X
Claims payment	X		X	X	X	X
Encounter data				X		X
Data analysis	X		X	X		X
Provider feedback	X		X	X		X
Peer review		X		X		X
Quality assurance	X	X	X	X	X	X

NOTE: MD indicates physician; Grp indicates group practice.

on medical services to the HMO itself. In Model 2, the HMO may also be responsible for utilization review for services covered by the medical fund (for example, specialty referrals and diagnostic testing). In Model 3, the HMO largely assumes the role of a broker; it markets benefits to employers, enrolls members, and pays claims for noncapitated services. Otherwise, the IPA or group is given complete responsibility for all utilization review and data analysis.

In the case studies, we have provided examples of one two-tier, Model 1 plan (Case 5), three three-tier, Model 1 plans (Case Studies 1, 3 and 4), and one three-tier, Model 3 plan (Case Study 2).

APPROACHES TO UTILIZATION MANAGEMENT AND QUALITY ASSURANCE

As previously noted, responsibility for specific aspects of an HMO's operations vary by control model. Understanding where the locus of control rests is particularly important when evaluating those cost-containment approaches that affect patient care decisions. For this analysis, we have divided utilization management into its underwriting benefits, delivery of health services, and quality assurance components.

Underwriting Benefits

Almost always, benefit design and development of underwriting guidelines remain the responsibility of HMO management, not providers. (An exception occurs when providers require the use of copayments for office-based care to control unnecessary demand for services.) These functions can be described as follows.

Enrollment criteria are underwriting guidelines by industry or service class and by group size. Premium pricing and marketing practices also affect enrollment patterns and are included in this subcategory.

There has been a growing body of literature on enrollment patterns in HMOs to study the issue of selection bias. These analyses have been prompted, in part, by employer concerns that HMOs have attracted a disproportionate share of young and presumably healthy employees. In an analysis of 21 studies on self-selection, Wilensky and Rossiter concluded that most of the recent studies have shown HMOs to be enrolling a lower risk population. However, only rarely have any studies examined the impact of enrollee continuity on utilization rates.[15]

Benefit design relates to (1) the extent of coverage for specific services, drugs, and supplies; (2) any required copayments, coinsurance and/or deductibles; (3) level of services offered (for example, for mental health, the availability of individual or group therapy); (4) number of visits per condition; (5) out-of-pocket maximums; and (6) lifetime dollar benefits. Federally qualified HMOs have historically offered a more comprehensive set of benefits than have nonqualified prepaid plans or exclusive provider arrangements that are indemnity-based. With the recent growth of nonqualified plans and the move away from community rating and defined benefit packages to experience rating and negotiated benefits, there has been increased emphasis on benefit design as a cost-containment mechanism within HMOs.

Delivery of Health Services

The delivery component of utilization management involves seven subcategories, as follows.

Utilization review is usually administered under the auspices of a medical director and includes one or more of the following services; (1) preadmission review; (2) concurrent hospital review; (3) second surgical opinions; (4) specialty and/or out-of-network referral authorizations; (5) high-cost case management; (6) retrospective review of services; (7) bill audit; and (8) remedial action for providers suspected of fraud or noncompliance with utilization review or referral procedures.

Clinical protocols or guidelines are used for medical decision-making. Formal protocols exist in writing and define the exact procedures to be followed for specific clinical conditions. There are also informal guidelines that represent a consensus of the participating providers about delivery of care. Protocols and guidelines may define, for example, when it is clinically appropriate for a patient with a specific condition to undergo a surgical or diagnostic procedure; they may also define the types of services to be rendered to a patient with a given medical condition and the appropriate setting where these services should be provided. The development of formularies to control the dispensing of pharmaceuticals also falls into this category.

Patient flow procedures are used to control the scheduling and timing of patient services across the entire HMO physician network. Included in this category are the assignment of patients to "gatekeepers" for primary care services, guidelines for scheduling of visits by patient class (for example, acute-care patients, physical examinations, and follow-up visits), time allocated per appointment, access to specialists and tertiary providers, maintenance of telephone lines, office hours, and facility location. Development of staffing ratios for professional and administrative personnel represents another form of control over patient flow.

Physician selection involves an assessment of a physician's technical capabilities and practice style. In medical groups and staff model HMOs, the selection process begins at the initial time of hire and continues through a probationary period. In IPAs, the process is more limited and often focuses on establishing criteria for physician participation, such as a medical license in good standing, adequate malpractice coverage, local medical staff affiliation, and board certification or eligibility. For some community-based IPA HMOs, participation is on an "every willing provider" basis, with the intent of providing as widespread a geographic distribution of physicians as possible.

Data analysis involves a review of financial and utilization trends by practice site, by primary care or specialty service, by member class (for example, Medicare, Medicaid, commercial group, and individual membership), and by employer group. Data analysis also involves a review of individual provider performance by various utilization and clinical measures; feedback of this information to participating providers allows them to judge their performance relative to the performance of their peers. In two-tier arrangements, the data analysis is typically performed by the HMO. In three-tier, Model 3 IPA or group model HMOs in which providers are capitated for some or all of their services, the data analysis is usually conducted by the IPA or the group. In this situation, many HMOs receive only limited encounter information back from providers; as a result, the HMOs may actually lack the data to evaluate how providers are performing financially under their capitated contracts.

Peer review, which can be classified as both a utilization management and quality assurance tool, occurs on both a formal and an informal level. On a formal level, peer review may involve provider feedback, performance evaluations, and disciplinary action. In many plans, the thrust of this activity is on detecting outlier behavior (that is, poor-quality services, excessive ordering of services, referral to nonnetwork providers, etc.). For all two-tier HMOs, the monitoring process is the responsibility of the medical director and/or the peer review committee at the HMO. Here the onus is on plan management to prove that a physician is not performing according to preestablished standards. Typically physicians participating in three-tier IPA or group model HMOs are not subject to formal performance evaluations by HMO management, as this responsibility is handed to the contracting physician entity.

There also is the informal aspect of peer review that occurs during rounds, surgery, case conferences, and consultations. Physicians practicing in group or staff settings are subject to informal peer review on a daily basis. They can observe their fellow physicians both in office and hospital settings, whereas in most IPAs the informal peer review process is limited to the hospital setting.

Physician financial incentives include both the basic method of provider payment (salary, fee-for-service, or capitation) and the use of bonuses, withholds, and sharing of surpluses and deficits with the plan.

The delivery components of utilization management vary markedly by practice setting. In Table B-1, we presented various control models based upon the design of the contractual arrangement between HMOs and physician providers (two- and three-tier arrangements). Here, the emphasis is on the locus of control rather than the underlying organization of the physicians contracting with the HMO. In Table B-2, we look at one type of HMO (three-tier, Model 3), in which the HMO has capitated the physician entity (IPA or group) and has delegated control over the delivery components of utilization management.

TABLE B-2 Provider-Based Utilization Management Activities

Activities	Utilization Management Approach (Three-Tier, Model 3 HMO)		
	Community-Based IPA (FFS/Capitated)	Multispecialty Group (FFS/Capitated)	Multispeciality Group (Capitated)
Formal utilization review			
Preadmission review[a]	***	*/**	*/***
Concurrent review[a]	**/***	*/**	*/***
Second surgical opinion[a]	*/***		
Referral authorization[a,b]	*/***	*	*
Case management[a]	*/***	*/**	*/***
Bill audit	*/**	*	*
Remedial/fraud	***		
Remedial/penalties	*		
Clinical protocols[c]	In UR	Yes	Yes
Formularies		*/***	*/***
Patient flow			
Primary care physician	*/**	*/**	*/***
Staff size	*/**	***	***
Scheduling visits		**/***	**/***
Length of appointment		***	***
Specialty referrals		**/***	**/***
Diagnostic services		**/***	**/***
Physician selection	*/**	***	***
Data analysis	*/***	**/***	***
Provider feedback	*/***	**/***	**/***
Peer review			
Formal procedures	*	***	***
Financial incentives	Yes	Yes	Yes

NOTE: *, Occasionally used as a utilization management technique; **, Frequently used as a utilization management technique; ***, Regularly used as a utilization management technique. FFS indicates fee-for-service; UR indicates utilization review.

[a]Includes preestablished utilization guidelines by procedure or diagnosis.
[b]Includes diagnostic procedures and out-of-network services.
[c]Includes both protocols and informal clinical guidelines.

In Table B-2, there are three general types of contracting entities: (1) a community-based IPA whose member physicians continue to practice primarily in a fee-for-service setting and who are reimbursed by the IPA on a discounted fee-for-service basis subject to a withhold; (2) a multispecialty group practice with fee-for-service that has both patients and multiple managed care (HMO, exclusive provider, and/or preferred provider) contracts; and (3) a multispecialty group that contracts exclusively with one HMO and that receives almost all of its income from prepaid services. As shown in Table B-2, the IPA relies heavily on formal utilization review procedures to modify continuing fee-for-service incentives. That is, because participating physicians continue to be reimbursed on the basis of the number and level of services provided, the IPA focuses its efforts on controlling unnecessary utilization and on monitoring billing practices by participating physicians. In this environment, the decision-making process for high-cost care is transferred in part from the individual physician to the utilization review team (that is, for decisions involving certain types of diagnostic testing, inpatient admissions, referrals to noncontracting facilities, and rehabilitative services).

Depending upon group size, the other two physician entities in Table B-2 may or may not have formal utilization review programs. The larger the multispecialty group, the more the need for a formal utilization review program to standardize procedures across sites. As described in the literature, the utilization review program used by Kaiser Permanente physicians in southern California includes preadmission and concurrent review; discharge planning; home health; patient education services; and retrospective review of admissions, length of stay, and level of care.[16] Some groups also have case management programs to coordinate care for certain categories of high-cost patients. Some may require authorizations for referrals outside the multispecialty group, and bill audit, when it occurs, is usually for outside services. Unlike IPAs, multispecialty groups are generally not concerned with remedial action for fraud or nonadherence to utilization review protocols, since poorly performing physicians will not be retained in the practice.

In IPAs, clinical protocols are built into the utilization review algorithms, with primary emphasis placed on the control of inpatient and high-cost specialty and diagnostic services. Usually, there is little attempt to influence routine decision-making in the ambulatory setting other than through the referral process and benefit design. In multispecialty group practices, physicians may be encouraged to adopt a specific practice "style." While the group may have developed formal clinical protocols for specific conditions or procedures, typically, the process involves little more than senior physicians serving as mentors for newly hired staff.

In terms of controlling patient flow, IPAs do not generally determine the scheduling practices of their participating physicians, other than requiring plan subscribers to sign up with a primary care gatekeeper. Whereas IPAs rely on formal utilization review programs primarily to control costs, group practices may control utilization through the patient flow process. As shown in Table B-2, multispecialty groups rely on scheduling of appointments, the length of the appointment, and access to specialty providers as utilization management controls.

Typically, IPAs place less emphasis on staff size and physician selection than do multispecialty groups. In fact, many IPA HMOs purposely seek to develop a large physician base to gain market acceptance. As a result, HMO patient volume varies significantly among participating providers. Multispecialty groups, on the other hand, determine staff size for primary care and specialty services on the basis of preestablished patient-physician or enrollee-physician ratios. Recruitment of additional staff generally occurs only when there is sufficient patient or membership volume to provide a patient base for new physicians.

In terms of data analysis, theoretically, all IPAs and groups develop utilization statistics. As will be discussed subsequently, the accuracy and timeliness of this information and the frequency with which it is supplied to management and to participating physicians differ markedly across individual IPAs and groups. One generalization, however, is that groups operating in the fee-for-service sector tend to have more detailed financial and utilization data, with procedure codes, than do prepaid group practices that do not routinely prepare patient bills.

Finally, while the peer review process exists in all three settings described in Table B-2, the thrust of the activity varies in the IPA versus the group settings. In the former, the emphasis is on detecting outliers, whereas in the latter there is additional emphasis placed on how well a given physician adopts a groups practice style and works cooperatively with his or her peers, as will be discussed subsequently.

Quality Assurance

Quality assessment is an evaluation of quality of care through structure, process, and outcome measures, as originally defined by Donabedian.[17] Quality assurance is quality assessment plus correction of identified deficiencies. Mosser[18] has defined quality assurance on three levels. On the first level, and in its broadest sense, quality assurance includes such diverse activities as credentialing of providers, evaluating physician performance, disciplining poor performers, continuing education, tracking malpractice claims, collecting grievance information, conducting member satisfaction surveys, performing facilities review, and establishing laboratory quality control. On the second level, quality assurance is defined as the process of measurement, problem correction, and reevaluation. On the third and narrowest level, it consists of focused problem correction in groups, performance feedback to individuals, and direct surveillance and corrective action.

State HMO licensure requires documentation of a utilization review and quality assurance program, as does eligibility for a Medicare risk contract and participation in prepaid Medicaid programs. The actual implementation of these programs varies widely, with many plans tending to focus on utilization review activities and to pay only very limited attention to quality assurance protocols.

OPERATIONAL PROBLEMS IMPAIRING UTILIZATION MANAGEMENT AND QUALITY ASSURANCE PROGRAMS

Utilization Management Programs

Many HMOs have discovered that their utilization management programs in concert with risk incentives have had only limited success in modifying physician practice patterns. The situation is particularly difficult when providers are reimbursed on a fee-for-service basis, either directly by the HMO or through the IPA or group (which itself may be capitated). Additionally, there are specific operational problems that have plagued the HMO industry and that affect implementation of utilization management programs. These problems can be broken down into four broad categories.

1. *Inadequate management information systems and claims processing procedures.* The first generation of commercially available HMO software typically handled an enrollment size of no more than 40,000-50,000 members and a limited number of HMO benefit packages. Software suitable for IPAs contracting with physicians on a fee-for-service basis (using discounts and/or withholds) often was inappropriate for group and staff model HMOs that used capitated arrangements, and vice versa. Moreover, most of the early software had limited flexibility in terms of report generation, particularly for any analysis of practice patterns on a provider-specific basis.

Since the early 1980s, a number of plans have seen their membership pass the 50,000-member threshold and have experienced significant claims processing delays because of system overload and software design. Some HMOs find that their software cannot accommodate the proliferation of new benefit packages, including high- and low-option plans, the development of vision, mental health, dental and drug riders, and so-called indemnity wraparounds or self-referral options. Existing software also may not handle various hospital and physician risk-sharing arrangements. At one carrier-sponsored HMO, for example, the claims processors had to manually calculate all hospital claims involving per diem payments; another had to send all hospital claims to an affiliated payer to be assigned diagnosis-related groups before calculating any payments. In some cases physician withholds have had to be calculated manually, while other HMOs cannot handle volume discounts.

As a result of inadequate or outmoded management information systems (MIS), many HMOs have suffered such problems as buildup in unprocessed claims or encounter forms; inability to implement various forms of reimbursement such as multiple per diems for hospitals and variable risk withholds for physicians; and failure to provide physician-specific utilization data on capitated and noncapitated services, on authorized and nonauthorized admissions and referrals, and on billing practices.

Currently, a number of HMOs across the country are in the process of defining business requirements for new MIS, while others are installing or have just installed new systems. To the extent that these systems can handle a multiplicity of benefit and reimbursement arrangements, some of the problems described in this section will eventually be resolved.

2. *Lack of data integrity.* Until recently, the focus of claims processing operations was on the turnaround time for paying providers rather than on any statistical review of utilization patterns. In many instances, the data were grouped so arbitrarily as to eliminate the possibility of extracting useful information for actuarial or statistical studies. For example, at one HMO (see Case Study 3), all claims had to be classified into three categories: inpatient, outpatient, and other. Information on service location was missing (for example, emergency room, physician's office, and nursing home). Moreover, when a primary care physician provided services on both a capitated and self-referral basis during the same visit, the services had to be recorded as two separate encounters; a third encounter could result from the same visit if there were any charges for medical supplies. Because the standard reports from the claims system showed such visits as multiple encounters, any analysis of individual physician practice patterns was unreliable. In fact, in Case Study 3, actuarial projections could not be derived from the claims system; rather, they had to come from the data base of an outside consultant. (This consultant provided estimates based upon avarage costs and utilization rates across a series of clients.)

Some of the data integrity issues will be obviated with the purchase of new HMO software; others are a function of data collection and processing procedures that are independent of software design. To the extent that HMOs do not audit the performance of claims processors to ensure accuracy and consistency in data entry, data integrity problems may continue to go unrecognized in a number of plans.

A related issue concerns the noncomparability of data across HMOs for standard utilization measures, such as physician encounters per 1,000 members and hospital admissions or days per 1,000 members.

Some group and staff HMOs do not routinely record certain types of services, such as physician hospital visits, while others do not receive or record encounter information for capitated primary care services. Other plans, as previously noted, may have inflated or deflated visit counts or may arbitrarily collapse service location codes because of the design of their data systems. Also, data on out-of-plan use is often incomplete.[19] Thus, any comparison of utilization trends across plans requires a knowledge of their data classification procedures.[20]

3. *Lack of an integral role for the medical director at upper level HMO management.*   Many HMO medical directors are frustrated by their lack of input into HMO operations and their inability to obtain adequate budgets for professional support staff with appropriate statistical, utilization review, and quality assurance experience. In some cases, medical directors cannot reduce or deny payment to providers who are suspected of unusual billing practices or provision of unauthorized services. Depending on the plan, this authority may rest with the chief financial officer, the controller, or the director of provider relations. In HMOs with outmoded MIS, medical directors have expressed concern about their inability to obtain detailed utilization reports because of the priority attached by plan management to producing financial reports. As a result, medical directors may be unable to document poor practice patterns, even though they are aware of their existence; as a result, the entire peer review process suffers.

4. *Lack of provider feedback.*   Provider relations suffer when there is a shortfall between the actual claims experience for an IPA and the projected experience used to calculate the IPA's capitation rate.   This problem worsens when the withholding rate proves insufficient to cover the deficit.   In control models in which the HMO processes all claims, IPA management cannot anticipate any shortfall and initiate corrective action unless timely utilization data are provided by the HMO. In Case Study 1, local physicians threatened to withdraw from the IPA unless the capitation rate was increased; without appropriate utilization data, the physicians refused to acknowledge that there had been any unnecessary provision of services or unusual billing practices.

The first three problems listed above are not unique to the HMO industry; indemnity carriers and Blue Cross and Blue Shield plans face the same concerns.   Increasingly, the fourth problem—lack of provider feedback—is an issue for carriers and Blue Cross and Blue Shield plans, now that traditional fee-for-service coverage is giving way to preferred provider and closed panel arrangements. However, it is the potential for underservice in HMOs that has led to congressional concern about quality assurance in HMOs.   However, as discussed in the case studies, many HMOs have failed to thrive precisely because the fee-for-service mentality continues to flourish in the prepaid sector.

Quality Assurance

In our experience, HMO management generally gives the highest priority to day-to-day marketing, underwriting, and financial operations and the lowest priority to programs, such as quality assurance, for which an immediate impact on plan performance is not evident. Additionally, given the understaffing and limited MIS capabilities in many HMOs, implementation of formal quality assurance programs may become problematic. For example, in certain plans, performance feedback to physicians is uneven because of inadequate data systems, poor data entry procedures, claims processing lags, and/or failure to classify claims data in a format useful to participating providers. Conversely, there may be little incentive for capitated IPAs, groups, and individual providers to supply timely or complete encounter data back to the HMOs, since their payment is generally based on the number of covered enrollees, not on the actual services rendered. As a result, the HMOs may be unable to determine actual utilization rates or to detect underservice.

Many HMOs have a two-stage approach to quality assurance. Initially, when signing up physicians (as individuals or through IPAs or groups), they use eligibility criteria to ensure the adequacy of the provider network. Thereafter, quality assurance generally consists of problem identification. The process may be fairly extensive, such as using target medical conditions or types of cases, such as hospital readmissions, as the basis for a periodic review of medical records. HMOs that conduct their own utilization review programs may also obtain feedback on provider performance from their staff. Alternatively, some plans may limit their quality assurance programs to tracking malpractice claims, grievance filings, and disenrollment rates by medical group or by primary care provider if they use individual gatekeepers.

In three-tier model plans, the HMO may require that participating groups or IPAs assume full responsibility for peer review. Network or group model HMOs typically require evidence of a functioning peer review program before they award a contract to a multispecialty practice. HMOs contracting with IPAs may require that a formal peer review system be in place, but since many IPAs lack a track record for judging physician performance, the adequacy of these programs cannot be assured.

Thus, operational reviews frequently disclose that there is a wide gap between quality assurance programs, as they are described in documents supplied to federal and state regulators, and as they actually exist within licensed health plans. Historically, structural measures have been notoriously poor indicators of both HMO performance and quality of care. For example, in California during the mid-1970s, licensing of prepaid health plans, with requisite filing of appropriate quality assurance protocols and provider contracts, did not prevent abuses in the state's prepaid Medicaid program. More recently, in the International Medical Centers, Inc. situation in Florida, structural measures failed to guarantee Medicare beneficiaries adequate access to medical services. The problem with structural measures was highlighted in a recent survey of HMOs in Ohio, as conducted by the Joint Commission on Accreditation of Health Care Organizations (JCAHO). In a review of six HMOs with Medicaid contracts, JCAHO surveyors found that none of the plans had fully implemented its quality assurance program.[21]

Because of the limited scope of existing quality assurance programs, federal legislation now mandates review of inpatient and outpatient services provided by HMOs with Medicare risk contracts. External peer review organizations have begun using medical records and target medical conditions as indicators of the appropriateness of treatment, accessibility to services, and timeliness of care provided. The possibility of sanctions resulting from these reviews is now providing the impetus for HMOs to improve their quality assurance programs. For example, of the 15 HMOs in California, Hawaii, and Arizona with Medicare risk contracts, only 3 had fully implemented their quality assurance programs at the time of their initial evaluation by California Medical Review Inc.[22] Some HMOs have also begun to seek voluntary accreditation from external review organizations, such as JCAHO. However, because of the limited disclosure associated with mandatory and voluntary reviews, subscribers signing up with HMOs still have limited information available for evaluating quality of care within a given program.

DESIGN AND USE OF PHYSICIAN INCENTIVES

In the preceding section, we looked at the operational problems impairing the administration of utilization management and quality assurance programs. As noted, structural and process measures are often an inadequate measure of plan performance. A similar situation exists for any evaluation of risk incentives. In this section we briefly describe the background on current concerns about risk incentives, the types of risk incentives that have been identified, and the factors that modify their impact on provider performance.

Background

In a report issued in July 1986, the General Accounting Office (GAO) identified three types of physician incentive plans with a potential risk of abuse for Medicare beneficiaries: (1) the Paracelsus or hospital model, in which a monthly bonus was paid to staff physicians on the basis of a favorable ratio of total hospital charges for Medicare patients to Medicare payments for those patients; (2) the Medical Staff-Hospital Joint Venture or the MeSH model, a theoretical model in which an annual bonus was to be paid to those physicians with a positive cost performance using targeted costs per discharge; and (3) the individual practice association model in which incentives, including primary care capitation arrangements, cover inpatient and outpatient services on an annual basis. The GAO report concluded by recommending that any incentive payment programs should average costs versus payments over a fairly large patient base to reduce incentives to undertreat individual patients; the GAO also recommended that the time period for calculating these incentives should be relatively long (1 year).

The Omnibus Budget Reconciliation Act of 1986 specifically prohibited hospitals, as well as HMOs with Medicare risk contracts, from using financial incentives to reduce or limit services provided to Medicare beneficiaries. Because of the widespread use of physician incentive payments by HMOs and CMPs, however, Congress delayed application of this provision to prepaid plans until April 1, 1989, pending further research. Subsequently, the Omnibus Budget Reconciliation Act of 1987 extended the delay to April 1, 1990, and new proposals in Congress make implementation unlikely.

To date, much of the published research on physician incentives has focused on documenting the range of arrangements that exist and the frequency with which they are used by plan model, plan age, plan size, and geographic location. With the exception of recent work by Mathematica Policy Research, Inc.[24] there has been little research on the effectiveness of quality assurance programs or the impact of financial incentives on utilization of services in HMOs.

Current Surveys Concerning Physician Incentives

Since the GAO report, there have been four additional studies on financial risk arrangements in HMOs: (1) the Group Health Association of America (GHAA) Survey mailed to GHAA member organizations in December 1986;[25] (2) a Blue Cross and Blue Shield Association Survey, using the GHAA survey instrument, was mailed in March 1987 to BC/BS plans that sponsored HMOs;[26] (3) a March 1987 survey mailed by Alan Hillman, to all 595 HMOs known to be in operation as of June 1986;[27] and (4) a survey of 215 federally qualified HMOs or CMPs, in combination with a review of documentation in the Office of Prepaid Health Care of the Health Care Financing Administration, was conducted by ICF, Inc. under contract with the U.S. Department of Health and Human Services.[28] The GAO has also conducted an additional study of physician incentives in response to a request by the Ways and Means Committee of the U.S. House of Representatives.

An analysis of the first three surveys revealed that consistent definitions were not used across the studies, leading to variations in findings as to the frequency with which these incentives have been used by various types of HMOs (that is, staff, group, network, IPA, and mixed or hybrid model plans.) In general, financial incentives were broken into four broad categories, as follows: (1) the basic approach to physician payment (that is, salary, capitation, and fee-for-service); (2) sharing of plan surpluses and/or deficits; (3) use of bonuses and/or withholds; and (4) distribution of funds by individual, group or combined individual-group performance.

While the three studies reported varying use of payment mechanisms and risk incentives by plan type, the single most important difference between the three related to the prevalence of financial incentives based on individual performance factors. The GHAA study found that 140 of 164 responding plans (85.4 percent) had some form of financial incentive for primary care physicians. Sixty percent of the plans reporting on the design of these incentives used some type of individual incentive; 11.2 percent reported exclusive use of individual incentives. The Hillman survey reported that two-thirds of all contractual arrangements (232 of 353) withheld a portion of payments to primary care physicians, but only 18 percent (38 of 211) of the HMOs held physicians at risk on an individual basis for deficits beyond the withhold. Although the ICF study did not separate reporting of withholds from other financial incentives, this study reported that 0.5 percent of responding HMOs relied solely on individual performance for the distribution of deficits and surplus funds. In a recent reconciliation of their findings, ICF and GHAA have concluded that in their common sample of 54 plans, individual physician incentives (including individual cost- or utilization-based withholds) were used in 20 percent of plans.[29]

Administering Physician Incentives

Often, there is a discrepancy between risk incentives as defined in physician contracts and as administered by either the HMO, the IPA, or the group. The failure to implement risk incentives, according to contract terms, may reflect a conscious policy decision by management and/or operational difficulties. For example, one large network model HMO has reported that each month it withholds 10 percent from "an actuarially generous" capitation payment to participating multispecialty groups. The groups, however, record this withhold amount on their accounts receivable and anticipate the return of the funds. In the event of a deficit in any of the group's accounts because of unanticipated referral or ancillary service costs, the HMO would still return the withhold to maintain a good working relationship with the group.

The converse of this situation occurs when physicians automatically assume that the withhold will not be returned. The ICF study reported on one IPA HMO in which the withhold amount was seldom returned; the medical director stated that the withhold was not perceived as a financial incentive by the physicians but as a discount or as a business cost comparable to denied or suspended claims in the fee-for-service environment. We also found in several of our reviews that physicians respond to loss of the withholds by changing their billing patterns. For example, physicians may attempt to compensate for the withhold loss by inflating the CPT codes for consultations and office and hospital visits and by unbundling routine services, such as charging for component parts of blood chemistry panels.

In our experience, certain HMOs cannot readily detect inappropriate billing practices by individual physicians because of inadequate claims processing systems. In other cases, HMOs may control upcoding and unbundling by specifying acceptable CPT codes for specific types of visits and/or procedures. Alternatively, HMO management may choose to ignore these billing practices, particularly when taking action may antagonize providers and lead to loss of their participation.

Sometimes risk incentives are short-circuited when an HMO cannot fulfill the terms of its contracts because of operational difficulties. For example, if an HMO has a claims processing backlog and cannot provide requested utilization reports according to a predefined schedule, the HMO may have to return all or part of the withholds, despite the existence of deficits in the physician accounts. For example, one carrier-sponsored HMO, described in Case Study 3, recently made a conscious decision to distribute 75 percent of all physician withholds despite deficits in existing risk pools and despite the knowledge that some primary care providers were self-referring excessively for specialty services not included in their own capitation rates. This management decision was based, in part, upon the fact that the HMO was unable to produce its utilization reports according to schedule and, in part, to placate participating physicians.

Finally, there are cases in which physicians may actually be unaware of any financial incentives related to effective utilization management. For example, in the situation described in Case Study 2, the salaried physicians were not informed during recruitment of a possible bonus based on plan performance. In this plan, utilization management was more a function of scheduling rather than of any financial incentives.

Thus, the issues to be addressed when reviewing the financial incentives within HMOs include the degree to which they have been fully implemented and the degree to which participating providers are fully aware of them. The Hillman, GHAA, and ICF survey instruments have focused on the design of contractual arrangements, but further research is needed to assess the ability of HMOs and CMPs to support these arrangements.

POLICY AND RESEARCH ISSUES

There is a whole body of literature involving analysis of utilization rates in HMO and fee-for-service settings. Another set of studies looks at utilization rates in different HMO settings (for example, comparisons of the performance of totally versus partly prepaid group practices and of IPAs versus totally or partly prepaid group practices).[30] There also has been a growing interest in utilization rates and outcomes for specific medical conditions in the two settings.[31]

To date, health services researchers have assumed that differing financial incentives are responsible for the lower utilization rates in prepaid versus fee-for-service settings and have focused little attention on how HMOs achieve these reductions.[32] The literature on the delivery component of utilization management in HMOs consists largely of anecdotal reports detailing controls in place at specific plans and case studies involving one or more components of a utilization management program at a single HMO, IPA, or multispecialty group practice. For example, a recent report in the *New England Journal of Medicine* described one physician's negative experience working in a for-profit, staff model HMO.[33] Other studies have reported on the use of referrals or the impact of provider feedback on ordering of diagnostic tests in specific plans.[34]

Our operational reviews suggest that the structure of utilization management and quality assurance programs and their actual implementation vary widely across plans. On-site evaluations of these programs are currently being conducted by mandatory and voluntary review organizations. Until the findings of these review organizations are made public, it will be difficult to generalize about which types of HMOs and which control models have implemented utilization management/quality assurance programs the most successfully. Moreover, if the findings from the reviews do not address where the responsibility for utilization management rests, it may be difficult to develop a policy response that can be used to ensure quality of care in HMOs.

It also should be stressed that a large number of HMOs are not subject to federally mandated review, as they do not participate in the Medicare risk program. As already noted, state licensing has tended to focus on structural measures, with on-site reviews across plans occurring infrequently or restricted to problem plans. Additionally, none of the voluntary or mandatory reviews is specifically designed to evaluate the impact of various types of risk incentives on provider performance.

The Hillman, GHAA, and ICF surveys described above looked at risk incentives from a structural perspective. Each of the three studies used the HMO as the unit of observation. The survey information on physician practices that is currently available from the American Medical Association, from state medical societies, and from the Medical Economics Company Inc. (Oradell, New Jersey) does not have sufficient detail to evaluate the financial impact of risk incentives by HMO plan type or control model. Thus, to better understand how financial incentives affect practice patterns, there may be a need to modify existing survey instruments or to undertake a separate study that focuses on primary care physicians with and without HMO affiliations. For HMO physicians, the future studies should evaluate (1) HMO model type, control model, geographic location, and enrollment; (2) the gross income of the primary care physician and overall patient volume, as compared with HMO patient income and volume; (3) the structure of HMO risk incentives and their financial impact on the responding physicians; and (4) the design and implementation of utilization management and quality assurance programs, as perceived by the responding physician.

The results of this survey can then be correlated with findings from outcome studies, consumer satisfaction surveys, and on-site reviews, as conducted by various regulatory agencies, peer review organizations, consumer or employer coalitions, and university-based research teams. Only then will it be possible to ascertain definitively which types of HMO financial incentives are the most problematic in terms of their impact upon quality of care. Until then, it is probably premature to develop legislation that eliminates the use of any particular form of financial incentives in the HMO setting.

CASE STUDIES
INTRODUCTION

The following case studies are not based on a representative sample of HMOs. We present them solely with the intent of showing the range of problems that may be encountered by HMOs when implementing utilization management programs. The background material at the beginning of each case study has been altered to maintain client confidentiality. All plans are defined as staff, group, or IPA, according to their operational characteristics, rather than their federal or InterStudy designation. The network category has intentionally been eliminated, as have any descriptors indicating location of the plan, plan age, nonprofit, or for-profit status. Size is defined by three categories: under 25,000, 25,000-49,999, and 50,000 and over. Also, any descriptors that might allow for identification of the plan, such as university affiliation, hospital ownership, Medicare risk status, or unique organizational characteristics, have been removed. However, the descriptions of the control type, the financial incentives, the design of the MIS, the role of the medical director, and the structure of the utilization management program are reported precisely as they were found in each of the plans.

CASE STUDY 1:
HOSPITAL-SPONSORED IPA

Background

In the mid-1980s, management of a hospital with 350+ beds decided to establish an IPA model HMO in order to contract with one of the major employers in the state; simultaneously, physician leadership at the hospital helped to set up an IPA, which was open to any active member of the hospital's medical staff. After the HMO became operational, membership climbed rapidly to the range of 25,000-49,999, with the growth exceeding original forecasts. However, the plan posted larger financial losses than anticipated because its operating and administrative procedures, along with its MIS, could not keep pace with the enrollment growth. The sponsoring hospital was forced to subsidize the health plan, both directly and indirectly, by underwriting the operating losses and by charging the plan a composite per diem that was actually below its own operating costs.

Eventually, the sponsoring hospital sought financial relief and asked the hospital system with which it was affiliated to take over the HMO. When the hospital system took over management of the HMO, it attempted to cut the financial losses through new reimbursement procedures and risk-sharing arrangements; as a result, there was a serious breakdown in provider relations.

Control Type

Three-tier, with the HMO controlling most services (Model 1).

Financial Incentives

Under the original risk model, physicians contracted with an IPA that was fully at risk for all inpatient and outpatient physician services, including outpatient mental health, ancillary, and in-area emergency services; durable medical equipment; prosthetic devices; and prescription drugs. The HMO allocated a flat monthly capitation rate per adult and per child member to the IPA; physicians submitted their claims directly to the HMO, with payment based on a predetermined fee schedule subject to a 20 percent percent withhold. The 20 percent withhold was used to fund an IPA reserve account, as well as to fund any deficits in a separate hospital fund.

The HMO also allocated a flat per-member, per-month amount to the hospital fund, which covered inpatient hospital and mental health services, same-day surgery, skilled nursing and home health care, and out-of-area emergency services. Providers rendering services covered by the hospital fund, including the sponsoring hospital, billed the HMO directly for their services according to prenegotiated rates. (There was no withhold for any services covered by the hospital fund.) Any deficits beyond the 20 percent physician withhold in either the IPA or hospital funds were the responsibility of the HMO, while any surplus in the hospital fund was to be allocated between the IPA reserve fund and the HMO on an 80-20 basis. The targeted utilization rate for all inpatient services was set at 350 days per 1,000 members; in 1985 and 1986, the actual hospital utilization, after adjusting for coordination of benefits, was approximately 300 days per 1,000 members.

While the IPA had historically operated at a loss because of overutilization in the outpatient setting, in 1985 and 1986, the plan was able to return the physician withhold because of the surplus in the hospital fund. Problems emerged, however, when the plan was taken over in 1987 and new management wanted to lower the targeted hospital utilization rate, to share surplus and deficits in the hospital withhold pool on a 50-50 basis, and to increase the per diem paid to the sponsoring hospital. The physicians recognized that they would no longer be able to anticipate a return of their withhold and asked the health plan to modify their capitation to reflect their actual utilization experience. The net result was a standoff between the doctors and the health plan.

Design of MIS System

The claims processing system was using "first-generation" software and was incapable of handling the volume of claims that were being received. As a result, there was an emphasis on rapid claims payment, without appropriate controls on data entry or claims review procedures.

There was no automatic linkage of the authorization files to the claims history files. Therefore, before any inpatient, emergency, durable medical equipment, or out-of-area claims were paid, they were sent to a nurse coordinator for approval. All other claims were entered directly into the claims system, and unless they were suspended for lack of a provider number or a duplicate payment, they were paid as billed according to the existing fee schedule. In other words, outpatient claims were paid without any automatic review of frequency of service, procedure coding, or consideration of whether the service was appropriate, given the diagnosis, age, or sex of the patient.

Utilization Management

Primary care physicians theoretically were to act as gatekeepers and to approve all specialty referrals and hospital admissions. In reality, patients continued to self-refer themselves to specialists. The primary care providers (PCPs) were not required to adhere to any protocols for authorizing the use of specialty or ancillary services, nor had any procedures been established for the management of high-cost patients.

PCPs were required to notify the HMO's medical director of pending hospital admissions for his approval. This procedure was generally well observed, because of the widespread recognition by IPA members of the financial impact of controlled hospital utilization on the IPA reserve fund. The surplus in the hospital fund, in effect, had allowed the IPA physicians to continue practicing on an "as usual" basis in the ambulatory setting.

With the HMO takeover, the physician leadership of the IPA was vehemently opposed to any changes in allocation of the hospital fund surplus and to the repricing of the hospital per diem. The IPA leadership believed firmly that participating physicians were delivering efficient care and did not want to use the withhold to cover IPA deficits. Meanwhile, HMO management believed that there was excessive utilization in the ambulatory setting. Neither side, however, had any documentation to support its argument, as the IPA did not collect claims data and the HMO had never produced any physician-specific data or developed any normative standards for evaluating physician performance in the outpatient setting.

Medical Director and Utilization Management Support Staff

The medical director reported that he had not been an integral member of top plan management but had been hired only part-time to oversee the nurse coordinators and to review pending hospital admissions. The utilization review staff did not have well-defined policies or procedures to guide them, particularly when adjudicating claims. As a result, claims payment was not consistent across reviewers (for example, the same services might be paid in some cases and denied in others).

Although the HMO had a written quality assurance plan, the nurses had little time to undertake chart audits or to review treatment plans for target conditions; instead, as much as 50 percent of their time was spent on clerical work associated with claims processing. While the nurse reviewers recognized that some IPA physicians regularly did not adhere to utilization review requirements, they did not have the authority to apply any penalties. Therefore, of approximately 100 physician infractions identified in 1987 involving the provision of medically unnecessary services or referrals to nonparticipating physicians, only two resulted in warning letters from the plan.

CASE STUDY 2:
GROUP-MODEL HMO

Background

In 1985, a multispecialty group practice, which contracts primarily with one group-model HMO, expanded its operations into two metropolitan areas where, historically, fee-for-service providers had been highly resistant to participation in any form of managed care (i.e., HMOs or preferred provider organizations [PPOs]). The move into the other communities was made at the request of several large public and private employers anxious to have an alternative to fee-for-service medicine. Membership at the new sites grew rapidly. At the end of 2 years, membership size far exceeded HMO projections, and the medical group found that they had outgrown their facilities at the two sites. Also, recruitment of additional professional and administrative staff was not feasible until the practice sites could be expanded (membership size cannot be specified, per client request).

To ensure appropriate levels of care at the expansion sites, group physicians began referring patients out on a fee-for-service basis into the community for primary, specialty, and ancillary services that ordinarily would have been provided in-house. Lacking contracts with most of the local specialists, the group was forced to pay for these referrals from its capitation fund on the basis of billed charges. Because of the lack of cost controls over these outside referrals, the group sustained operating losses at the expansion sites in 1986 and 1987.

Control Type

Three-tier, with delivery of services controlled by the medical group (Model 3).

Financial Incentives

With the exception of the medical director in each of the two sites and one practicing physician per site, the rest of the physicians at the expansion sites had no prior experience working for the group. The newly hired physicians had a 3-year probationary period before they became eligible for partnership benefits; in the interim they were paid a flat salary with no productivity incentives. Salary levels were based on specialty training, board certification, and prior practice experience. There also was a profit-sharing program in which partners were eligible to participate; theoretically, the new hires were eligible for a year-end bonus, but only if the group had a profitable year. However, knowing the operating losses sustained by the group, the medical directors generally did not include any mention of a bonus in salary discussions with new recruits.

Design of MIS System

The MIS in place at the original practice sites had been designed to support the group's own internal data needs. This system had not been built to track or adjudicate fee-for-service claims from outside providers, under the assumption that the amount of care provided in the fee-for-service sector would be very limited. (At its main site, outside physician bills were reviewed manually, with payment made according to prenegotiated rates and authorized services.) When the expansion sites were opened, the group purchased software to allow for tracking of referral and hospital authorizations and for collection of information on fee-for-service claims, using standard CPT codes. However, fee caps or fee schedules were not installed in the system, and clinical edits, which determine whether procedures had been appropriately billed given the patient's age, sex, or diagnosis, were not activated. Thus, as long as a preauthorization for a referral existed in the new MIS, claims from community-based physicians were paid, without questioning the need for billed services or the use of specific CPT codes.

Utilization Management

The primary factor controlling outpatient utilization at each of the practice sites was the scheduling process. Each salaried physician was scheduled for a set number of morning and afternoon patient sessions per week, with a predetermined number of time slots allotted for acute-care patients, continuing patients, and physical examinations. As membership soared, the primary care physicians were unable to schedule specialty care within the group or handle conditions requiring intensive, short-term follow-up care on a timely basis, given the overbooking that was already taking place. As a result, they began to refer out into the community cases that ordinarily could have been handled in-house.

When outside referrals were authorized, there was no dollar limitation placed on the services to be provided, nor was the level of care specified (that is, type of consultation or office visit, by CPT code). The only requirement was that certain laboratory and x-ray tests be performed at the groups facilities; additionally, any surgical procedures or hospital admissions required another preauthorization. Aggregate reports summarizing referral rates and costs, by group physician, were received monthly by the medical directors, as were summaries on the number of patients seen and billed charges from each outside provider. However, none of this information was provided to the group physicians or their support staffs. Thus, there was no consensus among the group physicians and the referral clerks as to which local providers were the most cost-efficient, in terms of future referrals.

Medical Director and Utilization Management Support Staff

Both of the medical directors devoted approximately 50 percent of their time to their clinical practices and appeared to have taken on the management role with some reluctance. Neither had worked with their medical staffs to develop referral protocols or had undertaken any educational efforts to make them aware of referral costs by specialty. Moreover, both medical directors were extremely fearful about undertaking any program that would antagonize local physicians; thus, they did not encourage any claims review that would result in fee cutbacks by eliminating billing abuses or by using a fee schedule. Rather, the intent of the medical directors was twofold: to initiate preferred provider contracting with the specialists identified as being the most cost efficient and to internalize the high-volume specialties as quickly as possible to control the dollar outflow. However, the plan's ability to recruit specialty staff was dependent, in part, on its ability to expand its existing facilities and/or develop new clinical sites.

CASE STUDY 3:
CARRIER-SPONSORED HMO

Background

In the mid-1980s, a carrier took over an existing IPA model HMO operation that had a number of start-up sites. The computer system that was in place was inadequate to handle the variations in benefit packages across sites, as well as the different payment mechanisms used to reimburse hospitals and physicians. Because of the losses sustained at most of the HMO sites and the costs associated with upgrading the HMO software and developing new products (that is, triple option or a point-of-service HMO), the carrier decided to evaluate the future of each HMO site. The following description relates to one of the sites with fewer than 25,000 enrollees.

Control Type

Three-tier, with control resting with the HMO (Model 1).

Financial Incentives

Participating primary care providers received a monthly age- and sex-adjusted capitation payment for a CPT-coded list of services; this payment was subject to a 20 percent withhold (that could be increased to 30 percent, under specific conditions). Primary care physicians retained the right to self-refer for services not covered under the capitation agreement. The individual PCPs were then grouped into pods or arbitrary physician incentive pools with a minimum of at least 1,000 members; the withholds of all PCPs in each pod were then combined. For each pod, there was a separate referral services budget to cover the costs for specialty, hospital, and ancillary services; this payment was based upon the number of members in the pod, adjusted for their age and sex mix.

Specialists were paid out of the referral services budget, according to the 70th percentile of usual and customary rates, subject to a withhold. Hospitals were paid according to diagnosis-related groups (DRGs) or discounted charges, but not per diems. During the calendar year, if there were deficits in the referral services fund, the overrun was to be made up first through withholds in the specialist pool and then through withholds in the primary care pool, and finally, any remaining deficits were the responsibility of the carrier. Individual stop-loss coverage from the carrier protected the PCP from responsibility for charges in excess of $7,000 per calendar year.

Despite the ability of the HMO to penalize physicians for poor performance, there was a strong fear by plan management of antagonizing primary care doctors and losing their participation in the plan. Thus, for calendar years 1986 and 1987, a corporate decision was made to return 75 percent of the physician withholds at each of the HMO sites, regardless of the extent of deficits in the referral services funds.

Design of MIS System

The hardware and software were inadequate to support membership size, leading to a backlog of claims in excess of 20 days for the HMO site as of December 31, 1987. Moreover, at any given time, the number of unentered claims and their dollar value were unknown. Once a claim was entered into the system, there were minimal edits to allow processors to detect inappropriate or unnecessary services or unusual billing practices by referral physicians.

From a statistical perspective, the information that came off the claims system was suspect. For example, if a PCP submitted a bill that included both capitated services and specialty care (for a self-referral), two encounter numbers had to be generated; if supplies, reimbursable on a cost basis, were also included in the billing, a third encounter form was generated. Thus, the reports on cost per PCP encounter werc unreliable. Another example related to classification of claims by location of service. All claims had to be grouped into one of three categories: inpatient, outpatient, or other. As a result, nursing home expenses could not be easily separated out from hospital expenses, while home health care expenses, for example, could not easily be separated from those for physical and occupational therapy. As reported by the executive director at the local site, the system was designed strictly to allocate costs to the pods and to calculate withholds.

Utilization Management

There were no data by pod on patient demographics and no analysis of utilization patterns within pods to determine where or why deficits were occurring. In effect, there was no way to evaluate the performance of individual PCPs, except in terms of expenditures for self-referrals and outside referrals. Yet, the physicians in the pod were supposed to be self-disciplining. Their contract, however, did not specify the mechanics of any review process, nor did it define how a poorly performing physician could be removed from a pod.

Medical Director and Utilization Management Support Staff

At the local level there was a part-time medical director who largely handled physician and hospital contracting. Utilization review was handled by three nurses who functioned as patient care coordinators. They received all incoming calls for the authorization of hospital admissions, and depending upon the case and available time, they were responsible for conducting on-site concurrent review. The three nurses were also supposed to authorize referrals for some 20 high-cost diagnostic tests and procedures, such as use of magnetic resonance imagers and lithotripters. However, a number of PCPs regularly ignored this requirement, knowing that the plan had no intent of closely monitoring their behavior. In fact, other than the initial credentialing process, there was no quality assurance program in place.

CASE STUDY 4:
CARRIER-SPONSORED HMO

Background

A carrier established an IPA model HMO which then contracted with a series of open panel IPAs. Each IPA was responsible for delivering care in one or two counties of the state. The HMO provided all marketing, administrative, enrollment, accounting, financial, claims processing, and

MIS services for the IPAs. Under its contract, it was also responsible for supplying the IPAs with necessary data and reports to enable the IPAs to perform peer review, to operate a quality assurance program, and to determine the status of withhold accounts.

Problems arose when one of the IPAs discovered that it was operating at a deficit and requested an increase in its monthly capitation rate. The physicians in this IPA were convinced that the deficits were attributable to three problems: (1) the HMO's use of outmoded actuarial information, leading to an underestimation of outpatient costs and a miscalculation of the capitation payment to the IPA; (2) the miscoding or misclassification of claims data, preventing a meaningful comparison between capitated payments and actual claims costs; and (3) the failure of the HMO to provide the IPA with detailed financial and utilization reports on a timely basis. This case study examines the experience of this one IPA.

Control Type

Three-tier, with control resting with the HMO (Model 1).

Financial Incentives

The HMO allocated to the IPA capitation on a per-member, per-month basis (not adjusted by age or sex), with the HMO processing all hospital and professional claims. Claims from participating IPA physicians were to be paid by the HMO according to the lesser of billed charges or a maximum fee schedule. This schedule was approximately 10 percent higher than the sponsoring carrier's schedule for its standard business. Twenty percent of all physician's fees were to be withheld and placed in a risk account.

The IPA required enrolled members to sign up with a primary care physician, but did not actively support a gatekeeper system. Patients could self-refer to participating specialists. Authorizations for hospital admissions could be requested by primary care physicians or treating specialists. Moreover, there were no built-in financial incentives for performing the gatekeeper function. For example, the IPA did not allocate any percentage of funds in the withhold to primary care physicians, but distributed the funds on a pro-rata basis across the entire IPA membership.

Design of MIS System

Only management reports, not claims processing procedures, were reviewed. By April 30 of each year, an annual financial accounting was due, showing all capitation payments to the IPA for covered services and all billed and paid services adjusted for incurred but not reported claims;

from this accounting, the HMO would determine whether any or all of the physician withhold would be available to the IPA for distribution to participating physicians.

The reports received from the HMO in April 1986 indicated that the IPA did not have an operational deficit, and, therefore, the 1985 withhold was returned and the amount of the withhold was decreased from 20 to 10 percent. IPA leadership continued to believe that the IPA was operating profitably until the end of the year, when the HMO reported a substantial deficit in the IPA account, requiring an increase in the withhold.

Apparently, during the year the HMO had experienced a buildup in unpaid claims, resulting in a miscalculation of the incurred but not reported claim and a restatement of the IPA's financial position. At the same time, the IPA was not receiving adequate information from the HMO to develop any estimates of its own performance. For example, while the HMO provided monthly totals on admissions per 1,000 members and the average length of stay per discharge, there was no financial information on average cost per patient-day or per discharge, by type of service, or by diagnosis. Detailed information on cost per patient visit and average cost per procedure was not provided to the IPA prior to the announcement of the IPA's operational deficit.

The capitation shortfall was attributed in part to the fact that the HMO was predicating utilization rates on statistics presented by outside actuarial consultants; however, the data classification system in place at the HMO did not correspond to that used by the outside consultants. For example, laboratory and x-ray costs were allocated differently in the two systems, resulting in an underestimation of the cost of outpatient services in the capitation payment.

Utilization Management and Support Staff

For all hospital admissions, the admitting physician was to call the utilization review department at the HMO for preauthorization. The appropriateness of the admission and the site (inpatient versus outpatient) was not questioned initially by the staff, but rather was reviewed retrospectively. Nurses at the HMO were responsible for conducting concurrent utilization review by phone and/or handling on-site reviews. An additional team of one physician and two nurses handled all psychiatric admissions.

For outpatient services, the claims were screened by processors at the HMO by using a series of routine edits to detect duplicate billings, noncovered services, medically outmoded services, and services covered by total charges. Otherwise, there were no screens to review the frequency of services or upgrading of procedure codes. Individual claims were not subject to special review unless physicians contested not getting paid for all services rendered. There were no reports issued on a regular basis (that is, monthly or quarterly) listing physicians who routinely billed for more services per visit or had higher costs per visit than the IPA average—or the average across all participating IPAs. There was no separate tracking of ancillary services with respect to volume and dollar amounts, by referring or treating physician.

Approximately every 6 months, on an "as-needed basis," there was a joint meeting of IPA leadership and the HMO medical director and review staff to resolve outstanding problems. Actions of that committee typically included a determination of which physicians were utilizing nonparticipating providers and/or failing to notify the HMO of inpatient admissions. The IPA was then authorized to levy a $100 fine against noncomplying physicians; over a 2-year period, approximately 12 fines were issued. Otherwise, the combined HMO-IPA review team, which theoretically was responsible for quality assurance activities, did not undertake any analysis of member grievances, incident reports, admissions by diagnosis, or mortality rates.

Medical Director and Utilization Management Support Staff

There was a nominal flow of information down to the IPA from the medical director and his support staff at the HMO. As a result, physicians participating in the IPA continued to practice under fee-for-service incentives. The medical director of the IPA, along with the leadership of the IPA, had never supported an active utilization management program. For example, using annual information produced by the HMO on the distribution of office visits by specialty, the medical director had never sought to review the practice patterns of individual physicians identified as being in the top 25 percent by cost per visit. He had not worked with IPA leadership to develop protocols to curb unnecessary ordering of ancillary services and diagnostic testing or to foster the use of outpatient surgery. Rather, the focus of the IPA's management—and the medical director—had been directed to renegotiation of the capitation payment to eliminate the IPAs operational deficit.

CASE STUDY 5:
PHYSICIAN-SPONSORED IPA

Background

A physician-owned IPA model HMO with under 25,000 members and a panel of more than 1,000 physicians had consistently reported operating losses since its founding in the mid-1980s. In 1987, it was reported to be out of compliance with the capital reserve requirements of the state's insurance department. Accordingly, the IPA sought to determine how best to obtain an immediate infusion of funds. Two primary sources had previously been identified: additional contributions from participating physicians or a loan from one or more local hospitals. However, the analysis revealed that the physicians were quickly becoming disenchanted with the plan and were unlikely to contribute additional monies, while the hospitals were not anxious to loan money unless the operational expenses of the plan could be brought under control.

Control Type

Two-tier, with control resting with the HMO (Model 1).

Financial Incentives

The physician shareholders in the plan each originally contributed between $600 and $1,750 to finance the plan's start-up. The HMO has operated on a discounted fee-for-service basis, with reimbursement predicated upon the 85th percentile of the customary and reasonable rates used by carriers operating in the local market. After the first full year's experience, these rates were reviewed and adjusted downward to control operating costs. In addition, the plan retained 20 percent of paid charges as a withhold; this withhold was not returned after the initial year of operation, but was returned after the second year as a good faith effort on the part of the IPA leadership.

There were no other incentives in this plan other than the discounted fees and the withhold. Participating physicians who were interviewed felt that the withhold had no impact on utilization patterns in terms of frequency of office visits, ordering of ancillary services, or use of referrals. In fact, with the discounted fee arrangement, some primary care physicians noted that it was more cost-efficient to refer difficult or time-consuming patients to a specialist in order to maintain the patient flow within their own offices.

Because of the failure of the withhold to control utilization, plan management is now considering a preestablished budget by practice type or specialty; under this approach, a percentage of the premium will be designated to cover specific services (for example, family practice, obstetrical care, surgery, and allergy), with a reserve fund created from the premium allocation. Payback of this withhold would be based upon the combined experience of the specialties covered under each withhold.

Design of MIS System

The claims processing section was originally under the jurisdiction of the chief financial officer, who had no previous experience with a claims operation. As a result, the operation was poorly managed and understaffed, resulting in low morale, high employee turnover, and periodic claims lags. As for the claims system, the existing hardware was adequate to support the membership size, but the software lacked the necessary edits to detect unusual physician billing practices as well as a flexible report writer to produce reports according to management specifications.

Utilization Management

The primary care physician functioned as a gatekeeper and in that capacity was responsible for completing referral forms for all specialty, ancillary, and hospital services. Once an authorization was entered into the system, all claims were automatically paid without review, except for emergency room visits, mental health services, physical therapy, speech and occupational therapy, out-of-area claims, and out-of-plan referrals.

Because the IPA was originally established by the leaders of several local medical societies and/or hospital boards and because these individuals collectively represented the medical establishment in their communities, there was a reluctance on the part of the nurse reviewers to challenge participating physicians regarding their practice patterns. This problem was further compounded by the fact that there were few or no data with which to document consistent patterns of overutilization of services or unnecessary admissions.

The plan had two medical directors; one was largely responsible for utilization review and the other was responsible for physician relations and for recruiting primary care physicians for outlying areas. To date, the approach to utilization management has been through gentle persuasion, rather than tightly written protocols. However, the failure of the plan to bring utilization rates down (for example, to lower hospital utilization under 375 days per 1,000 members for the under age 65 population) has resulted in a decision to implement a more stringent review process.

IPA Management

The same chief executive officer has remained in place since the plan was founded. However, within the first year of its operations, the plan lost its original chief financial officer, its director of management information systems, its director of claims, its nursing supervisor (who was responsible for quality assurance), and several other key administrative staff. There continues to be a high degree of tension between the physician leadership of the IPA and its lay management. One area of major conflict has been over underwriting practices. Plan management had established a policy of not accepting groups with fewer than 25 employees because of potential high utilization. However, the IPA board of directors overruled management and decreed that participating physician offices and families were eligible for HMO membership. The offering was also extended to members of the local medical societies. Despite evidence to show that the physician offices had been high utilizers, the IPA physicians continued to overrule plan management.

NOTES AND REFERENCES

1. Page, Leigh, "New Era in Utilization Review," *American Medical News*, Vol. 1, December 9, 1988, pp. 48-49. (See also Scheier, Ronni, "Medicine by the Book," *American Medical News*, January 6, 1989, pp. 1, 20).

2. U.S. General Accounting Office, *Medicare Issues Raised by Florida Health Maintenance Organization Demonstrations*, Report to Congress, GAO/HRD-86-97, Washington, DC, July 1986.

3. U.S. Congress, House, *Maintaining Medicare's HMOs: Problems, Protections, and Prospects*, Hearing before the Select Committee on Aging, 100th Congress, First Session, Washington, DC, June 11, 1987.

4. U.S. General Accounting Office, *Medicare: Physician Incentive Payments by Hospitals Could Lead to Abuse*, Report to the Chairman, Subcommittee on Health, Committee on Ways and Means, U.S. House of Representatives, GAO/HRD-86-103, Washington, DC, July 1986.

5. Trauner, Joan B., "The HMO Identity Crisis." *Best's Review 87*, April 1987, pp. 60-70.

6. The Group Health Association of America's 1988 analysis of HMO industry performance, using 1986 survey data, showed that 39.2 percent of 181 plans submitting financial data had a profit or surplus. Of the HMOs that we reviewed, 25 percent were profitable in 1986. See Group Health Association of America, Inc., *HMO Industry Profile: Financial Performance*, Vol. 3, Washington, DC, September 1988.

7. In a study of physician incentives in HMOs, ICF researchers noted that they were unable to check the consistency or accuracy of information supplied by the plans. They also noted that information on file at the federal Office of Prepaid Health Care (OPHC) was not always reliable; in some cases, financial incentive arrangements contained in applications for federal qualification had never become operational, and in other cases, design of incentives had changed without being reported to OPHC. ICF, Inc., *Final Report: Study of Incentive Arrangements Offered by HMOs and CMPs to Physicians*, Submitted to the Office of the Assistant Secretary for Planning and Evaluation, Department of Health and Human Services, Washington, DC, May 18, 1988, p. II21.

8. InterStudy, *The InterStudy Edge*, Excelsior, MN, Spring 1988, p. 54.

9. For a different approach, when traditional community- or foundation-based IPAs are contrasted with newer group-based IPAs, see Welch, W. P., "The New Structure of Individual Practice Associations, *Journal of Health Politics Policy and Law*, Vol. 12, Winter 1987, pp. 723-739.

10. ICF, Inc., *Final Report*, p. IV-6 (see note 7 above).

11. Gnessin, Alan M., "Physician Incentive Payment Systems and Risk Sharing Alternatives," in Group Health Association of America, Inc., *Physician Incentive Programs: Defining the Risk*, Washington, DC, October 28-30, 1987.

12. For a description of an HMO in which individual physician incentives are used within pods, see the statement by Jerome Beloff, Corporate Medical Director, Av-Med Health

Plan of Florida before the Physician Payment Review Commission, Washington, DC, July 15, 1988.

13. Gnessin, Alan M., "Physician Incentive Payment Systems and Risk Sharing Alternatives," 1987 (see note 11 above).

14. Wilensky, Gail R., and Rossiter, Louis F., "Patient Self-Selection in HMOs," *Health Affairs*, Vol. 5, Spring 1986, pp. 66-80. For a more recent study showing the impact of dependents' claims on health plan selection see Lairson, David R., and Herd, J. Alan, "The Role of Health Practices, Health Status, and Prior Health Care Claims in HMO Selection Bias," *Inquiry*, Vol. 24, Fall 1987, pp. 276-284.

15. Neipp, Joachim, and Zeckhauser, Richard, "Persistence in the Choice of Health Plans," *Advances in Health Economics and Health Services Research*, Vol. 6, 1985, pp. 47-72.

16. Borok, Gerald M., "Appropriate Utilization of Resources Program," *Quality Assurance and Utilization Review*, Vol. 2, May 1987, pp. 57-61.

17. Donabedian, Avedis, "Explorations in Quality Assessment and Monitoring," *The Definition of Quality and Approaches to Its Assessment*, Vol. I, Ann Arbor, MI: Health Administration Press, 1980.

18. Mosser, Gordon, "Quality Assurance in HMOs," Presentation to Management and Physician Orientation Program, Group Health Association of America, Inc., New Orleans, December 9-11, 1987.

19. For a discussion of 15 ways in which out-of-plan use may occur, see Mott, Peter D., "Hospital Utilization by Health Maintenance Organizations: Separating Apples from Oranges," *Medical Care*, Vol. 24, May 1986, pp. 398-406.

20. For a discussion of the process used by the Rand Corporation to impute mental health visits and expenditures at one large HMO (Group Health Cooperative of Puget Sound), see Wells, Kenneth, Manning, Willard Jr., and Benjamin, Bernadette, "Comparison of Use of Outpatient Mental Health Services in an HMO and Fee-for-Service Plans: Sensitivity to Definition of a Visit," *Medical Care*, Vol. 25, September 1987, pp. 894-903.

21. Joint Commission on Accreditation of Health Care Organizations, *Report of the Findings of the Joint Commission's Quality Assurance Evaluation and Medical Records Audits of Health Maintenance Organizations in Ohio under the Medical Assistance Program*, Submitted to the Bureau of Alternative Delivery Systems, Ohio Department of Human Services, December 1987.

22. Conversation with Jo Ellen Ross, Chief Executive Office, California Medical Review Inc., San Francisco, January 17, 1989.

23. U.S. General Accounting Office, *Medicare: Physician Incentive Payments*, Washington, DC, July 1986.

24. Mathematica Policy Research, Inc., *National Medicare Competition Evaluation, Final Analysis Report: The Structure of Quality Assurance Programs in HMOs and CMPs Enrolling Medicare Beneficiaries*, Washington, DC, February 1987.

25. Gold, Marsha and Reeves, Ingrid, "Preliminary Results of the GHAA-BC/BS Survey of Physician Incentives in Health Maintenance Organizations (HMOs)," Group Health Association of America, Inc., *Research Briefs*, Vol. 1, November 1987, pp. 1-15.

26. Findings from the BC/BS survey have been used to augment the GHAA survey, with duplications removed. For the BC/BS results, see Blue Cross and Blue Shield Association, "A Survey of Physician Financial Payment Arrangements in Blue Cross and Blue Shield Plan HMOs," Chicago, January 1987.

27. Hillman, Alan, "Sounding Board: Toward Full Disclosure of Referral Restrictions and Financial Incentives by Prepaid Health Plans," *New England Journal of Medicine*, Vol. 317, December 31, 1987, pp. 1743-1748.

28. ICF, Inc., *Final Report* (see note 7 above).

29. Memorandum from Lewin/ICF, Inc. and Group Health Association of America to Chris Bladen, Division of Health Financing Policy, U.S. Department of Health and Human Services, Washington, DC, June 24, 1988.

30. For a review of early research studies on utilization rates in HMO and fee-for-service settings and across HMOs, see Luft, Harold S., *Health Maintenance Organizations: Dimensions of HMO Performance*, New York: Wiley, 1981.

31. See, for example, Yelin, Edward H., Henke, Curtis J., Kramer, Jane S., Nevitt, Michael C., Shearn, Martin, and Epstein, Wallace V., "A Comparison of the Treatment of Rheumatoid Arthritis in Health Maintenance Organizations and Fee-for-Service Practices," *New England Journal of Medicine*, Vol. 312, April 11, 1985, pp. 962-967. Also see Quick, Jonathan D., Greenlick, Merwyn R., and Roghmann, Klaus J., "Prenatal Care and Pregnancy Outcome in an HMO and General Population: A Multivariate Cohort Analysis," *American Journal of Public Health*, Vol. 71, April 1981, pp. 381-390.

32. For a study that assumed that the differential use of diagnostic testing was due to its increased profitability to fee-for-service providers, see Epstein, Arnold M., Begg, Colin B., and McNeil, Barbara J., "The Use of Ambulatory Testing in Prepaid and Fee-for-Service Group Practices: Relation to Perceived Profitability," *New England Journal of Medicine*, Vol. 314, April 24, 1986, pp. 1089-1094.

33. Scovern, Henry, "Hired Help: A Physician's Experiences in a For-Profit Staff-Model HMO," *New England Journal of Medicine*, Vol. 319, September 22, 1988, pp. 787-790.

34. For an example of a discussion on referral patterns, see Piland, Neil F., White, Robert E., and Smith, Howard L., "Physician Referral Patterns: Implications for Group Practice," *GHAA Journal*, Vol. 7, Winter 1986, pp. 4-12. For an example of a discussion on provider feedback, see Berwick, Donald M., and Coltin, Kathryn L., "Feedback Reduces Test Use in a Health Maintenance Organization," *Journal of the American Medical Association*, Vol. 255, March 21, 1986, pp. 1450-1454. See also Braham, Robert L., and Ruchlin, Hirsch S., "Physician Practice Profiles: A Case Study of the Use of Audit and Feedback in an Ambulatory Care Group Practice," *Health Care Management Review*, Vol. 12, 1987, pp. 11-16.

Appendix C
Utilization Management in
Peer Review Organizations*

The utilization management procedures used by federal utilization and quality control peer review organizations (PROs) have been shaped by the financial incentives created by the Medicare prospective payment system (Ermann, 1988; Gosfield, 1989; Physician Payment Review Commission, 1988, 1989). The varieties and complexities of PRO review depart considerably from the types of prospective and retrospective review typical of the private sector.

- First, preadmission review by PROs is much narrower in scope than it is for most private programs. It focuses on only a handful of procedures rather than all elective admissions.
- Second, PROs perform little continued-stay review because Medicare's prospective per-case system for paying hospitals is thought to be sufficient to discourage needlessly long hospital stays.
- Third, Medicare does not provide for high-cost case management, although it is planning four demonstration projects to assess the method's value in the context of prospective hospital payment.

In addition, compared with most private review programs, PROs are required to perform a broader array of retrospective reviews of medical records to assess the quality and necessity of care. For example, they must examine a 3 percent random sample of Medicare admissions and

---

*The initial draft of this appendix was prepared by Alice G. Gosfield.

must also review specified samples of other cases: patient transfers among hospitals, length-of-stay and cost-per-case outliers, and readmissions within 15 or 31 days of a previous discharge. Moreover, if a reviewed provider or practitioner exceeds a predetermined denial rate (six cases or 5 percent of the cases reviewed in a quarter, whichever is greater), a more intense level of review may be initiated. Altogether, the required review activities for PROs cover about 25 percent of all Medicare discharges, a considerably higher percentage than the committee was aware of in private programs.

Beyond these differences in review foci in the PRO program, the essential distinctions between PRO review and private utilization management stem from two factors: (1) the direct relationship between the provider and payer in Medicare, and (2) the public law principles that guide PRO procedures.

In Medicare, the responsibility for initiating preadmission review lies with the hospital or physician, not the patient. Failure to obtain the relevant certification may lead to a penalty for the provider, not the patient. The provider is also responsible if the PRO denies payment based on retrospective review of the necessity of care.[1] Generally, in the private sector, a contractual relationship must exist between the payer and the provider in order for the patient to be "held harmless" (without financial liability) in similar circumstances.

An even more fundamental difference between PROs and private review is founded in the public nature of PROs. Their agendas, objectives, criteria, and results are public. The manner in which they operate is subject to federal regulation and published guidelines and is informed by public law principles, including principles of due process. PROs are required by the Health Care Financing Administration (HCFA) to seek physician comments on their review criteria, to provide their criteria to state medical organizations, and to send the criteria to anyone requesting them.

The Congress and the HCFA take a very directive role with the PROs. Each contract period is covered by an extensive scope of work that lays out the work expected. This scope of work is accompanied by an array of

---

[1] In 1972, Congress recognized that the burden of a retrospective claims denial under Medicare fell unfairly on the beneficiary who incurs Medicare costs as a result of orders and charges generated by the physician and hospital. Therefore, in Section 1879 of the Social Security Act (1972), Congress established that where services were denied as not medically necessary or custodial, if the patient did not know and had no reason to know the care would be denied, Medicare would pay for the unnecessary services, waiving the patient's liability. The burden would then fall on the hospital and physician, and a judgment would be made as to whether they knew or should have known that the services would be deemed medically unnecessary. If they did not have the requisite knowledge, they too would be indemnified by Medicare. More recently, physicians have been required to reimburse Medicare patients who have paid for care (for example, through coinsurance) that was later determined to be inappropriate.

federal regulations and other rules governing PRO activities. About half of the original group of PROs failed the evaluation by HCFA for their first contract period, and only 15 received automatic renewals.

In addition to regular performance monitoring by HCFA, a private contractor—the so-called Super-PRO—audits samples of each PRO's decisions and compares its judgments of appropriateness with those of the PRO. The Super-PRO tends to judge more care as being inappropriate than the PROs do. The Super-PRO also has reviewed a small selection of the review criteria used by PROs, but there was no provision for more systematic evaluation of the criteria (Physician Payment Review Commission, 1988). Despite this extensive oversight, the U.S. General Accounting Office recently issued a report noting the "extreme variation" in PRO organizational structure and activities (General Accounting Office, 1988).

The public aspect of PRO operations is also reflected in the legislative provisions both for physician and patient appeals of PRO determinations. For the attending physician, the process may include a predenial discussion with a review physician, a postdenial reconsideration by a specialist (if possible), and, in limited circumstances, appeals to administrative law judges and even judicial reviews. Patient access to administrative and judicial review of denials is more generally available. Federal PRO law establishes that the PRO's determinations are binding upon claims payment agencies (intermediaries and carriers) on the matters assigned to PROs. The degree to which a private review entity's determinations are binding on claims administrators varies, as described in Chapter 3.

Federal law establishes that PRO norms, criteria, and standards for review must be public and must reflect at least regional patterns of practice. The basis of the standards in the community standard of care is so presumed in the law that a specific malpractice exemption is provided to any practitioner or provider relying upon the PRO norms and criteria in treating patients or reviewing utilization. The law states that no practitioner and no provider can be held civilly liable under any law of the United States or of any state on account of action taken in reliance upon PRO norms, criteria, and standards, provided that he or she otherwise exercised due care. Enacted in 1972 and intended to discourage expensive defensive medicine and encourage cost containment, the provision was reenacted verbatim in the PRO law. Although this provision has never been construed by a court and is little known by the provider community, in the overall design of a public utilization management program it may well be instrumental in garnering physician conformity. It also sharply distinguishes PRO review from private sector review.

Another distinguishing feature of PRO review is its range of potential sanctions. The law provides that each provider and practitioner is obligated to render medically necessary services in an economical setting, meeting professionally recognized standards of quality. Failure to do so can subject an errant provider or practitioner to fines or exclusion from Medicare. This sanction authority has been increasingly used over the past few years. There are two types of sanctions: A substantial failure to comply in a substantial number of cases presents a basis to penalize a practitioner for persistent overutilization problems; a single gross and flagrant violation of the statutory requirements involving quality of care can also trigger a sanction. This type of approach to patterns of care and inclusion of providers and practitioners in an insurance program rarely exists even in the context of HMOs.

Finally, it cannot be ignored that since their inception in 1984, PROs have increasingly focused their attention on quality issues. Moreover, the Consolidated Omnibus Budget Reconciliation Act of 1985 (P.L. 99-272) gave PROs the authority, not yet implemented at the time of this writing, to deny payment when services fail to meet quality standards. PROs or similar organizations are now to review the quality of care in HMOs, and they are required to consider whether accreditation agencies and state licensing boards should be notified when a possible quality problem is identified.

REFERENCES

Ermann, Danny, "Hospital Utilization Review: Past Experience, Future Directions," *Journal of Health Policy, Politics and Law*, Winter 1988, pp. 683-704.

General Accounting Office, *Medicare PROs: Extreme Variation in Organizational Structure and Activities*, GAO/PEMD-88-10, Washington, DC, November 1988.

Gosfield, Alice, "PROs: A Case Study in Utilization Management and Quality Assurance," *1989 Health Law Handbook*, New York: Clark Boardman Co., Ltd., 1989.

Physician Payment Review Commission, *Annual Report to Congress*, Washington, DC, 1988.

Physician Payment Review Commission, *Annual Report to Congress*, Washington, DC, 1989.

Appendix D
Summary of Public Hearings*

The Institute of Medicine Committee on Utilization Management by Third Parties held a public hearing on June 6, 1988, at the National Academy of Sciences building in Washington, D.C. Speakers from 27 organizations made presentations to the committee. A question and answer session followed each panel of three speakers. Eight groups submitted written testimony without any oral presentation.

Each of the organizations represented fell into one of five categories or interest groups (Table D-1 lists the organizations by category):

- Practitioners and Organized Medicine
- Health Care Institutions, Associations, and Suppliers
- Patients, Consumers, and Public Health Organizations
- Insurers and Utilization Management Firms
- Trade Associations and Other Organizations

The testimony reflected diverse sets of interests and perspectives on utilization management. There were differences of opinion over the appropriate role of the physician (and/or medical profession) in utilization management; the validity of the criteria currently being used; the impact of various approaches on cost, quality, and administration of services; criticisms or shortcomings of utilization management; and suggestions about what is needed for the future.

---

*This summary was prepared by Eileen Connor.

TABLE D-1 Organizations Presenting Testimony at the Public Hearing on Utilization Management by Third Parties

---

Practitioners and Organized Medicine
    American Academy of Child & Adolescent Psychiatry
    American Academy of Otolaryngology
    American College of Physicians
    American College of Utilization Review Physicians
    American Dental Association
    American Medical Association
    American Psychological Association
    American Rheumatism Association
    Coalition to Preserve Quality (written only)
Health Care Institutions, Associations, and Suppliers
    American Hospital Association
    American Pharmaceutical Association (written only)
    Hospital Association of Pennsylvania (written only)
    National Association of Ambulatory Care
    National Association for Private Psychiatric Hospitals
    Mayo Clinic (written only)
Patient, Consumer, and Public Health Organizations
    American Public Health Association
    National Health Law Program
    Public Citizen-Health Research Group
Insurers and Utilization Management Firms
    ALTA Health Strategies, Inc.
    Blue Shield of California (written only)
    Celtic Life Insurance
    Health Care COMPARE
    Health Data Institute
    Health Management Strategies International, Inc.
    Iowa Foundation for Medical Care
    Quality Standards in Medicine, Inc. (written only)
    U.S. Administrators
Trade Associations and Other Organizations
    American Association of Preferred Provider Organizations
    Blue Cross and Blue Shield Association
    Group Health Association of America
    Healthcare Financial Management Association (written only)
    Health Insurance Association of America (written only)
    InterQual
    Joint Commission on Accreditation of Health Care Organizations
    National Association of Quality Assurance Professionals

Despite the differences of opinion, however, there was considerable agreement on the following:

1. Utilization management is dynamic; it is evolving; studying utilization management now is like trying to focus on a moving target.

2. There is a proliferation of external review entities in the marketplace with different criteria and a variety of approaches to managing utilization.

3. There are variations in medical practice.

4. Criteria for appropriate medical care are imperfect.

5. Resources are limited (There is disagreement as to how limited, that is, how much the United States is willing or able to devote to health.)

6. Utilization management highlights the quality and cost debate in health care.

7. There are potential dangers in utilization management by third parties.

8. Utilization management does not seem to influence physician practices. (There is disagreement on how, why, and if it is good or bad.)

9. Utilization management needs physician involvement. (There is disagreement on the type and amount of physician involvement.)

10. Current utilization management programs do little or nothing in the areas of outpatient and office practice and/or monitoring for underservice.

Appendix E
Summaries of Committee Site Visits to
Utilization Management Organizations*

Members and staff of the Committee on Utilization Management by Third Parties visited 12 organizations during the summer of 1988. The organizations visited included three independent companies, three insurance company subsidiaries, two third-party administrators, two peer review organizations (PROs) engaged in private review, and two health maintenance organizations (HMOs) (one staff model and one independent practice association [IPA]). The sites were selected to convey something of the variety that currently exists in utilization management. The following summaries and Tables E-1 through E-4 at the end of this appendix briefly describe important features of the organizations visited. Appendix F provides an analysis of client contracts that were obtained from seven of the organizations visited.

ORGANIZATION 1

Organization 1 is a relatively small, independent organization that handles about 3,000 cases a month. It is a privately held, for-profit organization whose leaders come from professional standard review organizations

---

*The summaries and tables in this appendix were originally drafted by Susan Sherman and edited by Bradford H. Gray. Each organization reviewed its summary for accuracy. Eileen Connor undertook further editing of the summaries and tables. The data provided were not independently verified.

(PSROs) and academic health centers. Clients are third-party administrators and insurers, and the company sees itself as applying not only its own review criteria but also as applying the more general coverage provisions of clients' benefit plans.

A "standard" list of procedures that normally should be done on an outpatient basis is used to guide decisions about the appropriateness of proposed inpatient care. The details of the list, however, may vary by client. Allowances for preoperative days also vary by client. Criteria are modified on an ad hoc basis as issues are raised by reviewers. The organization also performs prior review of the medical need for certain procedures, which are a mix of inpatient and outpatient services.

The organization's services are limited to utilization management and include preadmission review, second-opinion screening, high-cost and psychiatric case management, bill audits, claims review, retrospective utilization review, and physician adviser services for in-house review programs operated by insurance companies. Most reviews take place by telephone, and the information is entered into a computer. Some psychiatric case management and most retrospective reviews are conducted at the site of service. Data analysis and program evaluation capabilities are limited because the organization has only its own activity data, not claims data or medical records.

Although patients are responsible for seeing that the prior review process occurs, most calls actually come from hospital staff. All required information is obtained on the first call in an estimated 80 percent of cases. The process works best when the reviewer calls the physician's office after receiving notification of an impending admission. Incoming calls are answered by a receptionist who refers them to review nurses, who collect the information and approve the admission if the criteria are met. If the criteria are not met, the nurses are authorized to negotiate changes with attending physicians. Nurse reviewers are expected to use their own clinical judgment. (It is acknowledged that reviewers sometimes "feed" the criteria to attending physicians to facilitate admission of a patient that the reviewer feels should be admitted.) When nurse reviewers find themselves unable to authorize proposed services, cases are referred to physician advisers, who serve part-time but work from the organization's office. Appeals of denied certifications go to a second physician adviser.

Some clients request that all reviews be done by physicians. In these situations, referrals come to the organization's physician review unit from the client's nurse reviewers by telephone or facsimile machine. Incoming calls are answered by an intake coordinator who enters the information into the organization's data base and prints the referral form for distribution to the appropriate physician specialist. Faxed referrals are handled in a similar fashion. The physician reviewer will, if necessary or requested, call the client's nurse reviewer to discuss the case and then call the attending physician to make a certification decision. The physician reviewer will inform the attending physician of the decision. The final decision is also faxed to the client's nurse review office.

In the high-cost case management program, the patient calls the insurer or claims administrator, who validates health plan eligibility and then refers the case to the case management unit. For those clients where site-of-service case management is operational, preadmission review is conducted by telephone, while emergency admission and all continued-stay reviews are conducted at the site of the service. The monitoring of aftercare or alternative care is done by the nurse case managers and physician case managers in the office. Obviously, for those clients for which case management is telephone-based, all levels of review are conducted directly out of the organization's office. The case management program uses a team approach, with nurses and physicians working together in the same unit.

The organization believes in intensive involvement of physicians in the review process, in the importance of informal communication among physician advisers, and in seeking cooperative relations with providers. The office is small, and much of the monitoring, sharing of information, and revision of procedures or criteria tends to emerge from the informal communication among nurses and physicians. More formal communication occurs through regular, scheduled medical review committee meetings that assess the quality of decisions by physician reviewers and evaluate the need to change review criteria. The committee is made up of senior physicians who are not involved in initial reviews.

The staff emphasizes cooperation with attending physicians. Although they are willing to deny certification, they think that to deny cases "too readily will alienate doctors." Rather, they encourage behavior change through effective negotiating skills by nurse and physician reviewers. And they "will bend over backwards" to certify a case that they deem a necessary admission, regardless of criteria. Overall, they find physicians to be generally accepting of their programs. Most days saved are as a result of persuasion, not denial.

Cost savings are measured by hospital days saved; the organization believes that it is helping to reduce inpatient days per 1,000 lives for its clients. Except for the case management program, no data on quality and appropriateness of service or on patients and families are collected. Retrospective reviews are done for several clients. The organization believes that its biggest impact has been in influencing a switch of some inpatient procedures to outpatient procedures, including cataract surgery, myelogram, cardiac catheterization, hemorrhoid surgery, hernias, and bronchoscopies, and in diverting emergency and inappropriate psychiatric and chemical dependency treatment from inpatient to alternate forms of care.

The organization expressed concern about the adequacy of the clinical research base for some review criteria. There was also concern that some criteria developed by medical specialty societies include too broad a range of acceptable services. It was noted that refusing to allow a preoperative day may be self-defeating if the addition of such a day would shorten the overall length of stay.

ORGANIZATION 2

Organization 2 is a wholly owned subsidiary of a third-party payer and was incorporated in 1985. Clients are mainly those of the parent payer, but it is branching out to others. It covers about 1.12 million lives and reviews about 2,000 cases per month. Services include preadmission review; admission review and concurrent review for medical, surgical, and psychiatric cases; case management; second surgical opinion; disability review and workman's compensation review; and hospital bill auditing.

The organization has developed a detailed set of administrative policies and procedures and comprehensive clinical screening criteria. Nurse reviewers are guided through the decision-making process by a criteria manual, which lists procedures, gives conditions for certifying an admission, and assigns a rating to conditions denoting the likelihood of an admission for this condition. Nurses must apply the criteria in all cases and consult a physician adviser if the information given does not meet the screening criteria. They must document their reasons for approval or referral to a physician adviser. The organization emphasizes that it requires its nurses to have at least 5 years of clinical experience. Physician advisers are local and work from their own offices. Advisers may sometimes know the physicians they are reviewing.

The cost-effectiveness of services and the cost-benefit of programs are emphasized rather than simple cost savings. The staff believes that cost savings from utilization management will decrease after the initial impact has been achieved, except in the mental health field where there is a greater potential to achieve the desired goals. The staff expressed skepticism about most measures of cost savings used by other companies. In this organization, pricing is based on the client company's inpatient utilization.

The organization is becoming more concerned about reviewing appropriateness of care and may call in a physician adviser on cases in which the quality of treatment is questionable. There is an internal quality assurance program, and the organization is now undertaking an outcome-based program to evaluate the appropriateness of decisions made by review coordinators and physician advisers.

The review process is initiated by the patient, a family member, or the provider. The organization expects employers to educate employees about the program. The organization has a full-time account services representative to assist employers with that education. When nurse reviewers are notified that an admission is planned, they call the attending physician to get the reason for admission, other clinical information, the anticipated length of stay, and the treatment plan. About 90 percent of the time, the reviewer speaks to the physician's office staff for medical and surgical admissions. For psychiatric admissions, the attending physician is almost always called. If the admission is authorized, the nurse notifies the attending physician, the patient, and the hospital. At the end of the certified length of stay, the nurse reviewer calls to verify that the patient is being discharged. If the patient needs additional time in the hospital, then the continued-stay review process continues until the time of discharge. If the nurse reviewer cannot approve a case based on the criteria, he or she will refer the case to a physician adviser, who must call the attending physician or document that they have made a reasonable attempt to discuss the case. Most referred cases involve requests for extensions of length of stay. About 2 percent of the total cases are denied. Appeals can be made to a second and then a third physician adviser. Of the denied cases, about eight or nine have been appealed.

Organization 2 does not currently review for quality of care but may refer problem cases to a physician adviser for review. The company surveys patient satisfaction by sending out a postcard questionnaire, for which there is a 15 percent return rate. It has observed a sentinel effect on physician requests for admissions and lengths of stay. The organization believes that it has had its biggest impact on cutting preoperative days, shortening lengths of stay, and increasing consumer awareness.

The organization expressed the following concerns about its current processes. (1) Attending physicians may bill patients for their time spent on the telephone with reviewers, and these charges are not usually covered by insurance. (2) All of the physician advisers work out of their own offices. In addition, the medical director and physician adviser work at the organization's offices part-time. Physician adviser specialists are reluctant to make calls to physicians who work in the same metropolitan area. The organization's management believes it is necessary to have at least one physician adviser on staff to ensure accessibility and consistency. (3) Patients are often uninformed about their benefit coverage. It is possible for a reviewer to certify a procedure as medically necessary, but to have that procedure not be covered by the patient's benefit package. However, letters sent by the organization to the patient clearly state that the days certified are certified for medical necessity only, and there may be contractual exclusions and/or limitations on coverage of these services in their health plans.

ORGANIZATION 3

Organization 3 is a third-party claims administrator that began to offer utilization management services about 1 year before the site visit. It covers about 2.3 million lives and has about 700 medium-sized companies (5,000 to 15,000 employees) as clients. Services include preadmission review, continued-stay review, retrospective review, discharge planning, second-opinion surgery (focused on specific procedures using criteria-based waivers), case management, and outpatient surgery review. It also conducts hospital bill audits and offers health information services and referral services to preferred providers.

Because this company does claims administration, it has a vast amount of data on its program and its impact on patients and providers. It can track case histories of patients, review benefits packages of patients, check outcomes of care in terms of rehospitalizations, and measure savings in terms of costs. A variety of reports can be generated on every aspect of its utilization management activities, including reports on days approved and used by diagnosis, extensions, averages for days requested and days approved, variances, estimated savings, and readmissions. Audits are done on both hospital services and physician services. The company considers data analysis and reporting one of its four main functions (the others are utilization management itself, claims administration, and preferred provider referencing).

This company is very client-oriented. It markets its programs as a service to employers. It believes it offers an added benefit to employees, guiding them through the maze of health care services. Decisions are rendered on the medical necessity of services and the reasonableness of provider charges to clients.

To maintain the quality of the review process, Organization 3 monitors almost every activity of the nurse reviewers, and reviewer comparisons are made across time. Reviewers have 5 years of clinical experience and some review experience. They go through a 3-week training program. Physician advisers are local practitioners who spend about 3 hours a week conducting reviews out of their own offices. Their decisions are monitored to see how often they uphold a nurse reviewer's recommendation to deny certification.

Nurse reviewers are allowed to negotiate with providers and may use their own clinical judgments. The company uses the Health Data Institute Optimed system, but it believes that the review criteria are too liberal. It plans to switch to a system of its own. Reviewers are allowed to override criteria with a supervisor's permission. All of the review information, including the criteria, is programmed into the organization's computer system.

Patients are expected to trigger the preadmission review process.

About half of calls come from patients, and about half come from physicians and hospitals. If the patient or the hospital has made the initial call, the nurse reviewer will call the physician's office to confirm the diagnosis and treatment plan. If the nurse reviewer approves the admission, he or she assigns the case a length of stay (based on the Professional Activity Study Western Region at the 50th percentile minus 1 day). The reviewer calls back on the day before the expected discharge date to verify the discharge. If the case is to involve a surgical procedure, the reviewer determines whether a second surgical opinion is necessary. The opinion may be waived by the reviewer on the basis of criteria indicating that there are solid indications for surgery.

If a case does not meet criteria and the reviewer cannot negotiate a change with the attending physician, he or she refers the case to a physician adviser. Most referrals concern inpatient versus outpatient decisions. About 75 percent of the referred cases are denied by the physician advisers. Appeals may be made for consideration by a second physician adviser. Less than 1 percent of cases are appealed.

During its 1 year of utilization management experience, the company says that it has brought about an average 12.5 percent reduction in admissions, a 32 percent reduction in days of hospital care per 1,000 employees, and a 26 percent reduction in hospital costs per covered person for its clients. The company monitors quality and appropriateness of care and patient satisfaction by conducting retrospective chart reviews and by having reviewers make follow-up calls to all patients after they return home. This follow-up also allows the organization to confirm information given upon admission about diagnoses and treatment. The biggest area of impact is believed to have been in moving tonsillectomies and cataract surgery to outpatient settings.

Staff expressed concerns about how data are used, how impact is measured, and how savings are calculated. They expect to be able to track the appropriateness of their decision-making, outcomes of care, and impact in a much more sophisticated manner as they update and improve their own data base. A more sophisticated data base is necessary to enable the organization to modify its review criteria appropriately. It expects to use more restrictive criteria reviews in the future to further reduce lengths of stay and inpatient admissions, and the staff wants to use data to justify and monitor these changes. More retrospective review of cases is planned.

ORGANIZATION 4

Organization 4 is an independent review organization with origins in a staff model HMO. It was one of the earliest organizations to apply preadmission review in an indemnity context. The company views its business as a health care cost management business, and it serves a variety of clients—both insurers and employers. The goal is to get the most cost-effective care for the employers. It offers a full range of utilization management services.

The company strives to eliminate all inappropriate and unnecessary care. Reviews are concerned not only with inpatient versus outpatient surgery, presurgical days, and length of stay, but also with medical necessity of admissions, necessity of surgery, and necessity of expensive outpatient testing and procedures (for example, nuclear magnetic resonance imaging and lithotripsy). Criteria are developed by panels of outside physicians, who build protocols using existing criteria sets, specialty society guidelines, and their own clinical judgment. Some decisions (for example, those regarding outpatient surgery) are based on clients' benefit plans rather than the company's own criteria. Information used for medical necessity determination includes all available clinical data and also the narratives for x-ray and lab work.

This company is at the high-tech end of utilization management in both computerization and telephone systems. It strives for a paperless process from initial phone call until discharge, except in those instances in which case management is involved. The system captures 150 data elements, including clinical information beyond just diagnoses and procedures.

Calls for review come to an operator who directs each call to one member of a team of review nurses (the goal is to do this within 30 seconds), who enter data into the computer. The average call lasts less than 5 minutes. Nurses collect and enter data but can neither certify nor deny certification for cases. All cases are transmitted electronically to a member of the full-time medical staff for review. An estimated 25-30 percent of cases involve virtually automatic decisions (for example, admission for childbirth), and an estimated 60 percent present significant complexities for the reviewing physician to evaluate. The review physician calls the attending physician in virtually all mental health and catastrophic rehabilitation cases, 65-70 percent of medical cases, 40 percent of surgical cases, and 15 percent of obstetrical cases. As many as 20-30 percent of the initial negative decisions are appealed, first to another staff physician and then to an external consultant. The company reports utilization levels comparable to those of a staff model HMO.

The organization emphasizes internal quality control. Nurses are monitored through the computerized telephone system by supervisors and physician reviewers. Physicians' decisions are reviewed by a team supervisor, and a random 10 percent of cases are sent each month to members of external advisory panels for review. They prefer to report to clients on before-and-after utilization levels rather than on days of care averted.

ORGANIZATION 5

Organization 5 is a third-party administrator that has been doing utilization management since the early 1980s. It has about 40 clients, most with 5,000 or more employees, and covers about 600,000 lives. Its services include benefit plan design, preadmission review, concurrent review, discharge planning, case management, second surgical opinions, and preferred provider organization (PPO) management and referral, bill audits, and claims payment.

Though committed to cost containment, this organization also takes a strong pro-employee/patient stance. The staff seeks to eliminate care that is of questionable medical necessity. It believes that patient cost-sharing is an important element of cost containment but seeks to have employers also hold patients harmless for costs incurred when *providers* do not follow review requirements or when bill audits identify unnecessary services. It contends that it is on solid ground in making those decisions and will go to court to defend its judgments. It considers assisting clients with their benefits packages to be an integral part of its service. Staff are also directly involved in educating employees about utilization management. Physician advisers and nurse reviewers meet with employees, benefits personnel, and representatives of physicians and hospitals in the communities at key locations of new clients. The physician or nurse reviewer may spend up to 2 weeks at a client company holding small group educational sessions. The company's toll-free 800 telephone number is also open to all employees 1 month before services are to begin, to enable employees to call in for information.

As a claims payer, Organization 5 has extensive data on its review programs and on actual utilization. It offers clients a wide selection of standard reports and will prepare ad hoc reports as clients request.

The staff uses internally developed criteria that they base on InterQual and Professional Activity Study lengths of stay, but nurse reviewers and physician advisers can make exceptions based on clinical judgment. A medical advisory committee of physicians from across the country develops and modifies criteria. They hold that the burden is on the provider to show that services are necessary, not on the review organization to show that they are unnecessary.

In the preadmission review process, about half of the initial calls come from patients, and about half come from physicians' offices. Staff members say that they can get most of the needed information from patients and hospitals "without disturbing the physician." Nurse reviewers can certify cases immediately if they meet the criteria, or they can negotiate with providers' offices. If an attending physician challenges the nurse reviewer, the case goes to a physician adviser. About 1 percent of the cases are referred. Most referrals are handled by the medical director (who works at the organization's offices nearly full-time) and four other advisers. The advisers may call specialists for advice. A majority of the referred cases are denied. Appeals are made directly to employers through benefit plan grievance processes.

Savings are measured by days of care averted. The organization also monitors provider charges to evaluate whether they are within reasonable and customary rates according to its own and Health Insurance Association of America data. It can address quality of care to some extent through bill audits and through second opinions if the proposed service seems unusual. The organization solicits feedback by sending comment cards to patients who have gone through utilization management. It believes that its impact has been greatest from disallowing preoperative days, managing long-term-care cases, arranging transfers to lower levels of care, and getting concurrence to outpatient rather than inpatient care.

The leaders of this organization expressed the following concerns. (1) The preadmission review system is being evaded by patients who are admitted on an emergency basis for diagnostic workups only. They seek to have these patients discharged. (2) About half the hospitals they deal with do not cooperate with concurrent review. Patients may end up paying for services not certified for payment by the employee's benefit plan. (3) Staff described "rolling" laboratories, mobile labs that offer complete testing for patients and then submit big bills for comprehensive, unnecessary tests. Most of these claims are denied. (4) Many companies lack the baseline data needed to evaluate changes in costs.

The organization plans to do more outpatient reviews and focused reviews based on historical data. It is developing a data base with claims histories for each patient.

ORGANIZATION 6

Organization 6 started doing disability and rehabilitation management and workman's compensation review in the 1970s. It then moved into medical case management and, more recently, into prior review services. A subsidiary of an insurance company, it now offers preadmission review, continued-stay review, second surgical opinion referrals, discharge planning, disability and rehabilitation management, vocational rehabilitation, hospital bill and provider auditing, and case management. It covers 8.5 million lives for large and small companies, insurers, third-party administrators, and self-insured employers.

Because this company's program grew from case management, it emphasizes appropriateness of services and review of the entire spectrum of services a patient receives. The staff is very patient-oriented. For example, reviewers will arrange patient appointments for second opinions, and case managers will help identify new jobs for partially disabled employees through the vocational rehabilitation program. Case management is done face-to-face with patients. The company has more than 100 local offices for the case management program. Case managers typically make several visits to patients in their homes to monitor the services they are receiving.

The company also emphasizes data collection, auditing, and monitoring of their services. The size of the quality assurance staff is proportional to the volume at each service center. One to five quality assurance staff per site is the range. Every month the quality assurance staff reviews a 2 percent sample of preadmission review cases, examining 14 different elements such as timeliness, accuracy of data entry, and application of criteria. They also review a 5 percent sample of physician advisers' decisions for consistency. Physician advisers also review a sample of one another's cases each month to monitor accuracy and the appropriateness of the determination. The quality assurance staff also tracks second-opinion referrals and provider billing accuracy. The company also has a sophisticated telephone monitoring system that tracks call volume, duration, hold time, abandon rates, and turnaround time. Daily reports on telephone activities are reviewed by a supervisor, who also regularly evaluates reviewers on their telephone performance.

The company assesses the medical necessity of admissions and the appropriateness of the level of care. It does not accept responsibility for determining whether services are otherwise covered under a client's benefit plan. The staff does, however, remind callers to check the provisions of their benefit plan. The organization uses a modified version of InterQual to judge the medical necessity of services. It modifies the criteria on the basis of its own data and other information data on medical practice. A panel of physicians approves modifications. The inpatient and outpatient lists vary, depending on client benefit plans.

Nurse reviewers work in teams to serve particular clients. Nurse reviewers have hospital and review experience and are allowed to use their own judgment in conjunction with the organization's written criteria. They can negotiate with providers and can make exceptions to the guidelines. All nursing judgments must be accompanied by supportive documentation in the patient's file. An administrator of the company said "we don't want to keep [the nurses] on a ball and chain." Physician advisers use their own judgment to decide cases. They work in the company's office 1 day per week; one physician adviser is on-site each day. Management suspects that nurse reviewers are more aggressive than physician advisers in negotiating lower lengths of stays or use of outpatient care.

The organization's review process is intended to be paperless. The reviewer enters information into the computer system as it is obtained and as decisions are made. Paperless processing eliminates the need for participating employees to submit forms. Through computer linkages to claims entities, the organization also has the capability of notifying the payers that prior review obligations have been met.

Patients are expected to trigger the review process. Most calls come from patients, families, and hospitals, but the nurse reviewer must always contact the attending physician to obtain information about the admission. About 120 data elements are collected on each patient. If criteria are met, reviewers may approve the admission; they call back on the day prior to discharge to verify the discharge or conduct continued-stay review if further days are requested. About 5 percent of the cases are referred to physician advisers. The most contentious cases involve preoperative days, overnight stays for outpatient procedures, and requests for longer stays, in that order. Most referred cases are approved by the advisers. About 1-2 percent of all cases are ultimately denied. Appealed cases receive a second review by a specialist in the local area. The company also has a complaint resolution process.

The company sees an average reduction of 10 percent in their clients' hospital inpatient costs and a reduction of 18 percent in the ratio of days requested to days certified after it implemented review. The company does not review for quality of care, but when quality problems appear in continued-stay review, the case is referred to a physician adviser, who may counsel the attending physician. Repeat admissions are referred to the case management program. Provider profiling is planned for the future. It is difficult for the firm to measure the impact of its programs because it does not pay claims or have other access to information about final payment decisions.

The company expressed the concern that current utilization management programs are only shifting health care costs to the outpatient setting and suggested that utilization controls on outpatient services are needed. Products for outpatient reviews are currently being developed. The staff also believes that a number of diagnostic tests and procedures are being "abused" and need to be monitored. A methodology to track overused tests and procedures is being developed.

ORGANIZATION 7

Organization 7 is a subsidiary of a regional third-party payer. Its review program is based on a model developed by a study committee sponsored by the Robert Wood Johnson Foundation. It has been engaged in utilization management since 1985. The organization services 1.7 million subscribers (including dependents). It offers preadmission review, admission review (emergency and maternity cases), home health review, skilled nursing facility care review, intensive psychiatric review, continued-stay review, second surgical opinion, medical and psychiatric case management, discharge planning, medical audits, workman's compensation and disability management, consumer education, benefits analysis, and hospital bill auditing. It also markets software products to support health information systems.

The company has a strong local base. More than half of its clients are located in the area. The company is oriented toward serving the employees of its client companies. It sees utilization management as a service to employees, as part of the employees' benefit package. Several of the major figures in the company have backgrounds in benefits and insurance. The company routinely conducts employee education programs to describe the details of the review program. Company representatives attend client meetings and union negotiation sessions. It has received endorsements from major employee groups.

The company emphasizes service to the employee population and is concerned that people understand their treatment options. Changing practice patterns is viewed as an evolutionary process.

An effort is made to minimize interference with individual physician-patient relationships. Nurse reviewers can certify admission based on established criteria and accepted medical practice and can negotiate with attending physicians regarding the appropriate level of care. If that fails, cases are referred to physician advisers. The physician adviser contacts the attending physician. The company views one aspect of its patient advocate role as preventing situations in which patients may see themselves as caught in the middle between their physician and the review organization.

The review process covers the medical necessity of admissions and verification that proposed services are covered by the benefit plan. The company uses a modified version of Appropriateness Evaluation Protocol criteria as guidelines and negotiating tools, rather than absolute standards. Company leaders stated that the objective is to affect medical outliers and not to lead medical practice trends but to follow clinical consensus. The list of procedures subject to second opinion varies with the client benefit package. The firm's quality assurance team has developed a rapid assessment tool for selected procedures and diagnoses. This tool assists the staff in establishing and maintaining the clinical picture for a patient from admission to discharge.

Nurse reviewers are assigned to teams. They must have 5 years of clinical experience; most have more. Many continue to work a few hours a week at local hospitals. Nurse reviewers can certify cases, negotiate with attending physicians, override existing criteria, and waive second surgical opinions. They are encouraged to utilize their medical expertise and are provided with continuing education. The nurse reviewers spend about half their time educating patients about treatment options, resources, and other health matters as part of a patient consultation module.

The company currently has a contract with an independent physician adviser network that includes board-certified physicians with utilization management experience. Only about eight advisers are dealt with on a daily basis. The private physician group also reviews modifications in the company's written review criteria. The organization plans to phase out the use of this panel in favor of a team of on-site physician advisers.

Telephone calls from physicians, hospitals, or patients can trigger the preadmission review process; no forms are needed. About 3-5 percent of cases are referred from nurse reviewers to physician advisers. Appeals are handled by a special review committee.

Through 1987, the company reported a 21 percent reduction in hospital admissions per 1,000 subscribers and a 20 percent reduction in days per 1,000 subscribers. It collects data on quality of care and checks for provider noncompliance with review programs. The company has observed that it has had a sentinel effect on physicians and has virtually eliminated preoperative days. Client surveys track patient satisfaction, and a combination of retrospective review and data analysis is used to track outcomes of care.

The organization expressed several concerns. (1) It is sometimes difficult to explain to employers why patterns of care may differ among groups of employees. Regional differences in demographics, health problems, and other factors exist, but employers tend to see the lowest reported utilization as the appropriate utilization for all areas. (2) Physicians need more education on the availability and efficacy of outpatient care. (3) Some benefit plans do not include coverage for alternative treatments or treatment settings, and this inhibits their use.

ORGANIZATION 8

Organization 8 is an independent review organization that was started in 1982 by a physician with extensive PSRO experience. The organization now handles about 1 million employees and their dependents and does about 2,000 certifications per day. It offers preadmission review, continued-stay review, second surgical opinion, case management, disability review, and mental health services review. It also maintains a medical information telephone line.

The organization claims to have set the pattern for independent utilization management. As one of the earliest utilization management organizations, it claims to have developed the basic procedure of having nurses review admissions and refer more complicated cases on to physicians. However, it differs from most other organizations in that 40 percent of cases are reviewed by physicians. Nurse reviewers may only certify cases that meet the written criteria. Any cases that vary must be referred to physician advisers, who work full-time at the organization's office. On receiving a case, the physician adviser telephones the attending physician to discuss the case. Physician advisers use their clinical judgment to negotiate with providers. The organization claims to cut extra days per 1,000 lives for each client because of this extensive use of physician review. It stresses that the goal of utilization management is to make physicians accountable for their decisions and believes that accountability can only be attained through objective peer review. Physicians must be reviewed by physicians who are affiliated with the review organization for the program to succeed.

Physician advisers have clinical experience, and the organization sponsors continuing education. It also has made arrangements with a local hospital to allow the physician advisers to attend grand rounds at the hospital. Moreover, the head of the organization notes that physician advisers have contact with 10,000 admissions per year through preadmission and continued-stay reviews and are continually educated through this process. Nurse reviewers also have clinical experience. They receive a 6-week training program and continuing education sponsored by the organization.

The organization claims to be the only review organization that is operating at a profit. It has several million dollars in billings and has doubled its business in the past year.

The review process can be triggered by physicians, patients, or hospitals. Usually, the hospital calls the utilization management organization, and the nurse reviewer then calls the attending physician's office. Nurse reviewers approve about 60 percent of the cases. Most of these conform to the organization's criteria initially; in a small number of instances, even though the nurse reviewer is not supposed to negotiate, changes occur in the process of obtaining information. The company's criteria are a modified version of the InterQual criteria. Forty percent of cases are referred to physician advisers, who negotiate changes and ultimately approve about 98 percent of the cases that are referred to them. Sometimes physician advisers can approve a case based on information provided by a nurse reviewer, but usually the physician adviser contacts the attending physician to discuss the case. They deny about 1-2 percent of the cases. Appeals can be made to a second physician adviser. About 1 percent of denial cases are appealed.

The organization claims to cut their clients' inpatient health care costs by 20-40 percent. Because they conduct physician-to-physician review, they can intercede if they perceive quality problems in a case, but they cannot actually determine care.

The organization expressed the following concerns. (1) Its second opinion list is too inclusive. They could cut back on waiver rates if the list were more selective. Clients need to be educated to the fact that second opinions have a low return. (2) No information on review organization experience is getting into the medical literature. There is a lot of information and expertise that is not being made available to people in the health care field. (3) The organization does not favor regulation of review organizations because it feels it is one of the better companies. If all companies were regulated, it believes that this might cut its effectiveness and it would lose its competitive edge.

ORGANIZATION 9

Organization 9 is a staff model HMO. It has been in operation for more than 15 years and began conducting concurrent review about 1 year ago. The HMO has over 200,000 members, which is a large share of the HMO population in its area. It conducts concurrent review, discharge planning, and case management. Staff physicians authorize admission to the hospital, but this is an administrative and not a review process. The organization relies on its physician members to act as gatekeepers. It assumes that the admissions requested by its physicians are appropriate.

Because it is a staff model HMO, this organization has a great deal of influence over the utilization practices of participating physicians. Because physicians who work for the HMO are "sold on the HMO idea," it is possible to get physicians to adapt to new patterns of practice. The organization also emphasizes physician leadership in changing practice patterns. Generally, one physician moves to a new treatment or diagnostic approach and champions the idea to other physicians, who eventually adopt procedures reported by peers to be appropriate. The organization does not use financial incentives to get physicians to change their practice patterns because it believes that financial incentives can have adverse effects. It tracks referral patterns and will counsel physicians who have unusual practice patterns.

The organization reports to have been the first in the community to have cut preoperative days and the first to have implemented a 2-day length of stay for normal deliveries. It also asserts that it is the first HMO in its area to offer managed care services.

The organization contends that concurrent review is more effective with physician participation and that preadmission review is unnecessary in staff model organizations. The emphasis is on collaboration with the attending physician when conducting concurrent review and case management.

For emergency admissions, staff physicians judge whether the admission has been justified—usually within 48 hours of the admission. Nurse reviewers conduct concurrent review. Nurse reviewers work on-site in most hospitals. They review the patient's charts and discuss the patient's care with the attending physician and the patient. Reviewers use InterQual criteria and Professional Activity Study data as guides for their professional judgments. They communicate closely with the attending physicians. If a physician disagrees with a shorter length of stay, the reviewer may refer to a medical adviser from the same specialty group as the attending physician. Each medical department in the HMO has a utilization review committee; medical advisers are drawn from each specialty group. The medical adviser confers with the attending physician. Denial of coverage is rare. It would occur if a patient goes to a nonplan physician for services or if the patient received services in an emergency room when clinic services would have been appropriate. Appeals may be made in the form of a request for a second opinion. Physicians or patients may also file complaints, and there is an arbitration process through member services.

The nurse reviewers consider quality of care to be part of the review process. The organization conducts peer review within each department and has a quality assurance department that conducts studies on outcomes of care. Patient satisfaction surveys are also conducted. Although the utilization review program is "invisible" to patients, patients "appreciate" case management services. The physicians on the staff are generally cooperative and amenable to new utilization practices.

Leaders of the organization expressed concern over the difficulty in measuring cost savings from utilization management because the cost of health care is generally increasing. They added that effective physician leadership is essential for changes to be made in practice patterns.

ORGANIZATION 10

Organization 10 is a private, not-for-profit statewide PRO. About 60 percent of its business involves private contracts; it has 25 private clients, including third-party payers and self-insured companies. It does Medicaid review in 6 states, and private review in 50 states. The organization reviews about 1.5 million cases per year. About 250,000 of the cases are within the state, a figure that represents 60-80 percent of the discharges within the state. It offers preadmission review; concurrent and retrospective review; outpatient review; discharge planning; some quality-of-care reviews and fee reviews; physician profiling within the state; and long-term-care, chiropractic, obstetrical, and disability reviews. In addition, it does data processing for 10 other PROs.

The organization has developed a means to focus preadmission review based on retrospective review experience. On the basis of Medicare data, it has selected certain procedures for 100 percent review. And it selects certain physicians for 100 percent review. (If a physician has one case denied retrospectively, all cases will be reviewed for 3 months. This intensified review is considered to be a sanction.) The organization believes that focused preadmission review would be more efficient and just as effective as full review of all elective procedures, but finds that most private clients want 100 percent review of all procedures.

The organization reports a high level of cooperation from providers. Because it is a PRO, the physicians in the state are very familiar with its methods. It has been in operation since 1972 and operates on a statewide basis. The organization also claims to have a strong political base and a good relationship with the state medical society.

The peer review aspect of the program is emphasized. Peer review is believed to be the only means by which quality-of-care issues and treatment options can be encompassed in the review process. The organization is planning to expand its private review, particularly into other states. There is also a desire to do more outpatient office procedure reviews.

Physicians are responsible for initiating the preadmission review. If a patient calls, they tell the patient to have their physician call. Nurse reviewers receive the information, may ask questions, and can certify cases that meet their criteria. They are not allowed to advise attending physicians. The nurse reviewers use a modified version of InterQual criteria that was developed and approved by physician members of the PRO. Cases that fail the screens are referred to physician advisers. Nurses may choose the physician adviser to whom they refer a case. The PRO has about 23,000 physician members, but most reviews are conducted by about 200 physicians, who work out of their own offices. Physician advisers ordinarily make their decisions based on the information provided by the nurse reviewer and rarely contact the attending physician, unless the case has been appealed and is being reconsidered. Physician advisers make decisions based on their own clinical judgment, not written criteria. The organization has an internal validity committee that monitors reviewer and adviser decisions. Reviewers are held to a 95 percent accuracy standard; that is, the committee must agree with 95 percent of their decisions.

About 80 percent of the cases are approved by nurse reviewers; 20 percent get referred. About 1 percent are denied. Appeals take the form of reconsideration by one or two physicians, depending on the client. A second formal written appeal process is also available.

The organization believes that it has substantially cut inpatient days for its clients. It claims to have saved clients a total of $117 million on inpatient days since 1982. It evaluates quality of care in the review process and believes that this has had a substantial impact on physician behavior. It reports a 100 percent compliance rate, and physicians "fight" to stay off of intensified review. Of a total of 3,600, about 150 physicians are on the list at any one time.

The organization expressed concern about service underuse, which it is unable to track.

ORGANIZATION 11

Organization 11 is an IPA model HMO. It has been operating since 1974 and began preadmission review in 1981. It has 175,000 members and 2,000 participating physicians. Most activity is concentrated in the local area. The organization offers preadmission certification, preprocedure review, concurrent review, case management, retrospective claims audit, discharge planning, second surgical opinions, and some outpatient procedures review. It also reviews claims and conducts physician profiling.

The organization states its utilization management objectives as follows: (1) to monitor the medical needs of patients; (2) to monitor the level of care; (3) to ensure that appropriate resources are used; and (4) to develop and evaluate utilization data and identify potential utilization problems. It emphasizes education and physician cooperation but has strict sanctions for noncompliance. Physicians are fined $25 of the fee the first time, $50 the second time, and $100 the third time they fail to comply with the preadmission review program within 1 calendar year. Sanctions also are imposed for allowing unnecessary days of care (20 percent of hospital per diem for the first offense, 50 percent for the second offense, and 100 percent plus an appearance before the membership committee for the third offense) and referral to nonplan physicians (20, 50, and 100 percent of nonplan charges, respectively). In addition, time limits are set on referrals. Physicians are paid on a discounted fee-for-service system and split a surplus risk pool at the end of each year. The pool is accumulated from savings derived from hospital days saved.

The organization has a utilization review and quality assurance committee composed of five physicians who hold monthly meetings. They review physician utilization patterns and assess the utilization review program annually. They also conduct some special studies.

The preadmission review process can be initiated either in writing or by telephone. The IPA physician is responsible for beginning the process. Clerks take the preadmission calls and ask physicians (or their representatives) a series of questions from a one-page questionnaire. The questionnaires identify conditions for admission for a variety of disorders. The criteria are used by the state PRO. If the clerks receive a yes response to any of their questions, they give the questionnaire to one of two supervisors, who signs the form and authorizes the admission. The clerks can tell physicians that they will receive certification. The organization believes that this procedure is more efficient than having nurses handle the calls, because a vast majority of the admissions are routine.

Concurrent review begins on admission and continues every 2 days thereafter. Nurse reviewers work on-site at the hospital, review medical charts, and may negotiate with the attending physician. They use the

InterQual criteria and professional activity study lengths of stay for their region. Standards for any new procedures are developed by the firm's health care standards committee, which meets every 2 months. Medical necessity standards for about 12 medical procedures have been developed by the utilization review and quality assurance committee.

If criteria are not met, the nurse reviewer refers the case to one of the two supervisors or to the medical director, who is a full-time employee in charge of the utilization review program. The medical director then discusses the case with the attending physician. He may also ask two members of the utilization review and quality assurance committee to review the case. Denials are rare. Only the medical director can deny a case. Appeals may be made to the grievance committee. If a physician is sanctioned she or he may appeal to the utilization review and quality assurance committee and then to the HMO board of directors.

The organization has decreased its days of care from 560 days per 1,000 members in 1980 to 319 days per 1,000 in 1988. It believes that it has had an impact on quality of care. Reviewers use a generic quality screen developed by the utilization review and quality assurance committee on all discharges. The nurse reviewer conducts a retrospective chart review on cases that do not pass the screen. Quality problems are categorized into three levels of severity. If there is any potential harm associated with the quality discrepancy, the attending physician will be called before the utilization review and quality assurance committee. The physician is reviewed by three peers. The committee evaluates the case and recommends corrective action. Corrections can take the form of continuing education, intensified review of the physician's cases, or limiting the physician's services within the IPA. This process takes place only occasionally. The organization also monitors members and has a grievance committee that receives member complaints.

The organization expressed the concern that assigned lengths of stay can become a floor and that assigned days will be used even if they are not necessary. Therefore, reviewers do not assign specific lengths of stay.

ORGANIZATION 12

Organization 12 is a PRO that was begun by the state medical society in 1970. It started conducting private reviews in 1976; currently, more than half its business is private review. It covers about 600,000 employees. Reviews are conducted for 40-50 relatively small companies and for part of the CHAMPUS program. The organizations offers preadmission review, concurrent and retrospective review, second surgical opinion, case management, hospital bill certification, bill audit, claims administration, long-term-care review, workman's compensation reviews, discharge planning, substance abuse review, and quality reviews of hospital care.

Because it was one of the original PSROs, this organization claims to have set precedents in many programs. One strength is its historical and political base in the state. Leaders of the organization know the state, and providers in the state know them. Most nurse reviewers conduct reviews on-site in the hospitals. They claim to have strong support from the physicians. Ninety-five percent of the county medical societies participate in the PRO. The organization has a 23-member board made up of physicians, administrators, business representatives, and a consumer representative, and it also has five regional councils with the same composition. These representatives "have made a commitment to make the system work" and devote a good deal of volunteer time to the program.

The organization emphasizes cooperation with physicians and providers. It takes an educational approach to solving problems. Written agreements with each hospital allow private reviews on-site.

Physicians are responsible for initiating reviews. Most are very familiar with the process. The PRO also accepts information from a physician's designee. About 15 percent of admissions in the state are reviewed by nurses operating from the PRO office. These admissions are mostly in small rural hospitals. The remaining 85 percent of admissions are reviewed by nurse reviewers on-site. This provides a direct check on the diagnostic and clinical information reported by physicians.

Nurse reviewers can certify cases that meet the PRO criteria. Criteria were developed by an internal health care standards committee and cover intensity of service and severity of illness. Quality of care is considered in each review. There are guidelines for making exceptions to the criteria. Nurses have some authority to negotiate.

About 15 percent of the cases are referred to physician advisers. About 200 physicians serve as advisers, working part-time out of their own offices. They may certify or deny a case based on their own clinical judgment. They may decide on the basis of the record provided by the nurse reviewer, or they may call the attending physician. The organization denies slightly more than 3 percent of cases. Denial is a last resort. Appeals go to a second physician adviser. The patient or physician requesting the appeal may ask for a physician of the same specialty.

The organization claims to reduce client admissions rates by 10-15 percent. It claims to have had a dramatic effect on preoperative days, which used to be common practice and are now rare. Reviewers have criteria to screen cases for certain quality-of-care problem and can refer any case with a potential quality problem to an internal committee for review.

The organization expressed several concerns. (1) Some hospitals bill patients for care for which the PRO has denied certification. (2) Most medical admissions are emergency admissions, the necessity of which is evaluated only through concurrent review. (3) Sometimes it is difficult to get physicians to act as advisers in remote rural areas where the physicians all know each other. (4) Specialists who develop review criteria tend to be too generous.

TABLE E-1 Summary of Volume of Business at Sites Visited

Site	Number of Covered Lives or Employees	Average Number of Cases Reviewed	Reviewer to Population Ratio Nurse	Reviewer to Population Ratio Physician
1	70,000 lives (comprehensive review)	450 cases/mo	1:15,000	1:70,000
	2 million lives (case management)	550 cases/mo	1:285,000	1:400,000
	3 million lives (independent physician review)	2,000 cases/mo		1:850,000
2	1.1 million lives	2,000 cases/mo	1:16,000	1:16,000
3	2.3 million lives	NA	1:7,500	1:365,000
4	2 million lives	Up to 4,500 cases/mo	1:32,000	1:200,000
5	600,000 lives	NA	1:10,000	1:80,000-100,000
6	8.5 million lives	NA	1:20,000	1:180,000
7	1.7 million lives	NA	1:25,000-30,000	1:375,000
8	1 million employees	2,000 cases/day	1:5,000	1:125,000
9	235,000 lives	NA	1:47,000	1:47,000
10	NA	1.5 million cases/year	1:8,000	1:8,000
11	175,000 lives	NA	1:2,500	1:25,000
12	600,000 employees	NA	1:15,000	1:3,000

NOTE: NA indicates not available.

TABLE E-2 Profile of Nurse Reviewers

Site	Experience	Training	RN Staffing	Supervision
1	5 yrs	1:1 supervision	5 RNs; 1 RN director	Informal observation
2	5 yrs	FTE trainer; 2 wks; review all decisions for 1 month	25 RNs; 2 supervisors; 1 UM director; 1 trainer	Accuracy of work; consistency; number of cases/mo
3	5 yrs	3 wks	17 RNs; 2 supervisors; 1 manager	Telephone monitoring; listen, review 5 cases/wk; weekly meetings
4	1 yr and some UR	4 wks	81 RNs; 5 LPNs; 1 supervisor per team	Telephone monitoring; listen, report daily on telephone activity, productivity
5	5 yrs	4-6 wks; in-house CE	56 RNs; 7 supervisors	Telephone monitoring; listen, review a percentage of cases weekly
6	Clinical, UR	2 wk class; 2-3 wks in unit	53 RNs; 7 supervisors; 1 director	Telephone monitoring; biweekly evaluation
7	5 yrs	2 FT trainers; 4 wks; CE	130 RNs; 1 supervisor per team	Telephone monitoring; random sample of cases; meetings

8	Clinical, several yrs	6 wks; in-house CE	200+ RNs; 1 supervisor per team of 18 RNs; 1 manager/4 teams; 1 director	Telephone monitoring; referrals
9	Hospital experience	1:1 supervision	5 RNs; 1 supervisor	NA
10	5 yrs clinical	2 wks	76 RNs; 1 supervisor	MD advisers fill out questionnaire reviewing RNs; internal committee monitors decisions for 95% accuracy of documentation; application of criteria; referrals; turnaround time Medical director does random clerk review
11	Clinical	NA	7 RNs; 1 supervisor; 1 director	
12	3-yr med/surg, ICU or ER	Orientation, 1:1 supervision	40 RNs; 1 supervisor; 1 director	Telephone calls/hr; number of reviews/hr; sample of cases; appropriateness of referrals and consistency, number of cases/reviewer

NOTE: Abbreviations are as follows: RN, registered nurse; FTE, full-time equivalent; UM, utilization management; UR, utilization review; LPN, licensed practical nurse; FT, full-time; CE, continued education; MD, physician; ICU, intensive care unit; ER, emergency room; NA, not available.

TABLE E-3 Profiles of Physician Advisers

Site	Experience	Training	Physician Staffing	Payment	On- or Off-Site	Full- or Part-Time
1	Board-certified	On-site	Med dir +60[a]; 7 FTE MDs	Per case; incentive for more cases/hr	On-site; work together	PT
2	Board-certified; in practice	1-day orientation; ongoing contact with med dir	25 do most reviews; FT med dir	Per call; assume 15 min/call	Work in own offices; 1 MD adviser on-site; med dir on-site	PT; on call
3	Board-certified; UR experience; in practice	In UR	21 MD advisers; 1 PT director	By hr	Work in own offices	PT, 3 hrs/wk
4	Board-certified; in practice	Several days	18 MDs (10 FTE on med/surg; 2.5 psych); 1 FT dir	Salaried or by hr	On-site (consultants off-site)	PT; 60% more than 20 hrs/wk
5	Experienced and respected; most board-certified	Briefed and observed for a couple days	Med dir; 6 FTE med/surg; 4 psych	By hr	On-site	PT; 1 on-site at all times
6	Board-certified; UR; in practice	Manual; meet with director	6 MD advisers; 40 on call; 1 PT director	Per hr or per case	Some on-site; some in own office	PT
7	UR; PRO	Med dir trains on UR issues	8 MD advisers	Per case	1 on-site; rest off-site; in group	PT; 1 FT on-site

8	Clinical	CE in-house; attend grand rounds at local hospital	24 MD reviewers; 3 MD middle management; 1 FT director	Annual salary	On-site	FT
9	Clinical	1:1 supervision; CE	1 from each medical specialty; clinical supervisors; dept heads; med dir	Salary	On-site	PT
10	In practice	1 day	200 MD advisers; 1 PT med dir	$54.00/hr	Work in own office	PT
11	In practice	NA	5 MD reviewers; 1 med dir	$250.00/mo	Work in clinic	PT
12	Board-eligible; PRO credentialing process	1 yr of experience in hospital UR/QA	200 MD advisers; 1 PT med dir; 5 regional managers	By hr	Off-site	PT

NOTE: Abbreviations are as follows: med dir, medical director; PT, part-time; FT, full-time; MD, physician; UR, utilization review; FTE, full-time equivalent; CE, continuing education; QA, quality assurance; NA, not available.

[a]Most physician review time is not devoted to prior review but to a review contract with an insurer. Most reviews are done by about five physicians.

TABLE E-4 Case Managers

Site	Staffing	Patient Contact	Authority	Monitoring
1	1 RN	By telephone	Selects cases; identifies services	None
2	3 RNs; 1 supervisor	By telephone; site visits every 30-90 days	Develops care plan; negotiates for services	Supervisor oversees
3	7 RNs; 1 manager	By telephone; may visit; contract with home health agency for site visits	Selects cases; negotiates for services	Weekly meetings; staff discusses cases
4	9 RNs	Contract with home health agency for site visits	Identifies cases; compares costs	None
5	2 RNs	By telephone	Develop care plan; negotiate for services	Staff meetings and case conferences with MD advisers
6	258 nurse coordinators; 25 supervisors; 5 regional supervisors	RNs make site visits, work out of 130 local offices	Develop care plan; can negotiate for services	Supervisor evaluates RNs; regional supervisors evaluate random sample of cases; clients audit cases

7	8 RNs	1 initial visit; 1 follow-up visit 2-3 months after case terminated	Identify cases; negotiate for services	Monthly reports on cases
8	Physicians; 1 director	Contact with patients if care (home health) is planned for longer than 1 wk	Negotiates with provider for early discharge	None
9	10 RNs; 5 discharge planners; 1 supervisor	Site visits; provide services	May negotiate for alternative services	Med dir monitors all cases
10	None	None	None	None
11	7 RNs who do CM part-time; consider physician as case manager	None	RNs negotiate with MDs and hospital discharge planner for alternative services	Med dir oversees
12	1 coordinator who does CM part-time	Site visits; provide services	Puts together teams for each case; team develops care plan; provides care	Med dir oversees

NOTE: Abbreviations are as follows: RN, registered nurse; MD, physician; med dir, medical director; CM, case management

Appendix F
Analysis of Agreements Between Utilization Management Organizations and Their Clients*

To secure more information about the operation of prior review programs, requests were made to several organizations for copies of their contracts or agreements with their clients. Copies of seven agreements were obtained, and these were reviewed to assess how they dealt with various matters. The contracts that were reviewed may or may not be fully representative of those used in the industry. Also, on certain important matters such as appeals procedures, some contracts referred to appendixes or attachments that were not provided for review. Despite these limitations, several observations can be made about the content and specific approaches used in the contracts that were reviewed.

CONTRACTUAL DESCRIPTIONS OF PRIOR REVIEW SERVICES

Contracts for prior review services vary greatly in length. One reviewed contract was 28 double-spaced pages long and detailed the various steps that would be taken in conducting the services covered by the agreement. This contract, which is a standard form or generic agreement (as were several of the others that were reviewed), permits the client to select from among the utilization management company's services, which are described in detail (some of it repetitive) over 16 pages of the contract. At the other

---

*The initial draft of this appendix was prepared by Nathan Hershey.

extreme was a contract that described the company's services in fewer than four pages.

Notwithstanding the differences from contract to contract in the amount of detail about the organization's services (for example, the options available when an initial negative determination of medical necessity has been made), a reading of the contracts does not reveal substantial differences among organizations in the services themselves.

SOURCES OF CLINICAL CRITERIA AND STANDARDS

The review of contracts suggests that employers and other purchasers apparently have not required information about the sources of the clinical criteria and standards used by the organization with which they contract for review services. Little or nothing in the contracts describes the criteria or indicates their sources. One contract states that medical review will use "recognized norms and standards, of the medical need for and appropriateness of proposed, ongoing or completed medical care." Regarding hospital admission review, the most comprehensive and detailed contract stated only that the review firm will evaluate proposed admissions to certify "medical necessity and appropriateness under the [insurer's] benefit plan." Another contract refers to "guidelines mutually agreed upon" by the contracting parties. The most specific contractual statement about criteria stated that the review organization would use the *purchaser's* "accepted review criteria and guidelines as the framework for making appropriateness decisions." These guidelines included the 1986 InterQual ISD-A criteria (intensity of service, severity of illness, discharge, and appropriateness screens).

There may be extracontractual discussions and negotiations between the review organization and client regarding the criteria used to evaluate the necessity or appropriateness of care. However, these agreements, like most commercial contracts, state that the contract is the entire agreement between the parties and that the agreement cannot be modified, except by action of both of the parties.

DISTINCTION BETWEEN THE REVIEW DETERMINATION AND PURCHASER'S DECISION TO PAY FOR SERVICES

Most of the contracts that were reviewed contain specific language about the distinct roles of the review organization and the purchaser. The contractual agreements generally specify that the review organization makes no decision respecting benefits, although an adverse review decision often will be the basis for an adverse decision on benefits. Note the following disclaimer language in one contract:

> In performing the [review] services the [review organization] shall not determine a Participant's eligibility for benefits under the Group Contract. Group shall have final and sole authority for all benefit determinations.

Another contract states:

> Unless specifically agreed in writing to the contrary, the [review organization] shall have no authority to bind you to any of its assessments, recommendations, findings or certifications in respect to Medical Review, and you reserve the right to act based upon your own judgment with respect to any and all claims or issues reviewed hereunder.

Additional provisions in two contracts have relevance to the distinction between determinations of medical need and decisions about payment of benefits. In one agreement, stated performance standards for the review organization implicitly recognize that reviewers may occasionally certify days of hospitalization that do not meet the guidelines agreed to by the organization and its client; it states that "95% of all days certified by [the reviewers] shall be appropriately certified based on guidelines mutually agreed upon." This provision suggests that the client accepts that a small number of certifications will not meet the mutually agreed upon criteria in order to reduce the potential for conflict. It also recognizes implicitly that the exercise of clinical judgment by the review organization's physicians may sometimes result in decisions that do not fit the criteria, but it sets up penalties if this happens too often.

Another contractual provision covers a utilization management organization's obligation to assist its client organizations in specified circumstances. The organization agreed to

> provide [the client] its case records, staff and professional medical consultation in the event that legal action is taken against [the client] for benefits which have been denied or reduced when [the client's] determination is supported by [the review organization] . . . or if [the client] is otherwise sued as a direct result of [the review organization's] . . . activities.

One review organization's generic contracts, in addition to specifying that its advice pertains only to medical necessity and appropriateness, not to payment of benefit claims, further states that

> The decision or determination to obtain or deliver any health care service is always made only by the [health plan participant] and/or his or her physician, and any decisions made by the [review organization] . . . or the health benefit insurer . . . shall relate only to the obligation for payment for any such service under the terms of the . . . group insurance policy . . . .

INDEMNIFICATION AND LIABILITY INSURANCE COVERAGE

Concern about liability, which is at a high level in virtually all areas of insurance and health care delivery, is clearly evident in contracts for prior review services. One manifestation is the indemnification provisions that were present in all but one of the contracts reviewed. Generally accompanying these provisions are statements that the providers and purchasers of review services are independent contractors. Representative of these provisions is the following:

> No provision of this agreement is intended to create, nor shall it be deemed to create, a relationship between [the client] and [the review organization] other than that of independent contractors. In addition, neither of the parties hereto, nor any of their respective employees, agents, or contractors, shall be deemed to be, or shall represent themselves as being, the employer, employee, or representative of the other, except as specifically provided in this Agreement.

Some indemnification provisions are broad or general; others specify the matters to which they apply. One illustrative indemnification provision states:

> [The client] agrees that [the review organization] shall be held harmless by [the purchaser] from all liability due to decisions made by officers or employees of [the purchaser] concerning eligibility of any [individual] insured for benefits under the provisions of the policyholder or contract holder's health benefit program. [The review organization] agrees that [the purchaser] shall be held harmless for all liability arising from failure by [the review organization] to exercise due care in its review procedures, in rendering its decisions, and in reporting them to [the purchaser].

Another relatively specific provision that is accompanied by an indemnification clause of a general character applies to breaches of described confidentiality obligations that would involve liability on theories other than negligence. It provides, in part:

> Should legal action be brought against either party or its affiliates as a result of a breach of said confidentiality, the party causing said breach agrees to indemnify and hold harmless the other party and affiliates for any loss, cost, or damage, including reasonable attorney fees, arising therefrom.

Several of the contracts contain provisions describing or requiring liability insurance coverage. For example, one contract provides that the review organization "is responsible for maintaining during the life of this Agreement liability insurance sufficient to protect it from claims of personal injury or property damage which may arise from its activities under this Agreement." The same contract also obliges the organization to require its physician reviewers "to carry or otherwise be covered by insurance in amounts adequate to protect them against professional liability claims which may arise hereunder." Only one of the contracts that contained an insurance requirement specified the amount of coverage.

STAFFING AND PERFORMANCE CRITERIA

Purchasers of utilization management services seek more appropriate use of health services by those covered under their benefit plan. This is expected to translate into reduced benefit costs in comparison with costs in the absence of utilization management services. Among matters relevant to the successful functioning of a review organization are the composition and qualifications of its staff and the criteria by which its performance is to be measured.

Most of the contracts reviewed contain little detail regarding staff. Typical is such language as "appropriate staffing levels" and "services shall be performed by physicians, registered nurses or record technicians as appropriate." Generally, references to physicians are preceded by "licensed," and references to board certification are occasionally present in descriptions of appeal processes.

The contracts usually specify the time periods within which determinations of medical necessity, length of stay, and other decisions are to be made. These can become, in effect, implicit staffing requirements (unless the review organization has flexibility in deciding how many cases to review in detail), since they require the organization to review, make determinations, and communicate with benefit plan beneficiaries and/or health care providers. within stated time periods.

Provisions in several contracts related directly to performance criteria. One standard contract, in respect to a bill screening and audit service, one of the services that could be selected by the purchaser, states the following:

> [the review organization] guarantees that the savings from the [bill review and medical audit] will exceed fees paid to [the review organization].

Another, more complicated, provision focused on adherence to numerical standards in performance under the contract.

> [the review organization] shall maintain the following performance standards for initial certification, recertification and appeal referrals:
>
> (a) 95% of all days certified by [physician reviewers] shall be appropriately certified based on guidelines mutually agreed upon between [review organization and purchaser].
> (b) 85% of all referrals shall involve direct contact between the [physician reviewer] and the attending physician.
> (c) 85% of all referrals shall be resolved within (12) business hours of the initial contact by the [review staff].

This contract goes on to provide penalties for failure to meet these performance standards, based on a reduction in the monthly retainer fee for each percentage point below those mentioned in the contract, up to a stated maximum. No other contract reviewed made specific links between the review organization's activity and its compensation.

PROPRIETARY INFORMATION AND COMPETITION

Both providers and purchasers of prior review services recognize that they will, in the operation of a review program, learn much about each other's processes and practices. Almost all the reviewed contracts contained provisions to maintain the confidentiality of proprietary information, with legal recourse in the event of the breach.

Two contract provisions are particularly noteworthy because they illustrate the overlap of some review organizations and purchasers in terms of their knowledge of utilization control procedures. For example, a health insurer that provides review services for some insured groups but contracts services out for others may be concerned that its subcontractor will try to solicit the health insurer's clients. One contract provides in part:

> [the review organization] shall use its best efforts to avoid soliciting the sale of its services to then current [clients] of [the health insurer] except in any cases where a [client] elects not to obtain from [the health insurer] such services. In the event [the review organization] inadvertently solicits any party prior to having actual knowledge that such party is then a current [client] of [the health insurer], [the review organization] agrees to terminate such solicitation promptly upon its gaining such knowledge.

The potential clash of interests may run in the opposite direction. For example, another contract, recognizing that a purchaser of review services can gain information to enable it to enter the utilization management business, contains the following limitation:

> [the purchaser] covenants and agrees that for the full term of this Agreement, including any extensions thereof, neither it nor any of its subsidiaries or affiliates will compete with [the review organization], either directly or indirectly, by performing or rendering the same or similar services within the United States of America, as rendered or performed by [the review organization] pursuant to this agreement.

Appendix G
Glossary and Acronyms

GLOSSARY

Access: The ability to obtain needed medical care.

Admission Review: Assessment of the appropriateness of urgent or emergency admissions within a limited period after hospitalization.

Ancillary Services: Supplemental services such as laboratory, radiology, and physical therapy that are provided in conjunction with medical care.

Appropriate Care: Care which is clinically justified; sometimes used interchangeably with necessary care and sometimes used only to refer to whether the use of a particular site of care (for example, hospital) is justified.

Business Coalitions: Regionally based groups of employers and/or providers, insurers, and labor representatives who may disseminate information on health care issues, collect and analyze data, and provide other services for members.

Capitation: A fixed rate of payment to cover a specified set of health services. The rate is usually provided on a per member per month basis.

Claim: A bill for health services submitted to a health benefits plan for payment.

Coinsurance: The percentage of a covered medical expense that a beneficiary must pay (after the deductible is paid).

Concurrent Review: *See* Continued-stay review.

Continued-Stay Review: Assessment of the need for continued inpatient care for a hospitalized patient.

Cost-Sharing: The share of health expenses that a beneficiary must pay, including the deductibles, copayments, coinsurance, and extra bill.

Criteria: Bases for assessing the necessity or appropriateness of a medical service; explicit criteria are written.

Current Procedural Terminology (CPT): A listing of descriptive terms and identifying codes for reporting physician services and procedures.

Deductible: The amount of medical expense that must be incurred and paid by an individual before a third party will assume any liability for payment of benefits.

Discharge Planning: The process of ensuring that patients are discharged as soon as medically appropriate, with follow-up care planned and arranged as needed.

Effectiveness: Probability of benefit to patients from a specific medical service under average conditions of use.

Efficacy: Probability of benefit to patients from a specific medical service under ideal conditions of use.

Efficiency: Level of benefit from a fixed level of input *or* amount of input cost to achieve a defined level of benefit.

Encounter: In the health maintenance organization setting, generally refers to an outpatient visit to a physician or allied health professional.

Enrollee: Individual covered by a health benefit plan.

Feedback Approaches: Programs in which physicians' patient care decisions are reviewed based on medical records, claims, or other documents of care, with the results shared with the physician.

Fee-for-Service: A method of paying practitioners on a service-by-service rather than a salaried or capitated basis.

Gatekeeper: Primary care provider who is responsible for coordinating all medical treatment rendered to an enrollee of a health plan.

Group Model Health Maintenance Organization: A health maintenance organization that contracts with a primary care or multispecialty medical practice for delivery of health services.

Health Maintenance Organization (HMO): An entity that accepts responsibility and financial risk for providing specified services to a defined population during a defined period of time at a fixed price.

High-Cost Case Management: A process for identifying high-cost patients and facilitating the development and implementation of less costly appropriate courses of care.

Individual Practice Association (IPA):   Model Health Maintenance Organization: A health maintenance organization that contracts with private physicians who serve health maintenance organization enrollees in their offices, generally on a fee-for-service basis.

Insurer: Organization that bears the financial risk for the cost of defined categories of services for a defined group of enrollees.

Medical Necessity: The need for a specific medical service based on clinical expectations that the health benefits will outweigh the health risks; sometimes used interchangeably with appropriateness.

Network Model Health Maintenance Organization: A health maintenance organization that contracts with two or more medical group practices.

Outcome: The result of a medical intervention.

Outliers: Cases that are at the extremes of a distribution.

Peer Review Organization (PRO):   A physician-based organization that reviews the medical necessity and the quality of care provided to Medicare beneficiaries.

Per Diem: A negotiated daily payment for delivery of hospital services, regardless of the actual services provided; sometimes refers only to "room and board" charges (meals, routine nursing care, etc.), not ancillary services.

Practice Guidelines: Clinical recommendations for patient care.

Practice Patterns: Aggregate characteristics of a practitioner's use of medical resources over time.

Practitioner: One who practices medicine; may include physicians, chiropractors, dentists, podiatrists, and physician's assistants.

Preadmission Review: Assessment of the clinical justification for a proposed hospital admission.

Premium: An amount paid periodically to purchase health insurance benefits.

Prepaid Group Practice: A term used before the term health maintenance organization was coined to refer to multispecialty groups paid on a salaried or capitated basis.

Preservice Review: Assessment of the clinical justification for a proposed inpatient or outpatient service.

Prior Review/Authorization/Certification/Determination: Prior assessment by a payer or payer's agent that proposed services, such as hospitalization, are appropriate for a particular patient. Payment for services also depends on whether the patient and the category of service are covered by a benefit plan.

Professional Standard Review Organization (PSRO):   Medicare review organization that preceded the peer review organization.

Profile Analysis: Use of aggregate statistical data on an institution or practitioner to compare practice and use patterns, identify inappropriate practices, or assess other characteristics of practice.

Provider: An individual or organization that provides personal health services.

Quality Assessment: Evaluation of the technical and interpersonal aspects of medical care.

Quality Assurance: An organized program to protect or improve quality of care by evaluating medical care, correcting problems, and monitoring corrective actions.

Referral: An arrangement for a patient to be evaluated and treated by another provider.

Retrospective Utilization Review: Assessment of the appropriateness of medical services on a case-by-case or aggregate basis after the services have been provided.

Second-Opinion Program: An opinion about the appropriateness of a proposed treatment provided by a practitioner other than the one making the original recommendation; some health benefit plans require such opinions for selected services.

Self-Insurance: When an organization bears financial risk for hazards (for example, medical costs, and property damage) that the organization itself may experience.

Self-Referral: The process whereby a patient seeks care directly from a specialist without seeking advice or authorization from the primary care physician.

Site of Service: Location where care is provided, for example, an inpatient facility or home.

Staff Model Health Maintenance Organization: A health maintenance organization which provides health services through a multispecialty group practice, usually on a salaried basis.

Third-Party Administrator (TPA): Organization that processes health plan claims without bearing any insurance risk.

Third-Party Payer: An organization other than the patient (first party) or health care provider (second party) involved in the financing of personal health services.

Triple-Option Plan: An experience-rated program for an employer group in which a single insurance carrier, Blue Cross and Blue Shield plan, or health maintenance organization provides indemnity or service benefits in conjunction with various managed care or health maintenance organization plans.

Unbundle: Charging for individual services which ordinarily should have been covered under one procedure code.

Upcode: Using a procedure code which reflects a higher intensity of care than would normally be used for the services delivered.

Utilization Management: A set of techniques used on behalf of purchasers of health benefits to manage costs through case-by-case assessments of the clinical justification for proposed medical services.

Withhold: A portion of a capitated or fee-for-service payment to a contracting physician withheld by an HMO or similar organization during the year.   Depending on how revenues cover costs, the organization may retain or return some or all of the amount withheld.

ACRONYMS

AEP: Appropriateness Evaluation Protocol

BCBSA: Blue Cross and Blue Shield Association

CBO: U.S. Congressional Budget Office

CCMC: Committee on the Costs of Medical Care

CPT: Current Procedural Terminology

DHHS: U.S. Department of Health and Human Services

DRG: Diagnosis-related group

FFS: Fee-for-service

FMC: Foundation for Medical Care

GAO: U.S. General Accounting Office

GHAA: Group Health Association of America

HCFA: Health Care Financing Administration

HIAA: Health Insurance Association of America

HMO: Health maintenance organization

ICD-9:   *International Classification of Disease*

IMC: International Medical Centers Inc.

IOM: Institute of Medicine

IPA: Individual practice association

ISD-A: Intensity of service, severity of illness, discharge, and appropriateness screens

OBRA-86:   Omnibus Budget Reconciliation Act of 1986

PCP: Primary care physician

PPO: Preferred provider organization

PPS: Prospective payment system (for hospitals)

PRO: Peer review organization

TPA: Third-party administrator

Appendix H
Biographies of Committee Members

JEROME H. GROSSMAN, M.D., is the Chairman and Chief Executive Officer of New England Medical Center, Inc. He is also Chairman of the Institute for the Advancement of Health and Medical Care and Associate Professor of Medicine at Tufts University School of Medicine. He serves as Trustee/Director of several corporations and institutions, including The Boston Private Industry Council, Tufts Associated Health Plan, Wellesley College, and Arthur D. Little, Inc. Dr. Grossman joined the staff of Massachusetts General Hospital in 1966, where he served in a variety of positions. He came to the New England Medical Center in 1979. Dr. Grossman was one of the original staff of the Harvard Community Health Plan, where he developed the world's first automated medical record system, known today as COSTAR. From 1982 to 1987 Dr. Grossman served as Program Director of the Commonwealth Fund Task Force on Academic Health Centers. He is a member of the Institute of Medicine.

HOWARD L. BAILIT, D.M.D., Ph.D., is Vice President for Healthcare Management at AEtna Life & Casualty. From 1967 to 1983, Dr. Bailit was on the faculty of the University of Connecticut Health Center, where he served as Associate Dean and Professor and Head of the Department of Behavioral Sciences and Community Health. From 1983 to 1986, he was head of the Division of Health Administration at the School of Public Health, Columbia University. He was a consultant to the Rand Health Insurance Experiment and has served on many professional and governmental committees, including the National Center of Health

Services Research Study Section. Dr. Bailit has been a member of the Institute of Medicine since 1984.

ROBERT A. BERENSON, M.D., is a practicing internist with an office in Washington, D.C., and is cofounder and medical director of the National Capital Preferred Provider Organization. Prior to entering private practice in 1981, he served on the White House Domestic Policy Staff in the Carter Administration. Dr. Berenson is on the faculty of the George Washington University and Georgetown University Schools of Medicine. He has written extensively about health policy, particularly on issues related to physician payment and managed care.

JOHN M. BURNS, M.D., is Vice President, Health Management of Honeywell, Inc. From 1965 to 1981, Dr. Burns was engaged in private practice in St. Paul, Minn. He is board-certified in internal medicine and nephrology. He served as medical adviser to Northwestern Bell Telephone Company from 1967 to 1981. He was President of the Ramsey County (St. Paul, Minn.) Medical Society in 1982. Dr. Burns joined Honeywell in 1981.

RICHARD H. EGDAHL, M.D., Ph.D., is Academic Vice President for Health Affairs at Boston University, Director of the Boston University Medical Center, and until May 1989, was an active endocrine surgeon. As Academic Vice President he serves as the chief academic officer for the university's four health schools–the Schools of Medicine (including Public Health), Graduate Dentistry, Social Work, and Sargent School for Allied Health Professions. Since 1976, Dr. Egdahl has been the director of the Boston University Health Policy Institute and the Center for Industry and Health Care. He writes and speaks widely on industry's crucial role in changing the nation's health care delivery system. Dr. Egdahl is a member of many professional societies including the American Society for Clinical Investigation, American Surgical Association, American College of Surgeons, and Society of Medical Administrators. A member of the Institute of Medicine, he served on its Governing Council from 1981 to 1985. He serves on the editorial boards of a number of professional journals including the *New England Journal of Medicine*.

JOHN M. EISENBERG, M.D., M.B.A., is Sol Katz Professor of General Internal Medicine and Chief of the Section of General Internal Medicine at the University of Pennsylvania. He is also a Senior Fellow of the University of Pennsylvania's Leonard Davis Institute of Health Economics. He has served as President of the Society for General Internal Medicine and Vice President of the Society for Medical Decision Making. Dr. Eisenberg is a member of the Institute of Medicine and a commissioner on the Congressional Physician Payment Review Commission. He is presently Chairman of the American College of Physicians' Health Care Financing

Subcommittee, is a member of its Health and Public Policy Committee, and has served as a member of the College's Board of Regents. He has served as a member of the editorial boards of *Medical Care, Health Services Research*, the *Journal of General Internal Medicine*, the *Journal of Gerontology*, and *Medical Decision Making*. He also serves as consultant to the *Annals of Internal Medicine*. Dr. Eisenberg has published on topics such as physicians' practices, test use and efficacy, medical education, and clinical economics. His book, *Doctors' Decision and the Cost of Medical Care*, was published by Health Administration Press in 1986.

DEBORAH ANNE FREUND, Ph.D., is Professor of Health Economics and Chair of the Health Sciences and Administration Division in the School of Public and Environmental Affairs and Adjunct Professor of Medicine at Indiana University. She also serves as Director of Indiana University's Health Services Research Center. She is an expert on Medicaid case management programs and has written extensively on this topic as well as on HMOs and alternative reimbursement strategies. She is the chairperson of the Medical Care Section of the American Public Health Association, and also serves on the Board of Directors of the Association of University Programs in Health Administration. She serves as a member of three editorial boards: *Medical Care, Inquiry*, and *Health Policy*.

PAUL M. GERTMAN, M.D., is Chief Executive Officer of Clinical Information Advantages, Inc., a new company developing voice-entry, expert system software for practicing physicians. Dr. Gertman also is Chairman of the Board of U.S. Quality Systems, Inc., and of Health Systems Advantages, Inc. Prior to his current position, Dr. Gertman was Associate Professor of Medicine and Chief of Health Care Research at the Boston University School of Medicine, then Founder and President of the Health Data Institute, Inc., and most recently, Vice Chairman of the Board and Chief Scientist at Caremark, Inc. His principal scientific interests focus on measurement of quality and efficiency of medical care and on use of information systems technology in health care.

ALICE G. GOSFIELD, J.D., is an attorney from Philadelphia who has been working with hospitals and physicians on utilization management, quality assurance, and peer review issues since 1973. She has been a public member of the Statewide Professional Standards Review Council and a consultant to state and federal regulatory agencies on health law issues. She has lectured widely on PROs, PSROs, utilization management, and quality assurance for various organizations, including the National Health Lawyers Association, the American Medical Association, the American Academy of Hospital Attorneys, the American Medical Peer Review Association, the Blue Cross and Blue Shield Association, and the American

Bar Association. A member of the Executive Committee of the National Health Lawyers Association, she is Program Chairman for their seminar "Utilization Management, PROs and Quality Assurance: The Legal Pitfalls" and on the Planning Committee for the first National Health Lawyers Association-American Medical Association program on physician legal issues. Ms. Gosfield has published a book on PSROs and numerous articles on utilization management and quality assurance topics and is the editor of the *1989 Annual Health Law Handbook*, published by Clark Boardman, Ltd.

MICHAEL E. HERBERT, M.B.A., is President and Chief Executive Officer of Physicians Health Services, Inc., the holding company that owns Physicians Health Services of Connecticut, Inc., and Physicians Health Services of New York, Inc. Prior to becoming President of Physicians Health Services, he was Vice President of InterStudy, the national health policy research firm. Mr. Herbert is Treasurer and Director of the American Medical Care and Review Association, the national group that represents IPA HMOs, and is President of the Association of Connecticut HMOs. He is also a consultant to the federal government's Office of Prepaid Health Care, reviewing HMO applications for federal qualification and performing HMO compliance reviews.

NATHAN HERSHEY, LL.B., is Professor of Health Law in the Graduate School of Public Health, University of Pittsburgh, and has been a member of the Institute of Medicine since 1972. He is counsel to two law firms, Markel, Schafer & Means, Pittsburgh, Pa., and Post & Schell, Philadelphia, Pa. In 1986, he authored Fourth-Party Audit Organizations: Practical and Legal Considerations, which appeared in *Law, Medicine & Health Care*, and examined a variety of questions regarding the impact of private utilization management organizations on relationships among patients, providers, and payers.

NEIL HOLLANDER is Vice President of Corporate Health Strategies at Blue Cross of Western Pennsylvania. Prior to joining Blue Cross in Pittsburgh, Mr. Hollander was a Vice President and Executive Director with the Blue Cross and Blue Shield Association; Director, Bureau of Program Development, Division of Medical Assistance, New York State Department of Social Services; a senior Research Associate at the National Academy of Public Administration in Washington, D.C.; Assistant to the Representative for the Ford Foundation in Cairo, Egypt; and Program Planner for North American Rockwell. He is a member of the Editorial Advisory Board of *Same-Day Surgery*; Chairman, Managed Healthcare Services Committee for the Pittsburgh Program for Affordable Health Care. Mr. Hollander also serves on the boards of the Alpha Center in Washington, D.C., and

Keystone Health Plan West, is a Consultant to the World Bank, and is a Panel Member of the American Arbitration Association.

KAREN IGNANI, M.B.A., directs the activities of the American Federation of Labor and Congress of Industrial Organizations (AFL-CIO) on health care, pensions, and social security. Prior to joining the AFL-CIO, Ms. Ignani served as a professional staff member on the U.S. Senate's Labor and Human Resources Committee. Ms. Ignani also served as Research Director and then Assistant Director for the Committee for National Health Insurance and was a Health Care Research Analyst for the U.S. Department of Health, Education and Welfare. Ms. Ignani has authored a number of articles about organized labor's position on employee benefits issues and has represented the AFL-CIO on numerous panels all over the country.

CAROL ANN LOCKHART, Ph.D., is Executive Director of the Greater Phoenix Affordable Health Care Foundation. She is a member of the Physician Payment Review Commission, which is responsible for recommending changes to the Congress in the way Medicare pays physicians. Dr. Lockhart is a fellow in the American Academy of Nursing and has been involved in national and local manpower issues. She is coauthor of two books on labor relations in health care and is on the editorial boards of *Health Care Management*, University Press, West Yorkshire, England, and *Home Health Care Nurse*. She was previously a director in the Arizona Department of Health Services and Senior Research Associate at Boston University School of Public Health, as well as a Pew Foundation Fellow at Brandeis University.

ARNOLD MILSTEIN, M.D., M.P.H., is a Managing Director of the Wm. M. Mercer component of Marsh and McLennan and President of its National Medical Audit (NMA) subsidiary. NMA is a national physician-based consulting group that specializes in the design and evaluation of medical cost management programs for Fortune 500 companies and large carriers. Dr. Milstein is also the medical director of SuperPRO Project of the Health Care Financing Administration. He has published multiple book chapters and articles on health care control methods and is the editor of a nationally published column on utilization review decision-making. In 1987, *Business Insurance* selected him as one of 20 people who made a difference in employee benefits management in the past 20 years. Dr. Milstein is a board-certified psychiatrist and an associate clinical professor at the University of California, San Francisco.

ALAN R. NELSON, M.D., is a private practitioner of internal medicine and endocrinology in Salt Lake City, Utah, and was named President of the American Medical Association in June 1989. A graduate of Northwestern

University School of Medicine, Dr. Nelson is a Fellow of the American College of Physicians, and a member of the Endocrine Society. He is also active in clinical teaching and is Associate Clinical Professor of Medicine at the University of Utah School of Medicine. Throughout much of his career, he has been involved in medical peer review and quality assurance. He organized a statewide peer review program for the Utah Medical Association, and served as a consultant for the National Center for Health Services Research. In 1975, he was elected to the Institute of Medicine, and served on its Governing Council from 1984 to 1987. He was also a Commissioner of the Joint Commission of Accreditation of Hospitals from 1982 to 1986, and he has authored numerous papers and several book chapters on medical peer review. He was a member of the National PSRO Council from 1973 to 1977.

ROBERT PATRICELLI, LL.B., is President of Value Health, Inc., a managed health care company based in Avon, Conn. Value Health provides a range of cost-containment and quality assurance services in such areas as mental health and substance abuse, prescription drugs, podiatry, and review of high-cost medical and surgical procedures. From 1977 to 1987, he was Senior Vice President of Connecticut General Life Insurance Company and then Executive Vice President of CIGNA Corp. and President of its Affiliated Businesses Group, which included CIGNA's $1 billion health care businesses (HMOs, utilization review, and rehabilitation services). He also spent 8 years in the federal government, including service as Deputy Under Secretary for Policy in the U.S. Department of Health, Education and Welfare from 1969 to 1971. Mr. Patricelli served from 1984 to 1988 as Chairman of the U.S. Chamber of Commerce's Health Care Council and is currently Chairman of its Subcommittee on Mandated Benefits. He is a Member of the Board on Health Care Services of the Institute of Medicine, the Board of Directors of the Institute of Living (the nation's largest private psychiatric hospital), and the Board of the American Pharmaceutical Institute and is on the editorial advisory boards of *Health Affairs*, *HealthWeek*, and *The American Druggist*. He is a graduate of the Harvard Law School.

CYNTHIA L. POLICH, M.A., Vice President, United HealthCare Corp., a health services and supply company based in Minnetonka, Minn. Until July 1989, she was President of InterStudy, a nonprofit health care research firm in Excelsior, Minn. Her work has focused on identifying and developing innovative and effective methods to organize, deliver, and finance health and long-term care for the elderly. She is the author of many publications in the areas of long-term care financing, Medicare enrollment in HMOs, case management, and home health care. She is Past President of The Women's Health Leadership Trust, Past President of the Minnesota

Gerontological Society, a Board Member of Quality Quest, and Chair of Senator David Durenberger's long-term care advisory group.

DONALD M. STEINWACHS, Ph.D., is Director of the Johns Hopkins Health Services Research and Development Center and is Professor of Health Policy and Management in the School of Hygiene and Public Health. The Center is an interdisciplinary research group involving faculty principally from the School of Hygiene and Public Health and the School of Medicine. Dr. Steinwachs is also Director of the recently established Center on Organization and Financing of Care to the Severely Mentally Ill. His research has addressed a wide range of issues involving the effects of organization, financing, manpower, and technology on utilization, cost, and patient outcomes from care. He has a particular interest in the role of management information systems as a source of data for examining patterns of ambulatory and inpatient care, cost, and indicators of quality in defined populations. Dr. Steinwachs is currently President of the Association for Health Services Research and serves as a consultant to federal agencies and private foundations.

BRUCE S. WOLFF, LL.B., is a partner in the New York and Washington, D.C., offices of the law firm of Proskauer Rose Goetz & Mendelsohn, where he specializes in health care transactional and nonprofit institutional matters. From 1977 through 1979, he was Deputy Assistant Secretary for Legislation at the U.S. Department of Health, Education and Welfare and Special Assistant to the Secretary. He is a Past Chairman of the Committee on Medicine and Law of the Association of the Bar of the City of New York and of the Citizens Advisory Committee to the Medicaid Program of the District of Columbia. He is a frequent speaker on health care delivery and public policy matters.

Index

contingent nature of, 19
contractual descriptions of services,
282–283
criteria for assessment of care, 7–8,
79–85, 89, 159–160
definition of, 17–18, 170
employer/purchaser reactions to, 42,
108–110
enrollee/patient education on, 7,
103–104, 109
financial penalties for noncooperation in,
18–19, 104
focus of, 66, 89, 110
guidelines for conduct of, 108, 148
handling of attending physicians, 72, 74,
78
impact of programs, 91–116
initiation of, 42, 69–70
and inpatient hospital utilization, 92, 93,
96–97, 110
integration with benefit plan
administration, 66–69
liability in, 180
limitations of data on, 114
measures of impact, 112–113
for Medicare recipients, 14
multivariate studies of, 96–98
nurses' role in, 66, 71–73, 89
and outpatient/physician office services
use, 92, 97
and patient costs, comfort, and
convenience, 92, 104, 109
physician adviser role in, 66, 72, 73–78,
83, 86, 89
and physician-hospital relations, 106
and physician-patient relationship,
105–106
and provider-purchaser relations,
106–108
and quality of care, 4, 7, 102–103, 110,
115–116, 146, 149
refusals to authorize services, 19
reporting and feedback mechanisms,
86–87
responsibility for obtaining, 108
retrospective denial of claims following,
19, 98, 106
spillover effects of, 98, 101, 110
targeting of, 108
timeliness in handling of requests, 107,
108
trends in use of, 14

weaknesses in evidence on, 99–101, 145
see also Admission review;
Continued-stay/concurrent review;
Discharge planning; Preadmission
review; Second-opinion programs
Private employers
attitudes on high-cost case management,
133–134
education of employees on utilization
management requirements, 7,
103–104, 109, 151, 182
effects of prior review on, 108–110
expenditures for health benefits, 2
factors shaping decisions on prior
review, 109–110
health care cost-containment initiatives,
40–43
with insured health benefit plans, 2; *see
also* Health insurance plans
liability for utilization review, 109,
188–190
population covered by health insurance
plans through, 32
PRO review contracts with, 39
responsibilities in utilization
management, 6–7, 69–70, 150–151
self-insurance by, 2, 41, 60, 61, 182, 189
share of spending for health services, 40
Professional Standards Review
Organization (PSROs), 39, 59, 60,
66, 79, 93
Proprietary information, and competition,
7–9, 286–287
Prospective Payment Assessment
Commission, 102
Prospective reimbursement
employer support for, 41
see also Medicare
Prostatectomy, 46, 156
Provident Mutual, 15
Provider payments
controls on, 35
Psychiatric cases
health plan coverage for, 141 n.8, 149
high-cost case management for, 128, 138,
141 n.8

Q

Quality assurance
defined, 219
in high-cost case management, 140
in HMOs, 206, 216, 219–220, 222–224